Sixth Edition

Nursing Diagnosis and Intervention Pocket Guide

Revised by
Judith M. Wilkinson, MA, MS, RNC

ADDISON-WESLEY NURSING
A DIVISION OF
THE BENJAMIN/CUMMINGS PUBLISHING COMPANY, INC.

Redwood City, California • Menlo Park, California • Reading, Massachusetts
New York • Don Mills, Ontario • Wokingham, UK • Amsterdam • Bonn
Sydney • Singapore • Tokyo • Madrid • San Juan

Executive Editor: Patricia L. Cleary; *Acquisitions Editor:* Erin Mulligan; *Managing Editor:* Wendy Earl; *Production Editor:* Sharon Montooth; *Text Designer:* Brad Greene; *Cover Designer:* Bob Ting/Lillian Carr; *Copyeditor:* John Hammett; *Proofreader:* Karen Stough; *Compositor:* The Cowans; *Indexer:* William Richardson Associates; *Printer and Binder:* Banta Company

Library of Congress Cataloging-in-Publication Data

Wilkinson, Judith M., 1946–

Nursing diagnosis and intervention pocket guide. — 6th ed. / rev. by Judith M. Wilkinson.

p. cm.

Rev. ed. of: Care planning pocket guide / Janet Reiss Leder . . . [et al.]. 5th ed. c1993.

Includes bibliographical references and index.

ISBN 0-8053-9365-X

1. Nursing care plans—Handbooks, manuals, etc. 2. Nursing diagnosis—Handbooks, manuals, etc. I. Lederer, Janet Reiss, 1944– . II. Care planning pocket guide. III. Title.

[DNLM: 1. Nursing Diagnosis—handbooks. 2. Patient Care Planning—handbooks. WY 39 W686n 1995]

RT49.C37 1995

610.73—dc20

DNLM/DLc

for Library of Congress 95-5119

CIP

3 4 5 6 7 8 9 10–BA–99 98

Addison-Wesley Nursing

A Division of The Benjamin/Cummings Publishing Company, Inc.

390 Bridge Parkway

Redwood City, California 94065

Table of Contents

Preface

The *Nursing Diagnosis and Intervention Pocket Guide,* 6th edition, is an educational tool and practical guide designed to help nurses develop individualized nursing care plans. The content of the new edition has been expanded to include all nursing diagnoses approved by the North American Nursing Diagnosis Association through January 1995. The new edition includes diagnoses associated with medical, surgical, psychiatric, perinatal, and pediatric patient populations. A variety of special features contributes to the book's usefulness and makes it an indispensable tool for planning patient care.

New Features

NIC Priority Interventions—For each nursing diagnosis, NIC priority interventions ("treatments of choice" in NIC terminology) are given and defined. These are the interventions designated by the Nursing Interventions Classification of the Iowa Intervention Project (1993) as being "most obvious" for a particular nursing diagnosis. The Nursing Interventions Classification was developed and linked to the NANDA categories by a research team using a multimethod process that included the judgments of experts in nursing practice and research.

Assessment, Teaching, and Collaborative Nursing Actions—For ease in locating particular types of nursing actions, activities have been grouped under the headings ongoing assessments, patient teaching, collaborative activities, and other activities.

Suggestions for Use—Suggestions are given to clarify many of the nursing diagnosis labels and to advise how they can best be used.

Organization of Defining Characteristics—These cues have been categorized as "subjective" or "objective," as well as "major," "minor," and "critical."

Critical Paths—An up-to-date discussion of nursing diagnosis and critical paths is featured, along with an example of the format for a multidisciplinary care plan (critical path).

Care Planning Checklist—A checklist is provided to assist the practitioner in evaluating the finished care plan for completeness and suitability for the client. The checklist is found in Appendix E.

Other Features

Organized for easy use

The book is divided into two main parts: (1) Complete plans of care, written according to nursing diagnoses; and (2) a list of medical, surgical, psychiatric, perinatal, and pediatric conditions, each accompanied by suggested nursing diagnoses. This organization allows the nurse to begin the care planning process with either a medical condition or a nursing diagnosis.

Easy to individualize

Each nursing diagnosis has suggested related factors or risk factors that make it easy to individualize the care plan to the specific patient situation. Creative nurses will add specific outcomes, interventions, and related factors or risk factors in order to tailor the care plan to the individual patient.

Comprehensive

Each plan of care is comprehensive and allows nurses to select specific content according to the patient's condition and situation. Each plan includes (1) a definition of the nursing diagnosis, (2) defining characteristics, (3) the related factors or risk factors, (4) suggestions for use, (5) suggested alternative diagnoses, (6) expected outcomes and evaluation criteria, (7) NIC (Iowa Intervention Project) priority interventions, and (8) suggested nursing actions.

Audience

This pocket guide was developed to facilitate care planning for nursing students, staff nurses in a variety of settings, clinical nurse specialists, and staff development instructors.

Introduction

Background

In 1973, nursing diagnosis was formalized when the American Nurses Association mandated the use of nursing diagnosis in nursing practice. Invited clinicians, educators, researchers, and theorists from every area of nursing practice came together to offer labels for conditions they had observed in practice. From this beginning, the North American Nursing Diagnosis Association (NANDA) was established as the formal body for the promotion, review, and endorsement of the current list of nursing diagnoses used by practicing nurses. The NANDA membership convenes every two years. The current list of over 100 diagnoses (see inside front and back covers) will undoubtedly expand as nurses explore the breadth and depth of nursing practice. Appendix A contains a list of new diagnoses that have been received for development. NANDA has entered them into taxonomy at level 1.4, which means that they are of limited use. Because they are in a very early stage of development, it is not recommended that these diagnostic labels be used in clinical practice.

As the list of nursing diagnoses expanded, NANDA developed a classification system, Taxonomy I (see Appendix F), which "groups the diagnoses into classes and subclasses so that patterns and relationships among them can emerge" (1992, Taxonomy I, Revised, p. 1). The taxonomy is not a "final product." It is evolving, and work continues to address a number of issues: for example, the taxonomy categories overlap, and some diagnostic labels are more abstract than others. NANDA has been working with the American Nurses Association and other organizations to include the NANDA labels in other classification systems, for example the World Health Organization International Classification of Diseases (ICD), and in other nursing and nonnursing databases (see Appendix B). NANDA diagnosis-related articles are presently indexed in the Cumulative Index of Nursing and Allied Health and in the National Library of Medicine Medical Metathesaurus for a Unified Medical Language.

The importance of nursing diagnosis is supported both in professional literature and in clinical practice. Nursing diagnosis helps define the scope of nursing practice by describing conditions the nurse can independently treat. Nursing diagnosis highlights critical thinking and decision making, and provides a consistent and universally understood terminology among nurses working in various settings, including hospitals, the community, extended care facilities, occupational health facilities, and private practice.

Nursing Process in Relation to Nursing Diagnosis

The nursing process provides a structure for nursing practice and is, in fact, the essence of nursing. The nursing process is put to use continuously to plan and give nursing care. The nurse considers the patient as the central figure in the plan of care and confirms the appropriateness of all aspects of nursing care by observing the patient's responses.

Data collection (also called *assessment*) is the initial step in the critical thinking and decision making that lead to a nursing diagnosis. The nurse uses the definition and defining characteristics of the nursing diagnosis to validate the diagnosis. Once the nursing diagnosis and the related factors or risk factors are determined, the plan of care is created. The nurse selects the relevant patient outcome statements, including the patient's perceptions and suggestions for the outcomes, if possible. Not all outcomes apply to every situation, so only those that are specific to the patient are selected. After identifying the outcomes, the nurse works with the patient to determine which actions will help achieve the stated outcomes. Finally, after implementing the nursing actions, the nurse evaluates the care plan and the patient's progress. Is the nursing diagnosis still appropriate? Has the patient achieved the desired outcome? Are the documentation interval and the target date still appropriate and realistic? Are certain actions no longer needed? The individualized plan of care is revised as needed.

Standards of Care in Relation to Nursing Diagnosis

Nursing diagnosis care planning and standards of care are interrelated. Standards of care are developed for a group of patients about whom generalized predictions can be made. These standards direct a set of common nursing interventions for specific patient groups. Where there are written standards of care, nursing diagnosis care planning is not used to communicate routine nursing actions. Nursing diagnosis care planning is used for those exceptional patient problems that are not addressed in the standards of care.

Case Management and Critical Paths

Escalating health care costs and the demand for health care reform have brought about a restructuring of traditional care delivery systems and practice patterns. Two multidisciplinary clinical systems that have emerged are managed care and case management. The objectives of such systems include:

1. Achieving the following high-quality patient outcomes within an appropriate time frame:
   - Patient wellness
   - Patient/family self-care skills
   - Patient/family satisfaction
2. Establishing collaborative practice and improving service coordination and continuity of care
3. Using health care resources appropriately
4. Directing the contributions of all care providers toward the achievement of patient outcomes
5. Increasing job satisfaction and job enrichment for caregivers
6. Encouraging innovation and ongoing integration of advances in health care

Case Management

Case management is a system that uses health care professionals to coordinate care for high-risk, complex populations who may use a disproportionate share of health care resources. These are the unusual, uncommon cases seen in an agency—patients whose condition changes frequently and unpredictably, and whose needs cannot be addressed by a standardized plan or critical path. The case manager, often an advanced practice nurse, focuses on roles and relationships and provides a well coordinated care experience for patients and families in all settings in which the patient receives care.

Critical Paths and Managed Care

Managed care is used to standardize practice for the common, usual, most prevalent case types in an agency. For example, case types in a cardiac care unit might be "myocardial infarction" and "cardiac catheterization." A tool called a *critical path* has been developed to facilitate achievement of predictable client and family outcomes within a specified time frame. The critical path is a multidisciplinary plan of care that outlines crucial activities to be performed by nurses, physicians, and other health team members at designated times (see the figure on page xxviii). When the expected outcomes are not achieved within the anticipated time frame, a "variance" occurs, requiring analysis. Variances may arise from a variety of sources, including the institution, the practitioner, and/or the client.

In managed care systems, the critical path replaces the traditional nursing care plan for many clients. The critical path is a "standardized" plan for outcomes and care that can be predicted to occur. Some agencies have incorporated nursing diagnoses directly into the critical paths. Others use nursing diagnosis to name variances and develop an individualized plan for achieving revised outcomes.

Nursing Diagnosis Incorporated into Critical Path—As an example, when incorporating a nursing diagnosis into a critical path for a newly diagnosed insulin-dependent diabetic, the following nursing diagnosis would be a part of the preprinted multidisciplinary care plan:

Ineffective Management of Therapeutic Regimen related to limited information and limited practice of skill, as evidenced by verbalization of limited knowledge, inaccurate follow-through of instruction, and inaccurate performance on tests.

The expected outcomes might be that by day 3, the patient will recognize signs and symptoms of hypo/hyperglycemia, and by day 5, be able to self-inject the required dose of insulin.

Nursing Diagnosis Used to Name Variance—In this case, the critical path for a newly diagnosed insulin-dependent diabetic would not include a nursing diagnosis, but rather would list "teaching needs" for each day. On day 5, if the patient is unable to meet the outcome of self-injection, this variance would be identified and analyzed. At that point the nursing diagnosis of Ineffective Management of Therapeutic Regimen. . . might be used to individualize the nursing care for this patient's variance from the critical path.

In organizations using managed care, the *traditional* nursing care plan does not exist. However, the nursing process is important in planning and giving patient care via a multidisciplinary care plan, and nursing diagnoses are valuable in individualizing standardized critical paths to meet unique, individual patient needs. It is vital that today's nurse be well versed in using nursing diagnoses in order to work with the multidisciplinary team to effectively identify and address nursing care issues in restructured care delivery systems.

Components of Nursing Diagnosis Care Plans

This book is organized into two parts: "Plans of Care" and "Clinical Conditions Guide to Nursing Diagnoses." Information regarding these two parts, with some examples of how to use them, follows.

Plans of Care

Each plan of care includes a nursing diagnosis label, the label definition, major and minor defining characteristics, suggestions for use, suggested alternative diagnoses, related factors or risk factors, measurable patient outcomes and evaluation criteria, NIC priority interventions, and nursing actions. See the figure on page xvi.

NANDA organizes nursing diagnoses according to a conceptual framework found in Taxonomy I, Revised (see Appendix F). Since the goal of this text is to provide a ready reference for the practicing nurse, the nursing diagnosis care plans are organized alphabetically instead of by the taxonomy. Some of the titles were reworded as well, to set forth the key concept in the first word of the title. For example, Individual Coping, Ineffective is more easily found in an index when it is written Coping, Ineffective Individual.

All approved NANDA diagnoses are included as separate care plans. However, the author has modified the standard care plan format for select diagnoses, believing that these particular diagnostic categories are too broad for one care plan. For diagnoses listed below, therefore, care plans in this text include the related factors or risk factors, definition, and defining characteristics. From there, the nurse is referred to other care plans for patient outcomes and interventions.

Disuse Syndrome: Risk for
Tissue Integrity, Impaired
Tissue Perfusion, Altered: Renal, Cerebral, Cardiopulmonary, Gastrointestinal

Communication, Impaired: Verbal (2.1.1.1) (Y10.0)

Definition: The state in which an individual experiences a decreased or absent ability to use or understand language in human interaction (NANDA).

Definitions help verify diagnosis

Defining Characteristics

Major

Objective

Does not or cannot speak
Speaks or verbalizes with difficulty
Unable to speak dominant language

Minor

Objective

Absence of audible speech
Anatomic defect
Difficulty expressing thoughts verbally

Defining characteristics divided into "Major," "Minor," and "Critical"

Related Factors

Acute confusion
Aphasia
Developmental disability

Many possible "related factors" for each diagnosis

Suggestions for Use

Use this label for those who desire to communicate but are having difficulty doing so. If communication problems are caused by psychiatric illness or coping difficulties, a diagnosis of Fear or Anxiety may be more appropriate (Carpenito 1993, p. 229).

Clarification and suggestions for use of the diagnosis

Suggested Alternative Diagnoses

Anxiety
Coping, Defensive
Fear
Sensory/Perceptual Alterations: Visual, Auditory
Thought Processes, Altered

Cross references to diagnostic alternatives

Patient Outcomes and Evaluation Criteria

Include patient-specific target date, evaluation and documentation intervals, and any other patient-specific outcomes.

The patient will:

- Communicate needs to staff with minimal frustration.
- Communicate satisfaction with alternative means of communication.

Outcome statements measure progress

NIC Priority Interventions

Active Listening: Attending closely to and attaching significance to a patient's verbal and nonverbal messages.

Communication Enhancement: Facilitating interaction with a patient who has difficulty delivering or receiving verbal or nonverbal messages.

Guide to selecting the most important nursing actions

Nursing Actions

Target actions to problem etiologies. Individualize actions to meet the unique needs of each patient.

Ongoing Assessments

- Identify and document patient's primary language.
- Assess and document:
  - Patient's ability to speak, hear, write, read, and understand to establish communication between staff and patient, family and patient.
  - Patient's communication pattern to facilitate optimal two-way communication.
  - Patient's response to touch, spatial distance, and male/female roles that may influence communication.

Select from many nursing actions that help patient achieve outcomes

Thermoregulation, Impaired
Urinary Elimination, Altered

Components of the care plan are described under the following headings.

Nursing Diagnosis

The nursing diagnosis is a concise phrase or label that describes patient conditions observed in practice. These conditions may be actual or potential problems. Using NANDA terminology, potential problems are labeled *Risk for.* Appendix C contains a list of definitions of the "qualifier" words that are used in many of the diagnostic labels (eg, acute, altered, impaired). You should add other qualifying words as needed to make diagnoses precise and descriptive

Definition

The definition for each nursing diagnosis helps the nurse verify a particular nursing diagnosis. Most definitions were developed by NANDA and a few were adapted by the authors from NANDA and other sources.

Defining Characteristics

Defining characteristics are descriptors of patient behavior, either observed by the nurse or verbalized by the patient/family. After assessing the patient, nurses organize the defining characteristics into meaningful groups or patterns of information that alert them to the possibility of an existing patient problem. Usually, the presence of two or three defining characteristics verifies a nursing diagnosis.

In this text, all NANDA defining characteristics have been included. For some nursing diagnoses, NANDA has further refined the defining characteristics as "major" and "minor." According to NANDA, the major defining characteristics are present 80–100% of the time, while the minor characteristics are present at least 50% of the time. A patient must have at least one major defining characteristic in order to use a diagnosis. As research continues, more major and minor defining characteristics will undoubtedly be identified. "Critical" defining characteristics are those that *must* be present in order to use a diagnosis. The term *critical* is no longer applied to new diagnoses, but remains for those that were initially developed.

Related Factors

The related factors imply a link or connection to the nursing diagnosis. Such factors may be described as "related to," "antecedent to," "associated with," "contributing to," or "abetting." Related factors delineate what should change for the patient to return to optimal health. Correctly identified related factors help the nurse to select nursing actions appropriate to the desired outcome. As an example, for the diagnosis Activity Intolerance, the nursing actions for a patient whose related factor is arrhythmias would be very different from those needed for a patient whose related factor is chronic pain.

Risk Factors

Risk factors will be found only in the "risk for" nursing diagnoses. Unlike the related factors described above, a cluster of risk factors contributes to the patient's potential problem, and may be only partially influenced by nursing care. The risk factors are similar to related factors and defining characteristics in the development of the care plan. They describe events and behaviors that put the patient at risk and suggest interventions to protect the patient. As an example, an elderly patient might be diagnosed with Risk for Trauma, and exhibit the following risk factors: weakness, poor vision, balancing difficulties, slippery floors, and unanchored rugs. As an etiology, this cluster of risk factors suggests the need for interventions to prevent falls.

Suggestions for Use

For problematic labels, clarifying comments are included, along with suggestions for using the diagnosis or differentiating between it and similar diagnoses.

Suggested Alternative Diagnoses

Suggested alternative diagnoses are other nursing diagnoses that may be considered when identifying the patient's problem. If a review of the definition and defining characteristics indicates that they do not match the patient data, the nurse may refer to the list of suggested alternative diagnoses for other options. This is particularly helpful for the nurse unfamiliar with the nuances of each nursing diagnosis. Some nursing diagnoses have no suggested alternative diagnoses because of their specificity.

Patient Outcomes and Evaluation Criteria

Patient outcomes are statements of patient/family behaviors that are measurable, observable, and denote a desired goal. Patient outcome statements, like all components of the care planning process, are dynamic. Therefore, patient outcomes change frequently. Some are easily achieved and, once accomplished, can be deleted. Others may take longer to achieve and need periodic reevaluation. Measurable patient outcome statements are critical because they are used to evaluate patient responses to care and the success of the nursing care plan.

Not all patient outcomes listed will be appropriate for each patient. The nurse should be realistic when constructing patient outcome statements, because partial behavior change may be the only attainable goal. With shortened length of hospital stay, patient outcomes may be completed after discharge by nurses in the community setting. At time of discharge, the nurse may initiate discussion with the patient to determine patient/family outcomes still requiring completion, with referral to appropriate community resources.

Patient outcomes may be selected from this handbook or developed specifically for the patient/family situation. Use as few or as many patient outcomes as are necessary to help the patient achieve his/her goal. Prioritize outcomes with consideration given to length of stay, patient condition, and/or what the patient and family can reasonably accomplish.

For the patient outcomes selected or developed, always specify a target date and documentation interval. The *target date* is the estimated date by which the outcome will be accomplished. The date is individualized to the patient, and is flexible. The *documentation interval* designates how often documentation should occur for each outcome. This interval should be determined during initial assessment and may be changed as patient behaviors indicate the completion of a goal (outcome). For example, in the care plan for Fatigue, the documentation interval for the outcome "Patient demonstrates increasing ability to concentrate" could be specified as "q8 hours." This means that documentation must occur at least every eight hours until the outcome is accomplished.

NIC Priority Interventions

These are the interventions developed by the Iowa Intervention Project team as the "treatments of choice" for treating a particular nursing diagnosis (Daly, 1993). They are the most obvious interventions to effect problem resolution, but this does not mean that they are the only interventions to be used. A variety of interventions should always be considered.

In NIC terminology, the specific, detailed actions taken by the nurse (eg, taking vital signs, assessing for pallor, monitoring intake and output) are called *activities.* The Nursing Interventions Classification is an effort to categorize such nursing activities using standardized language. In NIC terminology, "interventions" are broad, general category labels. A set of these category labels has been developed by the Iowa Intervention Project research team, using a multimethod process (See Appendix D). These category labels were then linked to the NANDA diagnosis labels through a systematic process drawing upon the judgments of experts in nursing practice and research. In the same manner, the treatments of choice (referred to as "priority interventions" in this text) were identified.

The NIC treatments of choice (priority interventions) are really category labels that specify a *general* type of intervention. They direct the nurse to review *first* the nursing activities related to that label. In this book, many of the activities are found in the nursing actions sections. Other specific nursing activities can be found in the 1992 *Nursing Interventions Classification (NIC)* handbook. Following is an example of how the NIC priority interventions can guide care planning for the nursing diagnosis Fatigue:

1. In the care plan for Fatigue, note that the NIC priority intervention is "Energy Management." The definition of this intervention is shown as: Regulating energy use to treat or prevent fatigue and optimize function.
2. Look in the nursing actions section for the specific activities that would accomplish "Energy Management"—that is, those that specifically focus on regulating energy and treating/preventing fatigue, such as the following examples:
   - Plan activities with patient/family that minimize fatigue. Plan may include setting small, realistic, attainable goals for patient that decrease fatigue.
   - Encourage patient to identify measures that prevent or modify fatigue.
   - Discuss with patient/family ways to modify home environment to maintain usual activity level/social interaction and to minimize fatigue.
   - Plan activities to allow time for adequate rest.
3. Finally, review the rest of the nursing actions for Fatigue. There may be actions in addition to Energy Management that would be helpful for some clients, depending on their problem etiologies and individual needs.

You will be able to find effective nursing actions to deal with your patient's fatigue by using Steps 1, 2, and 3. However, you may wish to compare your chosen nursing actions to the research-based interventions listed in the 1992 *Nursing Interventions Classification (NIC)* handbook. In the handbook under the intervention label Energy Management, there are many specific nursing activities that accomplish Energy Management. Following are three examples:

- Encourage physical activity; for example, ambulation or performance of activities of daily living (ADLs), consistent with patient's energy resources
- Encourage an afternoon nap if appropriate
- Assist patient to schedule rest periods

Nursing Actions

Nursing actions should address the etiology of the patient's nursing diagnosis. The nursing actions listed for each care plan should be chosen only if they apply to the patient's condition and circumstance. Not every action will be appropriate for every patient. For example, it may be necessary to select only a few of the nursing activities at first and add others later as necessary. The nurse has the option to alter nursing actions to make them specific to the patient. This ensures an individualized plan of care. In certain instances, "q ___" or "specify plan" is included in the nursing action statement as a reminder to individualize the plan. A nursing order is not complete or useful without this specificity.

Ongoing assessments are grouped together, as are patient teaching and collaborative actions. Certain nursing actions require assessment of available laboratory values. Normal ranges for laboratory values vary with the clinical laboratory equipment used in different facilities, and the nurse may need to refer to other resources to evaluate the patient's results.

As the patient's condition changes, other interventions may be added, changed, or deleted. Frequent updating of this portion of the care plan is essential.

Clinical Conditions Guide to Nursing Diagnoses

The second part of this handbook is organized to help nurses focus their assessments when the patient's medical condition is known but the appropriate nursing diagnoses have not yet been established. In this section, medical, surgical, psychiatric, perinatal, and pediatric conditions are listed with associated nursing diagnoses and their related factors or risk factors. The suggested nursing diagnoses and related factors or risk factors are thought to occur frequently when the particular medical condition is present. Remember that not all of the nursing diagnoses will apply to each patient situation. Select only those nursing diagnoses that are confirmed by the assessment data collected. Furthermore, these lists should not be considered exhaustive. It is quite possible that a client with a particular medical condition will have nursing diagnoses that are not on the list. Because they represent unique human responses, nursing diagnoses cannot be predicted on the basis of medical condition alone.

The list of clinical conditions does not include unusual disease conditions, and it may be necessary to refer to a more general title. For example, the patient's medical diagnosis may be scleroderma. Since this condition occurs infrequently, the nurse should look under the general title Autoimmune Disorders and review the nursing diagnoses listed there.

How to Create a Nursing Diagnosis Care Plan

The following example shows how to use this book to create a care plan in a specific situation.

Mrs. B, a 75-year-old female, has been admitted to a surgical unit from the recovery room (postanesthesia recovery) following a hip pinning. Mrs. B's daughter, who is sitting at her mother's bedside, has provided the following history. Mrs. B lives alone in an upstairs apartment, which has been her home for the past 25 years. Her husband died 10 years ago as a result of Alzheimer's disease. She has many friends and is involved in community affairs at the local senior center where she volunteers her time two days a week for secretarial support. She loves to walk and to ride a bicycle. Her current hospital admission is a result of falling off her bicycle in front of her daughter's house. Mrs. B's postoperative medical orders include the following:

Foley catheter to gravity drainage
D_5 .2% NaCl with KCl 20 mEq to be infused over 8 hours
Advance diet, as tolerated
Vital signs qid
Morphine sulfate 1–2 mg, IV push, q15 minutes until comfortable to a maximum of 10 mg in 1 hour
Morphine sulfate 6–8 mg, IM q3–4 hours, prn pain
Phenergan 25 mg IM q4–6 hours, prn nausea
Monitor intake and output
CBC and electrolytes tomorrow in AM
Overhead trapeze to bed
Turn patient from back to unaffected side q1–2 hours
Pressure-reducing mattress overlay to bed to relieve pressure to bony prominences
Ambulate with assistance in AM and then qid
Turn, cough, and deep breathe at least q2 hours

Assessment

4:00 PM—The nurse's initial assessment following return from the recovery room indicates that the patient is sleeping comfortably, vital signs are within normal limits, and the operative dressing is dry and intact. Foley catheter is draining clear, amber urine. The IV is infusing at the prescribed rate; skin is warm and dry.

7:00 PM—Mrs. B's daughter has left the bedside to return home.

7:30 PM—The nurse enters Mrs. B's room to check her vital signs and finds Mrs. B attempting to climb out of bed "because I have to go to the bathroom." The nurse reminds Mrs. B that she is in the hospital and has a Foley catheter in place. Mrs. B's responses indicate that she is disoriented to place and time.

Diagnosis

The nurse's assessment of Mrs. B indicates that the most appropriate nursing diagnosis for Mrs. B is Risk for Injury. The definition of Risk for Injury is "a state in which the individual is at risk of injury as a result of environmental conditions interacting with the individual's adaptive and defensive resources." The risk factors identified from Mrs. B's assessment data are altered mobility, disorientation, pain medication, and change in environment.

The nurse next considers suggested alternative diagnoses:

Sensory/Perceptual Alterations
Tissue Perfusion, Altered: Peripheral
Skin Integrity, Impaired: Risk for

After review of the alternatives, the nurse determines that the most appropriate nursing diagnosis for Mrs. B is Risk for Injury related to altered mobility, disorientation, pain medication, and change in environment.

Patient Outcomes and Evaluation Criteria

The nurse next determines the measurable outcomes from the care plan, such as the following:

Patient will avoid physical injury.

The outcome is measurable and appropriate for Mrs. B's situation. The documentation interval for the outcome could be q8 hours, and the target date could be 1–2 days after surgery. The target date should be stated as an actual date (eg, 1/30). The documentation interval and target date should be reviewed at least daily to evaluate appropriateness.

Nursing Actions

Next, the nurse selects nursing actions. The NIC treatments of choice are: Fall Prevention and Safety Surveillance. Reviewing first the nursing actions specific to those treatments, the following may be selected for Mrs. B's plan of care:

Assess and document patient's motor and/or sensory deficit to determine safety needs of patient. Specify safety needs of patient: ___.

Reorient patient to reality and immediate environment when necessary.

Encourage patient to request assistance with activities. Use pressure reduction device, foot cradle, heel and elbow pads to prevent/inhibit skin injury.

All of the aforementioned interventions could be part of Mrs. B's care plan. Once an intervention is no longer applicable, the nurse should delete it from the care plan.

Depending on the assessment data, other nursing diagnoses could apply in this case study. This example demonstrates the process used to develop a care plan using nursing diagnostic statements, patient outcomes, documentation intervals, target dates, NIC priority interventions, and nursing actions.

Creating a Critical Path

Explained very simply, creating a critical path is a matter of combining the care plans from nursing, medical, and other services, and imposing a timeline upon the combined plan. All care and treatments are shown on the plan, and care is organized by days, weeks, or even hours and minutes, for example:

Day 1	*Day 2*	*Day 3*
Outcomes	Outcomes	Outcomes
Nursing interventions	Nursing interventions	Nursing interventions
Medical interventions	Medical interventions	Medical interventions

The timeline of a critical path is different for each institution, however, depending on the patient population. In some hospitals a herniorrhaphy might mean an overnight stay (and therefore a two-day critical path); in others it might be an outpatient procedure, with the critical path broken up into hourly segments. Therefore, standardized times cannot be given for the interventions on the nursing diagnosis care plans in this book. However, the care plans can be used when creating critical paths, the same as they are used in creating nursing diagnosis care plans.

1. Determine the nursing diagnoses your patient population (eg, herniorrhaphy patients) typically has preoperatively and postoperatively—or on day 1, day 2, and so on. Refer to the Clinical Conditions Guide to Nursing Diagnoses for ideas as needed.
2. Choose patient outcomes and nursing interventions for each day (or hour), just as you would for a traditional nursing care plan. The difference is that instead of a single care plan for a nursing diagnosis, you will have, essentially, a care plan for each day of the patient's stay in the institution.

Refer to the figure on page xxviii.

CRITICAL PATHWAY FOR CLIENT FOLLOWING LAPAROSCOPIC CHOLECYSTECTOMY

Expected length of stay: less than 24 hours

	DATE ______ PREOPERATIVE	DATE ______ 1st 24 hrs. following surgery
Daily outcomes	Client will verbalize understanding of preoperative teaching, including turning . . .	Client will • be afebrile. • have a dry, clean wound with well-approximated . . .
Tests and treatments	CBC Urinalysis Baseline physical assessment	Vital signs and O_2 saturation, neurovascular assessment, dressing and . . .
Knowledge deficit	Orient to room and surroundings. Include family in teaching.	Reorient to room and postoperative routine. Include family in teaching.
Psychosocial	Assess anxiety related to pending surgery.	Assess level of anxiety. Encourage verbalization . . .
Diet	NPO Baseline nutritional assessment	Advance to clear liquids . . .
Activity	OOB ad lib until premedicated for surgery	Provide safety precautions. Bathroom privileges . . .
Medications	NPO except ordered medications	IM or PO analgesics Antibiotics if ordered
Transfer/ discharge plans	Assess discharge plans and support system.	Probable discharge within 24 hours of surgery.

Plans of Care

Diagnostic labels, definitions, and defining characteristics are based primarily on the North American Nursing Diagnosis Association (NANDA) taxonomy. The first number following the label locates the diagnosis in the NANDA taxonomy. The second number locates the diagnosis in the proposed ICD-10 version of the taxonomy.

Suggested alternative diagnoses are provided for some labels. These should be considered if a label does not fit the patient data satisfactorily. The author's discussion and recommendations for using certain diagnoses are identified by the heading "Suggestions for Use."

Activity Intolerance (6.1.1.2) (Y50.0)

Definition: A state in which an individual has insufficient physiologic or psychologic energy to endure or complete required or desired daily activities (NANDA).

Defining Characteristics

Subjective

*Verbal report of fatigue or weakness
Exertional discomfort or dyspnea

Objective

Abnormal heart rate or blood pressure in response to activity
EKG changes during activity reflecting arrhythmia or ischemia

*Critical

Related Factors

Acute pain
Arrhythmia
Bedrest/immobility
Chronic pain
Imbalance between oxygen supply and demand
Sedentary life-style
Weakness

Suggestions for Use

Do not use this label if it is not possible to increase the patient's endurance.

Use this label only if the patient verbally reports fatigue or weakness in response to activity. Medical conditions (eg, heart disease or peripheral arterial disease) often cause Activity Intolerance. The nurse cannot independently treat medical conditions, so a diagnostic statement such as "Activity Intolerance related to coronary artery disease" is not very appropriate.

Activity intolerance often causes other problems, such as Self-Care Deficit, Social Isolation, or Sexual Dysfunction, and you can use it most effectively in conjunction with these other labels. You may specify Activity Intolerance by levels of endurance, as follows (from M. Gordon, *Nursing diagnosis: Process and application,* 2d ed., New York: McGraw-Hill, 1987, p. 147)):

Level I: Walks regular pace on level ground but becomes more short of breath than normal when climbing one or more flights of stairs.

Level II: Walks one city block 500 feet on level or climbs one flight of stairs slowly without stopping.

Level III: Walks no more than 50 feet on level without stopping and is unable to climb one flight of stairs without stopping.

Level IV: Dyspnea and fatigue at rest.

The following is an example of such a diagnostic statement:

Self-Care Deficit (Total) related to Activity Intolerance (Level IV).

Suggested Alternative Diagnoses

Fatigue (Activity intolerance is relieved by rest. Fatigue is not.)

Self-Care Deficit

Patient Outcomes and Evaluation Criteria

Include patient-specific target date, evaluation and documentation intervals, and any other patient-specific outcomes.

The patient will:

- (If infant) demonstrate increasing tolerance for ADLs/activity.
- Demonstrate ability to intersperse activity with appropriate rest periods.
- Identify activities that increase fatigue.
- Identify anxiety-producing situations that may contribute to activity intolerance.
- Participate in necessary physical activity.

- Report increased comfort while performing activities.
- Use safety measures to minimize risk for injury.
- Verbalize acceptance of limitations in strength and endurance.
- Verbalize understanding of need for oxygen, medications, and/or equipment that may increase tolerance for activities.

NIC Priority Interventions

Activity Therapy: Prescription of and assistance with specific physical, cognitive, social, and spiritual activities to increase the range, frequency, or duration of an individual's (or group's) activity.

Energy Management: Regulating energy use to treat or prevent fatigue and optimize function.

Nursing Actions

Target actions to problem etiologies. Individualize actions to meet the unique needs of each patient.

Ongoing Assessments

Assess and document:

- Emotional, physical, social, and spiritual response to activity.
- Increased pulse and respirations, dyspnea, cyanosis, pain, pallor, hemodynamic pressures, and diaphoresis as indicators of limited tolerance for activity q ____.
- Nutritional intake to ensure adequate energy resources.
- Patient's commitment to increasing frequency and/or range of activity.
- Physical limitations and level of tolerance to all activities q ____.
- Sleep pattern and number of sleep hours.

Patient Teaching

Instruct patient/family in:

- Use of equipment, such as oxygen, during activities.
- Use of relaxation techniques (distraction, visualization) during activities.
- Ways to identify and decrease anxiety-producing situations.

Collaborative Activities

- Administer pain medications prior to activity.
- Collaborate with occupational, physical, and/or recreational therapists to plan and monitor an activity program as appropriate.

Other

- Assist patient to focus on abilities rather than on deficits.
- Assist patient to identify preferences for activity.
- Avoid scheduling care activities during rest periods.
- Encourage patient to report onset of pain (severity, location, precipitating factors) that may inhibit activity. Document.
- Encourage patient to report activities that increase fatigue.
- Encourage patient to request pain medication prior to beginning activity, as necessary.
- Plan activities with patient/family that promote independence and minimize fatigue. For example:

  Contracting with patient regarding maintenance of or increase in activity. Contract is ____.

  Encouraging alternate periods of rest and activity.

  Including family in assisting patient with activities, as appropriate (specify).

  Keeping frequently used objects within easy reach.

  Providing positive reinforcement for increased activity.

  Providing safe environment by removing obstacles from ambulation area.

  Setting small, realistic, attainable goals for patient that increase independence and self-esteem. Specify goals ____.

- Plan care for the infant/child to minimize the oxygen needs of the body:

  Anticipate needs for food, water, comfort, and holding and stimulation, which will prevent unnecessary crying.

  Avoid environments low in oxygen concentration, eg, high altitudes, unpressurized airplanes.

  Minimize anxiety and stress.

  Prevent hyperthermia and hypothermia.

  Prevent infection.

  Provide adequate rest.

Activity Intolerance: Risk for (6.1.1.3) (Y50.1)

Definition: State in which an individual is at risk of experiencing insufficient physiologic or psychologic energy to endure or complete required or desired daily activities (NANDA).

Defining Characteristics

Presence of risk factors such as:

Subjective

History of previous intolerance
Inexperience with the activity

Objective

Deconditioned status

Risk Factors

See defining characteristics.

Suggestions for Use

Discriminate among Risk for Activity Intolerance, Fatigue, and Self-Care Deficit. See Activity Intolerance, suggestions for use.

Suggested Alternative Diagnoses

Fatigue (Risk for)
Self-Care Deficit (Risk for)

Patient Outcomes and Evaluation Criteria

Include patient-specific target date, evaluation and documentation intervals, and any other patient-specific outcomes.

The patient will:

- Complete desired/required daily activities.
- Describe plan for adapting to obstacles that inhibit activity.
- Identify risk factors that interfere with completing daily activities.

- Use safety measures to minimize risk for injury during activity.

NIC Priority Interventions

Emotional Support: Provision of reassurance, acceptance, and encouragement during times of stress.

Energy Management: Regulating energy use to treat or prevent fatigue and optimize function.

Nursing Actions

Target actions to problem etiologies. Individualize actions to meet the unique needs of each patient.

Ongoing Assessments

- Continually assess patient for development of actual intolerance to activity.

Patient Teaching

- Develop a realistic plan for adapting to patient's limitations.
- Explore with patient the specific consequences of inactivity.

Other

- Enlist family in efforts to support and encourage the patient's completion of activities.
- Identify the obstacles to activity.

Adjustment, Impaired (5.1.1.1.1) (Y02.0)

Definition: The state in which an individual is unable to modify his/her life-style/behavior in a manner consistent with a change in health status (NANDA).

Defining Characteristics

Major

Subjective

Verbalizes nonacceptance of health status change

Objective

Inability to problem solve or set goals

Minor

Objective

Extended period of shock, disbelief, or anger regarding health status change
Lack of future-oriented thinking
Lack of movement toward independence

Related Factors

Altered locus of control
Assault to self-esteem
Impaired cognition
Inadequate support systems
Incomplete grieving
Necessity for major life-style/behavior changes secondary to illness, traumatic events, and so forth
Pattern of dependence
Sensory overload

Suggestions for Use

This diagnosis is not specific enough to be clinically useful. If you use it, add clarifying phrases (for example, Impaired Adjustment: Inability to resolve anger over illness). When possible, use a diagnostic label that identifies the specific way in which adjustment is impaired (eg, Anxiety).

Suggested Alternative Diagnoses

The following are examples. Almost every NANDA label indicates some type of "impaired adjustment."

Coping, Ineffective Individual
Grieving, Dysfunctional

Patient Outcomes and Evaluation Criteria

Include patient-specific target date, evaluation and documentation intervals, and any other patient-specific outcomes.

The patient will:

- Acknowledge importance of life-style/behavior changes.
- Acknowledge value of independent behaviors.
- Demonstrate decreased anxiety and fear in independent activities.
- Follow agreed-on plan.
- Identify obstacles that hinder life-style/behavior changes.
- Identify personal strengths that will promote life-style/behavior changes.
- Verbalize feelings about the required life-style/behavior changes.

NIC Priority Interventions

Coping Enhancement: Assisting a patient to adapt to perceived stressors, changes, or threats which interfere with meeting life demands and roles.

Nursing Actions

Target actions to problem etiologies. Individualize actions to meet the unique needs of each patient.

Ongoing Assessments

Assess and document extent of patient's inability to solve problems and/or set goals.

Collaborative Activities

Refer patient to community agencies and/or support groups.

Other

- Encourage patient to meet and talk with others in similar situations to learn new ways to cope and to decrease isolation and fear.
- Include patient/family in a multidisciplinary conference to establish a plan of care. Plan may include:

  Assisting patient to identify obstacles that hinder life-style/behavior changes.

  Assisting patient to identify personal strengths that will help patient to achieve goals.

Assisting patient/family in reviewing necessary life-style/behavior changes and selecting one as an initial goal.

Providing continuity of patient care throughout patient assignment and use of care plan.

Setting realistic goals/limits. Prioritize goals/limits, and establish target dates.

- Provide a nonjudgmental environment in which patient/family can share concerns/anxieties/fears.

Airway Clearance, Ineffective (1.5.1.2) (Y26.0)

Definition: A state in which an individual is unable to clear secretions or obstructions from the respiratory tract to maintain airway patency (NANDA).

Defining Characteristics

Subjective

Dyspnea

Objective

Abnormal breath sounds, such as rales, rhonchi, crackles
Changes in rate or depth of respiration
Cough, effective or ineffective, with or without sputum
Cyanosis
Tachypnea

Related Factors

Decreased energy/fatigue
Perceptive/cognitive impairment
Tracheobronchial infection
Tracheobronchial obstruction
Tracheobronchial secretions
Trauma

Suggestions for Use

Use the key defining characteristics to discriminate carefully among this label and the two suggested alternative diagnoses.

	Key Defining Characteristics	
Nursing Diagnosis	*Present*	*Not Present*
Impaired Gas Exchange	Abnormal blood gases Hypoxia Changes in mental status	Ineffective cough Cough
Ineffective Breathing Pattern	Concerns the "appearance" of the patient's breathing: nasal flaring, use of accessory muscles, pursed-lip breathing Abnormal blood gases	Tachycardia, restlessness Ineffective cough Not caused by obstruction or aspiration
Ineffective Airway Clearance	Cough, ineffective cough Changes in rate or depth of respirations Usually caused by increased or tenacious secretions or obstruction (eg, aspiration	Abnormal blood gases

Suggested Alternative Diagnoses

Breathing Pattern, Ineffective
Gas Exchange, Impaired

Patient Outcomes and Evaluation Criteria

Include patient-specific target date, evaluation and documentation intervals, and any other patient-specific outcomes.

The patient will:

- Be able to describe plan for care at home.
- Be able to expectorate secretions effectively.
- Have a patent airway.
- Have pulmonary function within normal limits.

NIC Priority Interventions

Airway Management: Facilitation of patency of air passages.
Airway Suctioning: Removal of airway secretions by inserting a suction catheter into the patient's oral airway and/or trachea.

Nursing Actions

Target actions to problem etiologies. Individualize actions to meet the unique needs of each patient.

Ongoing Assessments

- Assess and document:

  Color, consistency, and amount of sputum.
  Effectiveness of oxygen administration q ____.
  Effectiveness of prescribed medications q ____.
  Trends in arterial blood gases (notify physician of abnormalities).

- Auscultate anterior and posterior chest q ____ to evaluate airway clearance.

Patient Teaching

- Explain proper use of supportive equipment (oxygen, suction, spirometer, IPPB).

- Inform patient and family that smoking is prohibited in room.
- Inform patient before initiating procedures to lower anxiety and increase sense of control.
- Instruct patient and family in plan for care at home (medications, hydration, nebulization, equipment, postural drainage, signs and symptoms of complications, community resources).
- Instruct patient in coughing and deep-breathing techniques, which facilitate removal of secretions.

Collaborative Activities

- Confer with respiratory therapist as needed.
- Consult with physician concerning need for percussion and/or supportive equipment.

Other

- Correlate all assessment data (patient sensorium, breath sounds, respiratory pattern, ABGs, sputum production), and document and report any changes.
- Encourage physical activity to promote movement of secretions.
- Maintain adequate hydration to decrease viscosity of secretions.
- Suction q ____. (Be sure to hyperoxygenate with ambu bag before and after suctioning ET tube or tracheostomy.)
- Suction the nasopharynx/oropharynx to remove secretions q ____.

Anxiety (9.3.1) (Y30)

Definition: A vague, uneasy feeling whose source is often nonspecific or unknown to the individual (NANDA).

Defining Characteristics

Subjective

Apprehension
Distress
Expressed concerns regarding change in life events
Fear of nonspecific consequences
Increased tension
Jitteryness, shakiness
Overexcitement
Painful and persistent increased helplessness
Regretfulness
Uncertainty
Worry

Objective

*Cardiovascular excitation
*Pupil dilation
*Superficial vasoconstriction
*Sympathetic stimulation
Extraneous movement (foot shuffling, hand/arm movements)
Facial tension
Focus on self
Glancing about
Increased perspiration
Increased wariness
Insomnia
Poor eye contact
Restlessness
Trembling/hand tremors
Voice quivering

*Critical

Related Factors

Interpersonal transmission/contagion
Situational/maturational crises
Threat of death
Threat to or change in environment

Threat to or change in health status
Threat to or change in interaction patterns
Threat to or change in role functioning
Threat to self-concept
Unconscious conflict about essential values/goals of life
Unmet needs

Suggestions for Use

Anxiety must be differentiated from Fear because the nursing interventions are different. When a patient is fearful, the focus is on removing or helping him/her to deal with the specific fear; when a patient is anxious, the nurse helps identify the cause of anxiety. Because the source of anxiety cannot always be identified, however, nursing care may also focus on helping the patient explore and express anxious feelings.

Because the level of anxiety determines the interventions, indicate in the diagnosis whether anxiety is moderate, severe, or panic-level. Panic may require collaborative interventions, such as medications. Mild anxiety should not be considered a problem, because it is a normal condition present in all human beings. Diagnose Anxiety only for patients who require special nursing interventions. Mild anxiety before surgery is a normal, healthy response.

Mild anxiety: Present in day-to-day living; increases alertness and perceptual fields; motivates learning and growth.

Moderate anxiety: Narrows perceptual fields; focus is on immediate concerns, with inattention to other communications and details.

Severe anxiety: Very narrow focus on specific detail; all behavior is geared toward getting relief.

Panic: The person loses control and feels dread and terror. A state of disorganization causes increased physical activity, distorted perceptions and relationships, and loss of rational thought. Panic can lead to exhaustion and death. (Stuart & Sundeen 1991)

Fear and Anxiety present diagnostic difficulty because they are not mutually exclusive. A person who is afraid is usually anxious as well. Many of the same signs and symptoms are present in both Fear and Anxiety: for example, increased heart and respiratory rate, dilated pupils, diaphoresis, muscle tension, and fatigue. The following comparisons may be helpful:

	Anxiety	*Fear*
Critical Defining Characteristic	Stimulation of the sympathetic nervous system	Ability to identify the object of fear
Type of Threat	Usually psychological (eg, to self-image); vague, nonspecific	Often physical (eg, to safety); specific, identifiable
Feeling	Vague, uneasy feeling	Feeling of dread
Source of Feeling	Unknown by the person	Known by the person

According to Carpenito (1993, p. 124), impending surgery may be the etiology for Fear, but most of the feelings about surgery relate to anxiety. Because the etiology (surgery) cannot be changed, nursing interventions should focus on supporting patient coping mechanisms for managing anxiety.

Suggested Alternative Diagnoses

Coping, Ineffective Individual
Fear

Patient Outcomes and Evaluation Criteria

Include patient-specific target date, evaluation and documentation intervals, and any other patient-specific outcomes.

The patient will:

- Demonstrate ability to continue necessary activities even though anxiety persists.

- Demonstrate ability to focus on new knowledge and skills.
- Identify those symptoms that are indicators of own anxiety.
- Report a decrease in somatic complaints.
- Report reduction in anxiety.
- Use anxiety-reducing techniques.

NIC Priority Interventions

Anxiety Reduction: Minimizing apprehension, dread, foreboding, or uneasiness related to an unidentified source of anticipated danger.

Nursing Actions

Target actions to problem etiologies. Individualize actions to meet the unique needs of each patient.

Ongoing Assessments

Assess and document patient's level of anxiety q ____.

Patient Teaching

Develop teaching plan with realistic goals, including need for repetition, encouragement, and praise of the tasks learned. Specify plan ____.

Other

- Encourage patient to verbalize thoughts and feelings to externalize anxiety.
- Explore with patient techniques that have, and have not, reduced anxiety in the past. Specify ____.
- Help patient identify events that have precipitated anxiety in the past.
- Help patient to focus on the present situation as a means of identifying coping mechanisms needed to reduce anxiety.
- Provide diversion through television, radio, games, and occupational therapies to reduce anxiety and expand focus.
- Provide positive reinforcement when patient is able to continue activities of daily living (ADLs) and other activities necessary to progress to optimal wellness.

- Reassure patient during interactions by touch and empathetic verbal and nonverbal exchanges, encourage patient to express anger and irritation, and allow patient to cry.
- Reduce excessive stimulation by providing a quiet environment, limited contact with others if necessary, and limited use of caffeine and other stimulants.
- Suggest alternative methods of reducing anxiety that are acceptable to patient. Specify ____.

Aspiration: Risk for (1.6.1.4) (Y23.0)

Definition: The state in which an individual is at risk for entry of gastrointestinal secretions, oropharyngeal secretions, or solids or fluids into tracheobronchial passages (NANDA).

Defining Characteristics

Presence of risk factors such as:

Objective

Decreased gastrointestinal motility
Delayed gastric emptying
Depressed cough and gag reflexes
Facial/oral/neck surgery or trauma
Gastrointestinal tubes, tube feedings
Hindered elevation of upper body
Impaired swallowing
Incomplete lower esophageal sphincter
Increased gastric residual
Increased intragastric pressure
Medication administration
Presence of tracheostomy or endotracheal tube
Reduced level of consciousness
Wired jaws

Risk Factors

See defining characteristics.

Suggestions for Use

Always use the most specific label for which the patient has the necessary defining characteristics.

Do not use Risk for Injury if the patient has the defining characteristics for Risk for Aspiration.

Suggested Alternative Diagnoses

Airway Clearance, Ineffective
Injury: Risk for
Self-Care Deficit: Feeding
Swallowing, Impaired

Patient Outcomes and Evaluation Criteria

Include patient-specific target date, evaluation and documentation intervals, and any other patient-specific outcomes.

The patient will:

- Demonstrate increased improvement in swallowing.
- Swallow independently without choking.
- Tolerate oral intake and secretions without aspiration.
- Tolerate enteral feedings without aspiration.

NIC Priority Interventions

Aspiration Precautions: Prevention or minimization of risk factors in the patient at risk for aspiration.

Nursing Actions

Target actions to problem etiologies. Individualize actions to meet the unique needs of each patient.

Ongoing Assessments

- Assess patient's lung sounds before and after feeding and before and after giving medication; document any adventitious sounds.
- Check gastric residual prior to feeding and giving medications.
- Evaluate patient for potential aspiration, including level of consciousness (LOC), tube placement, handling of secretions.

- Monitor tube feeding residual q ____.
- Verify placement of enteral tube prior to feeding and giving medications.

Patient Teaching

- Instruct family in feeding/swallowing techniques.
- Instruct patient in use of suction for removal of secretions.
- Review with patient and family signs and symptoms of aspiration and preventive measures.

Collaborative Activities

- Report any change in color of lung secretions that resembles food or feeding intake.
- Request occupational therapy consultation.

Other

- Allow patient time to swallow.
- Crush medications to facilitate swallowing.
- Have a suction catheter available at the bedside, and suction during meals as needed.
- Involve the family during patient's ingestion of food and meals:

  Evaluate family's comfort level.
  Provide support and reassurance.

- Place the patient in semi- or high-Fowler's position when eating whenever possible.
- Place patients who are unable to sit upright on their side, and elevate the head of the bed as much as possible during and after feeding.
- Provide positive reinforcement for attempts to swallow independently.
- Use a syringe, if necessary, when feeding the patient to facilitate swallowing.
- Vary consistency of foods to identify those foods more easily tolerated.

Body Image Disturbance (7.1.1) (Y61.0)

Definition: Viewing oneself differently as a result of actual or perceived changes in body structure or function. (NANDA: Disruption in the way one perceives one's body image.)

Defining Characteristics

Either (A) or (B) must be present to justify the diagnosis of Body Image Disturbance. The remaining defining characteristics may be used to validate the presence of (A) or (B).

Subjective

(A) Verbal response to actual or perceived change in structure or function

Depersonalization of part or loss by impersonal pronouns
Emphasis on remaining strengths and heightened achievement
Expressing feelings of helplessness, hopelessness, or powerlessness
Expressing negative feelings about body
Extension of body boundary to incorporate environmental objects
Focusing on past strengths, function, or appearance
Personalization of body part or loss by name
Preoccupation with change or loss
Refusal to accept change
Reporting changes in life-style
Verbalizing fear of rejection by or reaction of others

Objective

(B) Nonverbal response to actual or perceived change in structure or function

Actual change in structure or function
Change in ability to estimate spatial relationship of body to environment
Change in social involvement
Hiding or overexposing body part (intentional or unintentional)

Missing body part
Not looking at body part
Not touching body part
Showing reluctance to touch or look at affected body part
Trauma to nonfunctioning part

Related Factors

Chronic illness
Chronic pain
Congenital defects
Cultural or spiritual beliefs
Eating disorders (specify)
Pregnancy
Psychologic impairment (specify)
Situational crisis (specify)
Surgery
Treatment side-effects

Suggestions for Use

This label is related to Self-Esteem Disturbance but is specific to negative feelings about one's body or body parts. Although Body Image Disturbance is often caused by loss of a body part or actual body changes, the changes in structure or function can be perceived rather than actual. Patients on prolonged bed rest or who are dependent on machines (eg, dialysis, respirator) may experience distortion of body image. Eating disorders are often related to Body Image Disturbance.

Suggested Alternative Diagnoses

Nutrition, Altered: Less Than Body Requirements
Nutrition, Altered: More Than Body Requirements
Self-Esteem Disturbance

Patient Outcomes and Evaluation Criteria

Include patient-specific target date, evaluation and documentation intervals, and any other patient-specific outcomes.

The patient will:

- Acknowledge impact of situation on existing personal relationships and life-style.
- Acknowledge the actual change in body appearance.
- Describe actual change in function.
- Express willingness to consider life-style change.
- Express willingness to use suggested resources on discharge.
- Identify personal strengths.
- Maintain close personal relationships.

NIC Priority Interventions

Body Image Enhancement: Improving a patient's conscious and unconscious perceptions and attitudes toward his/her body.

Nursing Actions

Target actions to problem etiologies. Individualize actions to meet the unique needs of each patient.

Ongoing Assessments

- Assess and document patient's verbal and nonverbal responses to his/her body.

Collaborative Activities

- Assess need for assistance from social services department for planning care with patient/family and refer as needed.
- Offer to make initial phone call to appropriate community resources for patient/family.

Other

- Actively listen to patient/family, and acknowledge reality of concerns about treatments, progress, and prognosis.
- Assist patient in identifying personal strengths.
- Develop a plan of care with patient/family that identifies coping mechanisms and personal strengths and acknowledges limitations. Specify plan.
- Encourage patient to:

  Maintain usual daily grooming routine.
  Verbalize concerns about close personal relationships.

Verbalize consequences of physical and emotional changes that have influenced self-concept.

Wear clothing to enhance physical and emotional self-esteem.

- Encourage patient/family to air feelings and to grieve.
- Help patient identify alternative behaviors that are congruent with a change in personal relationships, life-style, and/or role performance.
- Provide care in a nonjudgmental manner, maintaining the patient's privacy and dignity.

Body Temperature, Altered: Risk for (1.2.2.1) (None)

Definition: The state in which the individual is at risk for failure to maintain body temperature within normal range (NANDA).

Defining Characteristics

Presence of risk factors such as:

Objective

Altered metabolic rate
Dehydration
Exposure to extremes in environmental temperatures
Extremes of age
Extremes of weight
Illness or trauma affecting temperature regulation
Immaturity of newborn's temperature-regulating system
Inability to perspire
Inactivity
Inappropriate clothing
Low birth weight
Medications (specify)
Sedation
Vigorous activity

Risk Factors

See defining characteristics.

Suggestions for Use

If the patient is at risk for both Hypothermia and Hyperthermia, then Risk for Altered Body Temperature is the appropriate label. If the patient is at risk for only an elevation in temperature, use Risk for Hyperthermia; for only decreased temperature, use Risk for Hypothermia.

Suggested Alternative Diagnoses

Hyperthermia
Hypothermia

Patient Outcomes and Evaluation Criteria

Include patient-specific target date, evaluation and documentation intervals, and any other patient-specific outcomes.

Temperature remains within normal limits for patient.

Patient/family will:

- Describe adaptive measures to minimize fluctuations in body temperature.
- Report early signs/symptoms of hypothermia/hyperthermia.

NIC Priority Interventions

Temperature Regulation: Attaining and/or maintaining body temperature within a normal range.

Vital Signs Monitoring: Collection and analysis of cardiovascular, respiratory, and body temperature data to determine and prevent complications.

Nursing Actions

Target actions to problem etiologies. Individualize actions to meet the unique needs of each patient.

Ongoing Assessments

- Assess patient for early signs and symptoms of hypothermia/hyperthermia.

- Evaluate home environment for factors that may alter body temperature.
- Monitor temperature q ___.

Patient Teaching

Instruct patient/family in measures to minimize temperature fluctuations.

For Hyperthermia

- Drink adequate fluids.
- Limit activity on hot days.
- Lose weight, if obese.
- Maintain stable environmental temperature.
- Remove excess clothing.

For Hypothermia

- Bathe in warm room, away from drafts.
- Increase activity.
- Limit alcohol intake.
- Maintain adequate nourishment.
- Maintain stable environmental temperature.
- Wear adequate clothing.

Instruct patient/family to recognize and report early signs and symptoms of hypothermia/hyperthermia.

For Hyperthermia

- Dry skin
- Headache
- Increased pulse
- Increased temperature
- Irritability
- Temperature above ___
- Weakness

For Hypothermia

- Apathy
- Cold, hard abdomen that feels like marble
- Disorientation/confusion
- Drowsiness
- Hypertension
- Hypoglycemia

- Impaired ability to think
- Reduced pulse and respiration
- Skin hard and cold to touch
- Temperature of less than 95F

Collaborative Activities

- Have social services meet with patient/family prior to discharge.

Other

- Maintain stable environmental temperature.

Bowel Incontinence (1.3.1.3) (Y20.0)

Definition: A state in which an individual experiences a change in normal bowel habits characterized by involuntary passage of stool (NANDA).

Defining Characteristics

Objective

Involuntary passage of stool

Related Factors

Decreased awareness of need to defecate
Loss of sphincter control

Suggestions for Use

Differentiate between this label and Diarrhea.

Suggested Alternative Diagnosis

Diarrhea

Patient Outcomes and Evaluation Criteria

Include patient-specific target date, evaluation and documentation intervals, and any other patient-specific outcomes.

The patient will:

- Be free of skin irritation to perianal area.
- Have fewer incontinent episodes.
- Regain voluntary control of defecation.

NIC Priority Interventions

Bowel Incontinence Care: Promotion of bowel continence and maintenance of perianal skin integrity.

Bowel Training: Assisting the patient to train the bowel to evacuate at specific intervals.

Nursing Actions

Target actions to problem etiologies. Individualize actions to meet the unique needs of each patient.

Ongoing Assessments

- Assess and document q ____.

  Condition of perianal skin after each episode of incontinence.

  Frequency of incontinent episodes.

Collaborative Activities

- Obtain order from physician to institute bowel-training program. (Program may include bulk-forming laxative; rectal suppository q day; digital stimulation; scheduled use of bedpan, commode, or bathroom.)

Other

- Protect patient's skin from involuntary stool (for example, use protective pad and ointments, frequently change bed linen).
- Provide bedpan or assist to commode q ___.
- Provide care in an accepting, nonjudgmental manner.
- Provide privacy for patient.

Breast-Feeding, Effective (Potential for Enhanced) (6.5.1.3) (None)

Definition: The state in which a mother-infant dyad/family exhibits adequate proficiency and satisfaction with breast-feeding process (NANDA).

Defining Characteristics

Major

Subjective

Contentment of infant after feeding

Objective

Ability of mother to position infant at breast to promote a successful latch-on response

Appropriate infant weight patterns for age

Effective mother-infant communication patterns (infant cues, maternal interpretation or response)

Regular and sustained suckling/swallowing at breast

Minor

Subjective

Maternal verbalization of satisfaction with the breast-feeding process

Objective

Adequate infant elimination patterns for age

Eagerness of infant to nurse

Signs and/or symptoms of oxytocin release (letdown or milk-ejection reflex)

Related Factors

Basic breast-feeding knowledge

Infant gestational age of more than 34 weeks

Maternal confidence

Normal breast structure

Normal infant oral structure
Supportive resources

Suggested Alternative Diagnoses

None

Patient Outcomes and Evaluation Criteria

Include patient-specific target date, evaluation and documentation intervals, and any other patient-specific outcomes.

- Mother and infant will maintain effective breast-feeding for as long as planned.

NIC Priority Interventions

Lactation Management: Promotion of successful breast-feeding and weaning through information and support.

Nursing Actions

Target actions to problem etiologies. Individualize actions to meet the unique needs of each patient.

Early Postpartum

Ongoing Assessments

- Confirm that infant has follow-up appointment with pediatrician.
- Observe for correct breast-feeding technique.

Patient Teaching

- Discuss breast-feeding schedule, usually a "demand" time every $1^1/2$ to 3 hours. Instruct mother to rest during/between feedings.
- Discuss ways to enhance milk supply:
  Drinking plenty of fluids.
  Getting enough rest.
  Nursing frequently.
  Using alternate breast at start of each feeding.

- Instruct mother in usual breast-feeding norms, eg, increased frequency of nursing in first weeks of life, baby's elimination patterns, uterine contractions during nursing.
- Provide anticipatory guidance for potential problems such as maternal fatigue; breast engorgement; sore, cracked nipples; inadequate milk supply; multiple births.
- Provide written materials for continued self-care at home.

Collaborative Activities

- Make referrals to appropriate community resources, such as Nursing Mothers' Council, La Leche League, other nursing mothers.

Other

- Promote maternal confidence by providing positive feedback.

Home Care

Ongoing Assessments

- Assess breast-feeding technique within first 5–7 days after birth.
- Confirm infant's elimination pattern.
- Explore mother's breast-feeding plans, eg, duration, return to work, introduction of solid foods, weaning; provide anticipatory guidance.

Patient Teaching

- Discuss mother's need to check with physician prior to taking any medication while breast-feeding.
- Provide instruction regarding breast engorgement, cracked and sore nipples, manual expression, infant appetite spurts, supplemental feedings.

Collaborative Activities

- Encourage mother to enlist/request available resources for assistance, eg, family, public health nurse, pediatrician, La Leche League, Nursing Mothers' Council.

Other

- Discuss impact of breast-feeding on family dynamics.
- Discuss setting priorities that

  Delegate meal preparation.
  Increase mother's rest.
  Minimize care of house.

- Promote maternal confidence by providing encouragement, praise, and reassurance.

Breast-Feeding, Ineffective (6.5.1.2) (Y53.0)

Definition: The state in which mother, infant, or child experiences dissatisfaction or difficulty with the breast-feeding process (NANDA).

Defining Characteristics

Major

Subjective

Unsatisfactory breast-feeding process (stated)

Minor

Subjective

Perceived inadequate milk supply

Objective

Actual inadequate milk supply
Arching and crying at the breast
Fussiness and crying within the first hour after breast-feeding
Inability of infant to latch onto maternal breast correctly
Insufficient emptying of each breast per feeding
Insufficient opportunity for suckling at the breast
No observable signs of oxytocin release
Nonsustained suckling at the breast
Observable signs of inadequate infant intake

Persistence of sore nipples beyond the first week of breast-feeding
Resistance to latching on
Unresponsiveness to other comfort measures

Related Factors

Inadequate sucking reflex in infant
Infant anomaly
Infant receiving supplemental feedings with artificial nipple
Interruption in breast-feeding
Knowledge deficit
Maternal anxiety or ambivalence
Maternal breast anomaly
Nonsupportive partner/family
Prematurity
Previous breast surgery
Previous history of breast-feeding failure

Suggestions for Use

Discriminate among this label and the suggested alternative diagnoses. This label focuses on the mother's satisfaction with the breast-feeding process, and includes an actual or perceived inadequate milk supply.

Diagnosis	*Cues (Defining Characteristics)*
Ineffective Breast-Feeding	Dissatisfaction with feeding process
Ineffective Infant Feeding Pattern	Inability of infant to suck or poorly coordinated suck-swallow response
Interrupted Breast-Feeding	Mother wishes to maintain lactation; unable to put baby to breast for some feedings (eg, illness or working)

Suggested Alternative Diagnoses

Breast-Feeding, Interrupted
Infant Feeding Pattern, Ineffective

Patient Outcomes and Evaluation Criteria

Include patient-specific target date, evaluation and documentation intervals, and any other patient-specific outcomes.

Baby will gain ____ grams/day or ____ grams/week.

Mother will:

- Describe increasing confidence with breast-feeding.
- State satisfaction with breast-feeding.

NIC Priority Interventions

Lactation Management: Promotion of successful breast-feeding and weaning through information and support.

Nursing Actions

Target actions to problem etiologies. Individualize actions to meet the unique needs of each patient.

Ongoing Assessments

- Assess mother's breast-feeding techniques and infant's ability to latch on and suck effectively.

Patient Teaching

- Instruct mother in breast-feeding techniques that increase her skill in feeding infant. Consider relaxation techniques, comfortable positioning, stimulating rooting reflex, stimulating infant to continue to feed, alternating breasts, and gradual increase of time on breast.
- Instruct mother in breast-pumping techniques to maintain milk supply during interruptions or delays in infant suckling reflex.
- Instruct mother in need for adequate rest and intake of fluids.

Collaborative Activities

- Make referrals to appropriate community resources, such as Nursing Mothers' Council, La Leche League, Public Health Department.

Other

- Have mother express enough milk to relieve engorgement, allowing nipples to evert.
- Increase number of nursings on demand for a crying, wakeful infant.
- Increase number of scheduled nursings for the sleepy infant of low birth weight.
- Offer food and fluids to mother during day and evening prior to breast-feeding times.
- Provide privacy for mother and infant.
- Recognize “time-out” behaviors in premature infant.
- Reinforce successful behaviors.
- Schedule infant activities to conserve energy prior to breast-feeding.
- Schedule rest periods as needed.
- Use ____ nipples.

Breast-Feeding, Interrupted (6.5.1.2.1) (Y53.0)

Definition: A break in the continuity of the breast-feeding process as a result of inability or inadvisability to put baby to breast for feeding (NANDA).

Defining Characteristics

Major

Objective

Infant does not receive nourishment at the breast for some or all of feedings

Minor

Subjective

Maternal desire to maintain lactation and provide (or eventually provide) breast milk for her infant's nutritional needs

Objective

Lack of knowledge regarding expression and storage of breast milk

Separation of mother and infant

Related Factors

Abrupt weaning of infant

Engorgement

Maternal medications that are contraindicated for the infant

Maternal obligations outside the home

Maternal or infant illness

Prematurity

Sore/cracked nipples

Suggestions for Use

Because this label represents a situation rather than a response, there is little the nurse can do to correct the interruption (eg, the need for the mother to work). Therefore, this label might function best as an etiology (eg, Risk for Ineffective Breast-Feeding related to Interrupted Breast-Feeding secondary to mother's employment). Also see suggestions for use for Ineffective Breast-Feeding.

Suggested Alternative Diagnoses

Breast-Feeding, Ineffective

Infant Feeding Pattern, Ineffective

Patient Outcomes and Evaluation Criteria

Include patient-specific target date, evaluation and documentation intervals, and any other patient-specific outcomes.

Mother will:

- Choose and demonstrate preferred technique for expression of milk.
- Describe safe storage techniques for expressed milk.
- Maintain lactation for as long as desired.

Baby will:

- Latch on and suck effectively at the breast.
- Receive mother's milk.

Mother and baby will maintain effective breast-feeding for as long as planned.

NIC Priority Interventions

Bottle Feeding: Preparation and administration of fluids to an infant via a bottle.

Emotional Support: Provision of reassurance, acceptance, and encouragement during times of stress.

Lactation Management: Promotion of successful breast-feeding and weaning through information and support.

Nursing Actions

Target actions to problem etiologies. Individualize actions to meet the unique needs of each patient.

Ongoing Assessments

- Assess family's ability to support lactation/breast-feeding plan and cope with life-style changes.
- Confirm readiness for transition to breast (infant's stability when outside the isolette, infant's coordination of sucking/swallowing/breathing, mother's willingness to try).
- Consider a feeding flow sheet to facilitate assessment: document infant's state, oxygen needs, positioning, time at breast, total nursing time, daily weight, stool pattern.

Patient Teaching

Assist working mother to maintain lactation by including the following teaching:

- Display/demonstrate variety of breast pumps, providing information about costs, effectiveness, and availability of each.
- Educate infant caretaker (storage and thawing of milk, no bottle feedings in the 2 hours prior to mother's return home).
- Instruct mother in chosen breast-pumping method.

- Provide information about lactation, breast-milk expression (manual and electric pump), collection, and storage.
- Provide information to enhance milk volume (adequate rest, regular expression of milk, increase mother's intake of fluid, especially toward the end of the work week).
- Provide mother with written/pictorial references for positioning infant.

Other

- Assist mother in setting realistic goals for herself.
- Assist mother and premature infant with transition to breast:

  Encourage skin-to-skin contact for mother and infant, using cover blanket over infant to maintain body temperature.

  Help infant open mouth wider.

  Position baby with one hand supporting head and other free to manipulate breast; ear, shoulder, and hips of infant should be aligned so that mother's nipples do not become sore.

  Provide privacy.

- Assist working mother to maintain lactation and effective breast-feeding:

  A few days before mother's return to work, introduce baby to bottle (someone other than mother, when mother is not present, when baby is hungry, in a different place than usual place for breast-feeding).

  Develop schedule for expression and storage of milk at work.

- Establish support network to ensure that mother has help with day-to-day lactation/breast-feeding problems as they occur.
- Provide anticipatory guidance for potential problems (eg, engorgement, pain, leaking, diminished milk production, feelings of disappointment/anger, depression, guilt, inadequacy).
- Time at breast will be longer than at bottle, but not to the point of infant's exhaustion; once latched on, allow infant

to nurse until baby stops sucking and swallowing. Switch baby to other breast and repeat until suck/swallow stops, then switch back.

- If abrupt weaning is necessary, assist mother to:

  Introduce bottle feeding.
  Manage breast discomfort.
  Verbalize feelings about sudden change in plans.

Breathing Pattern, Ineffective (1.5.1.3) (Y26.1)

Definition: The state in which an individual's inhalation and/or exhalation pattern does not enable adequate pulmonary inflation or emptying (NANDA).

Defining Characteristics

Subjective

Dyspnea
Shortness of breath

Objective

Altered chest excursion
Assumption of 3-point position
Change in depth of respirations
Fremitus
Increased anterior-posterior diameter
Nasal flaring
Premature infant
Pursed-lip breathing/prolonged expiratory phase
Tachypnea

Related Factors

Anxiety
Chronic or acute pain
Decreased energy/fatigue
Musculoskeletal impairment

Neuromuscular paralysis/weakness
Perception/cognitive impairment

Suggestions for Use

Do not use this label if the condition cannot be treated by independent nursing actions. Consider, too, that the ineffective breathing pattern may be a symptom of another problem, such as Anxiety. Differentiate carefully among this and the suggested alternative diagnoses. Also see suggestions for use for Airway Clearance, Ineffective.

Suggested Alternative Diagnoses

Activity Intolerance
Airway Clearance, Ineffective
Gas Exchange, Impaired

Patient Outcomes and Evaluation Criteria

Include patient-specific target date, evaluation and documentation intervals, and any other patient-specific outcomes.

The patient will:

- Demonstrate effective breathing pattern.
- Demonstrate optimal breathing while on mechanical ventilator.
- Request breathing assistance when needed.

Pulmonary function is within normal limits for patient.

Patient/family will be able to describe plan for care at home.

NIC Priority Interventions

Airway Management: Facilitation of patency of air passages.
Respiratory Monitoring: Collection and analysis of patient data to ensure airway patency and adequate gas exchange.

Nursing Actions

Target actions to problem etiologies. Individualize actions to meet the unique needs of each patient.

Ongoing Assessments

- Assess and document:

  Cyanosis q ____.

  Effect of medication on respiratory status.

  Location and extent of crepitus over rib cage.

  Presence or absence of breath sounds (anterior and posterior), noting rales, rhonchi, and diminished breath sounds q ____.

  Respiratory pattern, including rate, depth, and rhythm q ____.

- Observe and document bilateral chest expansion of patient on ventilator.

Patient Teaching

- Inform patient and family:

  About relaxation techniques to improve breathing pattern. Specify.

  About the plan for care at home (medications, supportive equipment, signs and symptoms of reportable complications, community resources).

  That smoking is prohibited in room.

  That they should notify the nurse at onset of ineffective breathing pattern.

Collaborative Activities

- Confer with respiratory therapist to ensure adequate functioning of mechanical ventilator.
- Report changes in sensorium, breath sounds, respiratory pattern, ABGs, sputum, and so on, as needed or per protocols.

Other

- Correlate all assessment data (patient sensorium, breath sounds, respiratory pattern, ABGs, sputum, effect of medications) and document.
- Encourage slow abdominal breathing during periods of respiratory distress.

- Give pain medications to allow optimal respiratory pattern according to the following schedule (specify schedule).
- Have patient turn, cough, and deep breathe q ____.
- Inform patient before beginning intended procedures to lower anxiety and increase sense of control.
- Maintain low-flow oxygen by nasal cannula, mask, hood, or tent. Specify flow rate: ____.
- Position for optimal breathing (specify).
- Reassure patient during periods of respiratory distress.
- Synchronize patient's breathing pattern with ventilator rate.

Cardiac Output, Decreased (1.4.2.1) (Y21)

Definition: A state in which the blood pumped by an individual's heart is sufficiently reduced that it is inadequate to meet the needs of the body's tissues (NANDA).

Defining Characteristics

Major

Subjective

Dyspnea
Fatigue

Objective

Arrhythmias
Cold, clammy skin
Color changes in skin and mucous membranes
Decreased peripheral pulses
Jugular vein distention
Oliguria
Orthopnea
Rales

Restlessness
Variations in blood pressure readings

Minor

Subjective

Shortness of breath
Vertigo
Weakness

Objective

Gallop rhythm
Syncope

Related Factors

Cardiac anomaly (specify)
Drug toxicity
Dysfunctional electrical conduction
Hypovolemia
Increased ventricular workload
Ventricular damage
Ventricular ischemia
Ventricular restriction

Suggestions for Use

This label does not suggest independent nursing actions. The nurse can neither conclusively diagnose nor definitively treat this problem. For patients with physiologic decreased cardiac output, you may find it more useful to use a label that represents a human response to this pathophysiology (eg, Activity Intolerance related to Decreased Cardiac Output). If the patient is at risk of developing complications, write them as collaborative problems (eg, Potential Complication of M.I.: Cardiogenic Shock).

Suggested Alternative Diagnoses

Activity Intolerance
Self-Care Deficit

Patient Outcomes and Evaluation Criteria

Include patient-specific target date, evaluation and documentation intervals, and any other patient-specific outcomes.

The patient will:

- Demonstrate increasing tolerance for physical activity.
- Describe the required diet, medications, activity, and limitations.
- Identify reportable signs and symptoms of worsening condition.
- Maintain hemodynamic stability. (Specify normal limits for blood pressure, pulse, pulse pressure, respirations, and hemodynamic parameters.)
- Report a decrease in severity and frequency of pain.

NIC Priority Interventions

Cardiac Care: Limitation of complications resulting from an imbalance between myocardial oxygen supply and demand for a patient with symptoms of impaired cardiac function.

Cardiac Care, Acute: Limitation of complications for a patient recently experiencing an episode of an imbalance between myocardial oxygen supply and demand resulting in impaired cardiac function.

Nursing Actions

Target actions to problem etiologies. Individualize actions to meet the unique needs of each patient.

Ongoing Assessments

- Assess and document:

  Blood pressure, presence of cyanosis, respiratory status, peripheral perfusion, mental status, and urine output.

  Dysrhythmias q ____. Correlate effects of laboratory values, oxygen, medications, activity, anxiety, and/or pain on the dysrhythmia.

  Patient's tolerance to activity, by noting onset of shortness of breath, pain, palpitations, or dizziness.

Presence of fluid overload, by assessing presence of dependent edema, weight gain, and decreased urine output. Auscultate lungs for adventitious sounds.

Patient Teaching

- Explain purpose of administering oxygen per nasal cannula or mask.
- Instruct patient and document instruction in nurse's notes.

  Regarding maintenance of accurate intake and output.

  In use, dose, frequency, and side-effects of medications.

  To report and describe palpitations and pain onset, duration, precipitating factors, site, quality, and intensity.
- Instruct patient/family in plan for care at home, including activity limitations, diet restrictions, use of therapeutic equipment, and reportable signs and symptoms.
- Provide information on stress-reduction techniques such as biofeedback, progressive muscle relaxation, meditation, exercise.

Collaborative Activities

- Confer with physician regarding parameters for administering/withholding blood pressure medications.

Other

- Correlate baseline vital signs with current vital signs and assess for changes in blood pressure, pulse (rate, rhythm, quality), and respirations and hemodynamic parameters.
- Correlate patient's blood pressure with blood pressure medications administered. Withhold blood pressure medications when there is a drop in blood pressure and notify physician.
- Change patient's position to flat or Trendelenberg when blood pressure is in a range lower than normal for patient. Document patient's response to position change.
- For sudden, severe, or prolonged hypotension, establish intravenous access for administration of intravenous fluids and/or medications to raise blood pressure.
- Maintain patient's appropriate/required activity level. Specify.

Caregiver Role Strain (Actual/Risk for) (3.2.2.2) (None)

Definition (Actual): A caregiver's felt difficulty in performing the family caregiver role (NANDA).

Definition (Risk for): A caregiver is vulnerable for felt difficulty in performing the family caregiver role (NANDA).

Defining Characteristics

Major

Does not have sufficient resources to provide the care needed

Feels that caregiving interferes with other important roles in his/her life

Feels loss because the care receiver is a different person than before caregiving began or, in the case of a child, that the care receiver was never the child the caregiver expected

Feels family conflict around issues of providing care

Feels stress or nervousness in his/her relationship with the care receiver

Feels depressed

Finds it hard to perform specific caregiving activities

Worries about the care receiver's health and emotional state, having to put the care receiver in an institution, and who will care for the care receiver if something should happen to the caregiver

Related Factors/Risk Factors

Developmental

Caregiver not developmentally ready for caregiver role, eg, young adult needing to provide care for a middle-aged parent

Developmental delay or retardation of the care receiver or caregiver

Pathophysiological

Addiction or codependency
Caregiver health impairment
Discharge of family member with significant home care needs
Illness severity of the care receiver
Premature birth/congenital defect
Unpredictable illness course or instability in the care receiver's health

Psychosocial

Care receiver exhibits deviant, bizarre behavior
Caregiver is female
Caregiver is spouse
Caregiver's marginal coping patterns
Marginal family adaptation or dysfunction prior to the caregiving situation
Past history of poor relationship between caregiver and care receiver
Psychological or cognitive problems in care receiver

Situational

Caregiver's competing role commitments
Complexity/amount of caregiving tasks
Duration of required caregiving, inadequate physical environment for providing care, eg, housing, transportation, community services, equipment
Family/caregiver isolation
Inexperience with/lack of knowledge of caregiving skills
Lack of respite and recreation for caregiver
Presence of abuse or violence
Presence of situational stressors that normally affect families, such as significant loss, disaster or crisis, poverty or economic vulnerability, major life events, eg, birth, hospitalization, leaving home, returning home, marriage, divorce, employment, retirement, death

Suggestions for Use

None

Suggested Alternative Diagnoses

Coping, Ineffective Family: Compromised
Coping, Ineffective Family: Disabling
Family Processes, Altered

Patient Outcomes and Evaluation Criteria

Include patient-specific target date, evaluation and documentation intervals, and any other patient-specific outcomes.

Caregiver will:

- Acknowledge impact of situation on existing life-style/role performance.
- Balance competing family and personal needs.
- Ensure provision of appropriate level of care.
- Express increased ability to cope with changes in family structure and dynamics.
- Express willingness to identify and use available resources and social supports.
- Identify personal strengths, social supports, and community resources.
- Obtain appropriate assistance/care through caregiver's efforts.

NIC Priority Interventions

Caregiver Support: Provision of the necessary information, advocacy, and support to facilitate primary patient care by someone other than a health care professional.

Nursing Actions

Target actions to problem etiologies. Individualize actions to meet the unique needs of each patient.

Ongoing Assessments

- Assess care receiver for signs of emotional and/or physical neglect or abuse.

- Assess caregiver for signs of increasing role strain (eg, depression, anxiety, increased use/abuse of alcohol/drugs, frustration, helplessness, sleeplessness, lowered morale, physical and/or emotional exhaustion, and personal health problems).
- Assess family's adjustment and coping.

Patient Teaching

- Facilitate coping and adjustment by teaching caregiver and care receiver how to (Chilman 1988):

  Deal with pain, incapacitation, and illness-related symptoms.
  Deal with hospital environment and disease-related treatments/procedures.
  Establish and maintain workable relationships with the health care team.

- Suggest caregiver education and training groups.

Collaborative Activities

- Make referrals as needed for counseling and support during times of stress or crisis.
- Refer for necessary assistance with preventive, supervisory, and instrumental caregiving (eg, VNA, respite care, hospice care, day treatment, secondary caregivers).
- Report signs of care receiver physical/emotional neglect or abuse to authorities.

Other

- Acknowledge that the work of the caregiver is both physical and mental and includes (Bowers 1987):

  Anticipatory caregiving (making decisions based on possible future needs of care receiver, eg, place of residence).
  Instrumental caregiving (direct, hands-on care).
  Preventive caregiving (taking action to prevent illness, injury, or complications, eg, altering the physical environment, preparing meals).
  Protective caregiving (protecting care receiver from threats to self-image, identity, and change in relationship with caregiver).

Supervisory caregiving (arranging for and monitoring care, eg, making appointments, arranging transportation, communicating with health professionals).

- Arrange for parent(s) of chronically ill child to receive training in areas of child development and education and compliance-related behavior problems.
- Assist caregiver to identify problems or concerns with caregiving (eg, lack of knowledge/skill/emotional readiness for caregiving, lack of social support, financial burden, caregiver response to care receiver's mental deterioration, disruptive behavior, impaired social functioning, increasing need for physical care).
- Develop a plan of care with caregiver that identifies coping mechanisms, personal strengths, social supports, and acknowledged limitations. Consider including the following:

Assistance with household tasks.
Family therapy.
Self-help and mutual support groups for information, advocacy, and emotional support.

- Explore with caregiver the possibility of institutional care (now or in the future) and feelings associated with institutionalization.
- Explore with caregiver/care receiver past and current closeness, shared activities, and confiding in one another as indications of emotional investment and commitment to the role.
- Facilitate family's adjustment to illness of family member by assisting them to (Chilman 1988):

Develop a flexibility regarding future goals.
Grieve for the loss of pre-illness family identity.
Maintain a sense of mastery over their lives.
Move toward acceptance of changes.
Pull together during short-term crisis.

- Promote self-care by care receiver, as appropriate, to encourage relief for caregiver.

Communication, Impaired: Verbal (2.1.1.1) (Y10.0)

Definition: The state in which an individual experiences a decreased or absent ability to use or understand language in human interaction (NANDA).

Defining Characteristics

Major

Objective

Does not or cannot speak
Speaks or verbalizes with difficulty
Unable to speak dominant language

Minor

Objective

Absence of audible speech
Anatomic defect
Difficulty expressing thoughts verbally
Difficulty forming words or sentences
Disorientation
Hearing deficit
Medical regimen/disease process interfering with ability to make audible sounds (eg, CVA, ET tube, tracheostomy)

Related Factors

Acute confusion
Aphasia
Developmental disability
Inability to speak or speak clearly
Intubation
Primary language other than English
Psychologic impairment (specify)
Tracheostomy

Suggestions for Use

Use this label for those who desire to communicate but are having difficulty doing so. If communication problems are caused by psychiatric illness or coping difficulties, a diagnosis of Fear or Anxiety may be more appropriate (Carpenito 1993, p. 229).

Suggested Alternative Diagnoses

Anxiety
Coping, Defensive
Fear
Sensory/Perceptual Alterations: Visual, Auditory
Thought Processes, Altered

Patient Outcomes and Evaluation Criteria

Include patient-specific target date, evaluation and documentation intervals, and any other patient-specific outcomes.

The patient will:

- Communicate needs to staff with minimal frustration.
- Communicate satisfaction with alternative means of communication.
- Demonstrate increasing ability to express needs to staff and family.
- Demonstrate increasing understanding of spoken words and gestures.
- Demonstrate understanding of need to change method of communication to express needs to staff and family.

NIC Priority Interventions

Active Listening: Attending closely to and attaching significance to a patient's verbal and nonverbal messages.

Communication Enhancement: Facilitating interaction with a patient who has difficulty delivering or receiving verbal or nonverbal messages.

Nursing Actions

Target actions to problem etiologies. Individualize actions to meet the unique needs of each patient.

Ongoing Assessments

- Identify and document patient's primary language.
- Assess and document:

  Patient's ability to speak, hear, write, read, and understand to establish communication between staff and patient, family and patient.

  Patient's communication pattern to facilitate optimal two-way communication.

  Patient's response to touch, spatial distance, and male/female roles that may influence communication.

Patient Teaching

- Explain to patient why he or she cannot speak.

Collaborative Activities

- Consult with physician regarding need for speech therapy, if appropriate.

Other

- Encourage attendance at group meetings for interpersonal contact. Specify group ____.
- Encourage frequent family visits to provide stimulation for communication.
- Encourage patient to communicate slowly and to repeat requests.
- Encourage patient's communication with staff and family by giving frequent positive reinforcement to patient.
- Encourage patient's self-expression in any manner that provides information to staff/family to ensure that patient's needs are being met.
- Establish one-to-one contact with patient q ____.
- Give clear and simple directions, which will avoid overwhelming choices that may add to the patient's confusion. For example, take patient by the arm, saying, "Walk with me now."

- Involve the patient and family in development of communication plan. Communication plan is ____.
- Provide care in a relaxed, unhurried, nonjudgmental manner.
- Provide continuity in nursing assignment to establish trust and reduce frustration.
- Reassure patient that frustration and anger are acceptable and expected.
- Speak slowly, distinctly, and quietly, facing the patient.
- Use family/significant person or hospital translator, as appropriate. Specify name, phone number, and relationship.
- Use flash cards, pad/pencil, gestures, pictures, foreign language vocabulary lists, and the like to facilitate optimal two-way communication.

Constipation (1.3.1.1) (None)

Definition: A state in which an individual experiences a change in normal bowel habits characterized by a decrease in frequency and/or passage of hard, dry stools (NANDA).

Defining Characteristics

Major

Subjective

Reported feeling of pressure in rectum
Reported feeling of rectal fullness

Objective

Decreased activity level
Decreased frequency of defecation
Hard, forced stools
Palpable mass
Straining at stool

Minor

Subjective

Abdominal pain

Back pain

Headache

Objective

Appetite impairment

Interference with daily living

Use of laxatives

Related Factors

Decreased activity

Decreased fluid intake

Decreased motility (secondary to aging, multiple sclerosis, Hirschsprung's disease, and so on)

Dietary changes

Medications (specify)

Painful defecation

Suggested Alternative Diagnoses

Constipation, Colonic

Constipation, Perceived

Patient Outcomes and Evaluation Criteria

Include patient-specific target date, evaluation and documentation intervals, and any other patient-specific outcomes.

The patient will:

- Demonstrate knowledge of bowel regimen necessary to overcome the side-effects of medications.
- Describe dietary requirements necessary to maintain usual bowel pattern.
- Pass stool of usual consistency for patient.
- Report presence of optimal bowel pattern.
- Report the passage of stool with a reduction of pain and straining.

NIC Priority Interventions

Constipation/Impaction Management: Prevention and alleviation of constipation/impaction.

Nursing Actions

Target actions to problem etiologies. Individualize actions to meet the unique needs of each patient.

Ongoing Assessments

- Gather baseline data on bowel regimen, activity, and medications. Document patient's usual pattern.
- Assess and document:

  Color and consistency of first stool postoperatively.
  Frequency, color, and consistency of stool q ____.
  Passage of flatus.
  Presence of impaction q ____.
  Presence or absence of bowel sounds and abdominal distention in all four quadrants q ____.

Patient Teaching

- Inform patient of possibility of medication-induced constipation.
- Instruct patient in bowel elimination aids that will promote optimal bowel pattern at home.
- Teach patient the effects of diet (eg, fluids and fiber) on elimination.
- Instruct patient in consequences of long-term laxative use.
- Stress the avoidance of straining during defecation to prevent change in vital signs, dizziness, or bleeding.

Collaborative Activities

- Consult with dietitian for increase in fiber and fluids in diet.
- Request a physician's order for elimination aids, such as dietary bran, stool softeners, and laxatives.

Other

- Encourage patient to request pain medication prior to defecation to facilitate painless passage of stool.

- Encourage optimal activity to stimulate patient's bowel elimination.
- Provide privacy and safety for patient during bowel elimination.
- Provide care in an accepting, nonjudgmental manner.
- Provide fluids of patient's choice ____ (specify).

Constipation, Colonic (1.3.1.1.2) (Y20.1)

Definition: The state in which an individual's pattern of elimination is characterized by hard, dry stool, which results from delay of passage of food residue (NANDA).

Defining Characteristics

Major

Subjective

Painful defecation

Objective

Decreased frequency of defecation
Hard, dry stool
Palpable mass
Straining at stool

Minor

Subjective

Abdominal pain
Appetite impairment
Distended abdomen
Headache

Related Factors

Change in daily routine
Chronic use of medication and enemas
Decreased activity

Decreased fluid intake
Emotional disturbances
Fear of moving bowels in hospital environment
Hypokalemia
Immobility
Lack of privacy
Less than adequate amounts of fiber and bulk-forming foods in diet
Metabolic conditions such as hypothyroidism

Suggestions for Use

None

Suggested Alternative Diagnoses

Constipation
Constipation, Perceived

Patient Outcomes and Evaluation Criteria

Include patient-specific target date, evaluation and documentation intervals, and any other patient-specific outcomes.

The patient will:

- Demonstrate knowledge of bowel regimen necessary to overcome the side-effects of medications.
- Describe dietary requirements (eg, fluids and fiber) necessary to maintain usual bowel pattern.
- Pass stool of usual consistency and frequency for patient.
- Report presence of optimal bowel pattern.
- Report the passage of stool with a reduction of pain and straining.

NIC Priority Interventions

Constipation/Impaction Management: Prevention and alleviation of constipation/impaction.

Nursing Actions

Target actions to problem etiologies. Individualize actions to meet the unique needs of each patient.

Ongoing Assessments

- Gather baseline data on bowel regimen, activity, and medications. Document patient's usual pattern.
- Assess and document:

  Frequency, color, and consistency of stool q ____.
  Passage of flatus.
  Presence of impaction q ____.
  Presence or absence of bowel sounds and abdominal distention in all four quadrants q ____.

Patient Teaching

- Inform patient of possibility of medication-induced constipation.
- Instruct patient in maintaining high-fiber, bulk-forming foods in diet; increasing physical activity; and increasing fluid intake to promote optimal bowel function at home.
- Stress the avoidance of straining during defecation to prevent change in vital signs, dizziness, or bleeding.

Collaborative Activities

- Consult with dietitian for increase in fiber and bulk-forming food in patient's diet.
- Request a physician's order for elimination aids, such as dietary bran, stool softeners, and laxatives.

Other

- Encourage optimal activity to stimulate patient's bowel elimination.
- Encourage patient to request pain medication prior to defecation to facilitate painless passage of stool.
- Provide care in an accepting, nonjudgmental manner.
- Provide fluids of patient's choice (specify).
- Provide privacy and safety for patient during bowel elimination.

Constipation, Perceived (1.3.1.1.1) (Y20.2)

Definition: A state in which an individual makes a self-diagnosis of constipation and ensures a daily bowel movement through the use of laxatives, enemas, and suppositories (NANDA).

Defining Characteristics

Major

Subjective

Expected passage of stool at same time every day

Objective

Expectation of daily bowel movement, with resulting overuse of laxatives, enemas, and suppositories

Related Factors

Cultural/family health beliefs
Faulty appraisal of normal bowel function
Impaired thought processes

Suggestions for Use

None

Suggested Alternative Diagnoses

Constipation
Constipation, Colonic

Patient Outcomes and Evaluation Criteria

Include patient-specific target date, evaluation and documentation intervals, and any other patient-specific outcomes.

The patient will:

- Acknowledge dependence on use of laxatives, enemas, and

suppositories.

- Describe dietary regimen that will more naturally regulate bowel function.
- Verbalize understanding of need to decrease use of laxatives, enemas, and suppositories.

NIC Priority Interventions

Bowel Management: Establishment and maintenance of a regular pattern of bowel elimination.

Nursing Actions

Target actions to problem etiologies. Individualize actions to meet the unique needs of each patient.

Ongoing Assessments

- Assess patient's expectation of normal bowel function.
- Observe, document, and report requests for laxatives, enemas, and/or suppositories.

Patient Teaching

- Instruct patient and family in diet, fluid intake, activity, exercise, and the consequence of overuse of laxatives, enemas, and suppositories.

Collaborative Activities

- Initiate a multidisciplinary care conference involving the patient/family to encourage positive health-seeking behaviors.

Other

- Assist patient to identify realistic use of laxatives, enemas, and suppositories.
- Discuss with patient/family the patient's perceived need to utilize aids for defecation.
- Explore with patient the need to change diet and fluid intake.
- Provide support to patient when behavior change occurs.

Coping, Defensive (5.1.1.1.2) (Y02.2)

Definition: The state in which an individual experiences falsely positive self-evaluation based on a self-protective pattern that defends against underlying perceived threats to positive self-regard (NANDA).

Defining Characteristics

Major

Subjective

Denial of obvious problems/weaknesses
Projection of blame/responsibility
Rationalization of failures

Objective

Grandiosity
Hypersensitivity to slight or criticism

Minor

Subjective

Difficulty in reality testing perceptions

Objective

History of difficulty in establishing/maintaining relationships
Hostile laughter or ridicule of others
Lack of follow-through or participation in treatment or therapy
Superior attitude toward others

Related Factors

Situational crisis (specify)
Psychological impairment (specify)

Suggestions for Use

None

Suggested Alternative Diagnoses

Adjustment, Impaired
Communication, Impaired
Coping, Ineffective Individual
Denial, Ineffective
Thought Processes, Altered

Patient Outcomes and Evaluation Criteria

Include patient-specific target date, evaluation and documentation intervals, and any other patient-specific outcomes.

The patient will:

- Acknowledge specific problems/conflicts that interfere with social interactions/relationships.
- Demonstrate decrease in defensiveness.
- Participate in treatment program.

NIC Priority Interventions

Self-Awareness Enhancement: Assisting a patient to explore and understand his/her thoughts, feelings, motivations, and behaviors.

Nursing Actions

Target actions to problem etiologies. Individualize actions to meet the unique needs of each patient.

Ongoing Assessments

- Assess degree of defensiveness/denial that interferes with self-assessment.

Patient Teaching

- Teach patient alternative behaviors to obtain positive regard through group therapy, individual therapy, role playing, and role modeling.

Collaborative Activities

- Refer to appropriate community resources.

Other

- Assist patient in recognizing negative coping behaviors.
- Identify and discuss the subjects, situations, and people that trigger negative coping behaviors.
- Include family in treatment as needed.
- Provide feedback in a supportive environment on how behavior is being perceived by others.
- Provide reality testing during times of grandiose behavior, denial of obvious problems, and projected blame/responsibility.

Coping, Family: Potential for Growth (5.1.2.2) (None)

Definition: A state in which a family member(s) has effectively adapted to patient's health challenge and now exhibits desire and readiness for enhanced growth in regard to self and in relation to the patient (adapted from NANDA).

Defining Characteristics

Subjective

Family member begins to recognize growth potential of crisis in relation to own goals, priorities, or relationships

Family member requests information about support groups

Family member verbalizes need to enhance quality of life

Objective

Family member promotes and evaluates care for patient

Related Factors

Sufficient achievement of patient's basic health care needs, enabling goals of self-actualization to surface

Suggestions for Use

None

Suggested Alternative Diagnoses

None

Family Outcomes

Family member(s) will:

- Develop a plan for personal growth.
- Evaluate and change plan as needed.
- Identify and prioritize personal goals.
- Implement plan.

NIC Priority Interventions

Family Support: Promotion of family interests and goals.

Nursing Actions

Target actions to problem etiologies. Individualize actions to meet the unique needs of each patient.

Other

- Assist family member(s) in developing a plan for personal growth. Plan may include investigation of employment opportunities, school, support groups, enrichment activities, and exercise.
- Assist family member(s) in identifying and prioritizing personal goals.
- Encourage family member(s) to compare initial response to the crisis with current situation and to recognize change.
- Provide an opportunity for family member(s) to reflect on impact of patient's illness on family structure and dynamics.
- Provide emotional support and availability to family member(s) during implementation, evaluation, and revision of plan.

Coping, Ineffective Family: Compromised (5.1.2.1.2) (Y00.0)

Definition: A state in which a usually supportive family member/close friend provides ineffective comfort/support that may be needed by the patient to manage or master adaptive tasks related to his/her health challenge (adapted from NANDA).

Defining Characteristics

Subjective

Family expresses a lack of knowledge needed for effective assistive or supportive behaviors

Family expresses preoccupation with own reaction (eg, fear, grief, guilt, anxiety) to patient's illness or disability or to other situational or developmental crises

Patient expresses concern/complaint regarding family members' response to her/his health problem

Objective

Family attempts to assist with patient care but is unsuccessful

Family displays emotional lability

Family displays rigid role boundaries

Family member interferes with necessary medical/nursing actions

Family member overassists or overprotects patient

Family member underreacts—eg, withdraws, ignores, minimizes, refuses to assist

Family members are divisive and form unsupportive coalitions

Family verbal interaction with patient is absent or decreased

Related Factors

Chronic illness or disability

Developmental crisis (specify)

Economic problems

Inadequate or incorrect information or understanding by family member/close friend
Lack of mutual decision-making skills
Patient's diminished support of family member/close friend
Shift in family's normal power structure
Situational crisis (specify)
Temporary family disorganization and role changes
Temporary preoccupation of family member/close friend with own emotional conflicts and personal suffering
Unrealistic expectations/demands

Suggestions for Use

Caregiver Role Strain focuses on the needs of the caregiving family member, whereas Ineffective Family Coping: Compromised focuses more on the needs of the patient. This diagnosis is similar to Altered Family Processes. For severe malfunction or for abusive or destructive situations, use Ineffective Family Coping: Disabling, which can be differentiated by the following defining characteristics:

Denial of existence or severity of illness of a family member
Despair, rejection
Desertion
Abuse (child, spousal, elder)

Suggested Alternative Diagnoses

Caregiver Role Strain (Actual/Risk for)
Coping, Ineffective Family: Disabling
Family Processes, Altered
Parental Role Conflict
Parenting, Altered

Family Outcomes

Include patient-specific target date, evaluation and documentation intervals, and any other patient-specific outcomes.

The family will:

- Acknowledge needs of family unit.
- Acknowledge needs of patient.

- Begin to demonstrate effective interpersonal skills.
- Express increased ability to cope with changes in family structure and dynamics.
- Express unresolved feelings.
- Identify conflicting coping styles.
- Participate in developing and implementing a treatment plan.
- Use more flexible problem-solving strategies.

NIC Priority Interventions

Family Involvement: Facilitating family participation in the emotional and physical care of the patient.

Family Mobilization: Utilization of family strengths to influence patient's health in a positive direction.

Family Support: Promotion of family interests and goals.

Nursing Actions

Target actions to problem etiologies. Individualize actions to meet the unique needs of each patient.

Ongoing Assessments

- Assess interaction between patient and family; be alert for potential destructive behaviors.

Patient/Family Teaching

- Discuss the common responses to health challenges, eg, anxiety, dependency, depression.
- Discuss with family effective ways to demonstrate feelings.
- Provide information about specific health challenge and necessary coping skills.
- Teach the family those skills required for care of patient. Specify.
- Teach, role model, and reinforce communication skills, which may include active listening, reflection, "I" statements, conflict resolution.

Collaborative Activities

- Explore available hospital and community resources with family.

- Initiate a multidisciplinary patient care conference, involving the patient/family in problem solving and facilitation of communication.
- Provide continuity of care by maintaining effective communication between staff members through nurse report, patient care conferences, and care planning.
- Refer family members to appropriate support systems to encourage attention to needs of self.
- Request social service consultation to help the family determine posthospitalization needs and identify sources of community support.

Other

- Assist family in identifying personal strengths.
- Assist family in identifying behaviors that may be hindering prescribed treatment.
- Assist family in realistically identifying the needs of patient and family unit.
- Assist family members in assuming new roles.
- Assist family with decision-making and problem-solving.
- Encourage family to express concerns to help plan post-hospital care.
- Encourage family to identify needed role changes to maintain family integrity.
- Encourage family to participate in patient's care.
- Encourage family to recognize changes in interpersonal relationships.
- Encourage family to verbalize feelings.
- Encourage family to visit patient whenever possible. Provide privacy to facilitate family interactions.
- Explore impact of conflicting coping styles on family relationships.
- Promote an open, trusting relationship with family.
- Provide structure to family interaction. Consider:

  Content of interaction.
  Length of visiting time.
  Staff support during visit.

Which family member(s) will visit, based on patient's treatment plan.

Coping, Ineffective Family: Disabling (5.1.2.1.1) (Y00.1)

Definition: Behavior of a significant family member that disables his/her own capacity, as well as the patient's capacity to perform effectively tasks essential to either person's adaptation to the health challenge (adapted from NANDA).

Defining Characteristics

Subjective

Distortion of reality of patient's health problem, including extreme denial about its existence or severity

Objective

Abandonment

Aggression/hostility

Agitation

Decisions and actions by family that are detrimental to economic or social well-being

Depression

Desertion

Disregarding patient's needs

Family member displaying illness signs of patient

Impaired individualization

Impaired restructuring of a meaningful life for self

Inability to make decisions and solve problems

Intolerance

Neglectful care of patient in regard to basic human needs and/or illness treatment

Neglectful relationships with other family members

Patient displaying helpless, inactive dependence

Psychosomatic symptoms
Rejection of patient

Related Factors

Child sexual/physical abuse
Chronically unresolved feelings (specify hostility, anxiety, guilt, despair, and so on)
Emotionally disturbed family member
Highly ambivalent family relationships
Substance-abusing family member
Use of violence to manage conflict

Suggestions for Use

This label is appropriate when there is severe malfunction, or for abusive or destructive situations. It represents a more dysfunctional situation than does Altered Family Processes or Ineffective Family Coping: Compromised. The diagnostic label Caregiver Role Strain focuses on the needs of the caregiving family member, whereas Ineffective Family Coping: Disabling focuses more on the needs of the patient and/or the family unit. The label Risk for Violence should be used when the abusive behavior is potential rather than actual.

Suggested Alternative Diagnoses

Caregiver Role Strain (Actual/Risk for)
Coping, Ineffective Family: Compromised
Parenting, Altered
Violence, Risk for: Self-Directed or Directed at Others

Family Outcomes and Evaluation Criteria

Include patient-specific target date, evaluation and documentation intervals, and any other patient-specific outcomes.

The family will:

- Acknowledge needs of family unit.
- Acknowledge needs of patient.
- Begin to demonstrate effective interpersonal skills.
- Demonstrate ability to resolve conflict without violence.

- Express unresolved feelings.
- Identify and maintain intrafamily sexual boundaries.
- Identify conflicting coping styles.
- Participate in effective problem solving.
- Participate in treatment plan.

NIC Priority Interventions

Family Support: Promotion of family interests and goals.

Family Therapy: Assisting family members to move their family toward a more productive way of living.

Nursing Actions

Target actions to problem etiologies. Individualize actions to meet the unique needs of each patient.

Ongoing Assessments

- Assess interaction between patient and family, being alert for potential destructive behaviors.

Patient/Family Teaching

- Discuss how violence is a learned behavior and can be transmitted to offspring.
- Discuss with family effective ways to demonstrate feelings.
- Teach the family those skills required for care of patient. Specify.
- Teach, role model, and reinforce communications skills, which may include active listening, reflection, "I" statements, conflict resolution, and nonviolent methods of expressing anger.

Collaborative Activities

- Initiate a multidisciplinary patient care conference, involving the patient/family in problem solving and facilitation of communication.
- Provide continuity of care by maintaining effective communication between staff members through nurse report, patient care conferences, and care planning.
- Refer family/individual members to support groups, psychiatric treatment, social services (eg, chemical depen-

dence programs, Parents United, Incest Survivors Anonymous, child protective services, battered wives' shelters).

- Report indications of physical/sexual abuse as directed by law to appropriate authorities.

Other

- Assist family in realistically identifying the needs of patient and family unit.
- Assist family in recognizing the problem, eg, managing conflict with violence, sexual abuse.
- Encourage family participation in all group meetings.
- Encourage family to express concerns and to help plan posthospital care.
- Explore impact of conflicting coping styles on family.
- Provide structure to family interaction. Consider:

  Content of interaction.
  Length of visiting time.
  Staff support during visit.
  Which family member(s) will visit, based on patient's treatment plan.

Coping, Ineffective Individual (5.1.1.1) (Y02)

Definition: A state in which an individual is unable to problem solve or use adaptive behaviors to meet life's demands and roles (NANDA).

Defining Characteristics

Subjective

*Verbalization of inability to cope or inability to ask for help
Change in usual communication patterns
Expressing unrealistic expectations
Reported substance abuse
Verbal manipulation

*Critical

Objective

*Inability to problem solve
Alteration in societal participation
Destructive behavior toward self and others
Evidence of physical/psychologic abuse
High illness rate
High rate of accidents
Inability to meet basic needs
Inability to meet role expectations
Inappropriate use of defense mechanisms

*Critical

Related Factors

Personal vulnerability in a maturational crisis (specify)
Personal vulnerability in a situational crisis (specify)

Suggestions for Use

This label represents a more chronic or long-term pattern than does Impaired Adjustment. It is less specific than the label Defensive Coping. Many labels represent failure to cope (eg, Risk for Violence, Hopelessness). Always use the most specific label that fits the patient's defining characteristics.

Suggested Alternative Diagnoses

Adjustment, Impaired
Anxiety
Fear
Grieving, Dysfunctional
Post-Trauma Response
Violence, Risk for: Self-Directed or Directed at Others

Patient Outcomes and Evaluation Criteria

Include patient-specific target date, evaluation and documentation intervals, and any other patient-specific outcomes.

The patient will:

- Demonstrate interest in diversional activities.

- Identify personal strengths that may promote effective coping.
- Initiate conversation.
- Participate in activities of daily living.
- Participate in decision-making process.
- Use patient's verbal and nonverbal expressions applicable to situation.
- Verbalize plan for either accepting or changing the situation.

NIC Priority Interventions

Coping Enhancement: Assisting a patient to adapt to perceived stressors, changes, or threats which interfere with meeting life demands and roles.

Decision-Making Support: Providing information and support for a patient who is making a decision regarding health care. Specify estimated date of completion. Specify frequency.

Nursing Actions

Target actions to problem etiologies. Individualize actions to meet the unique needs of each patient.

Ongoing Assessments

- Assess aggressive behaviors.
- Assess potential for self-destructive behaviors, and document.

Collaborative Activities

- Initiate a patient care conference to review patient's coping mechanisms and to establish a plan of care.
- Involve hospital resources in provision of emotional support for patient and family.

Other

- Assist patient in developing a plan for accepting or changing situation.
- Assist patient in identifying personal strengths.
- Encourage patient to:

  Be involved in planning care activities.
  Demonstrate feelings.

Express concerns and help solve problems.
Initiate conversations with others.
Participate in activity.
Request family visitation whenever possible.

Decisional Conflict (specify) (5.3.1.1) (Y02.1)

Definition: State of uncertainty about course of action to be taken when choice among competing actions involves risk, loss, or challenge to personal life values (NANDA).

Defining Characteristics

Major

Subjective

Verbalizing uncertainty about choices
Verbalizing undesired consequences of alternative actions being considered

Objective

Delaying decision making
Vacillating between alternative choices

Minor

Subjective

Displaying signs of distress or tension (eg, increased heart rate, restlessness, increased muscle tension)
Focusing on self
Verbalizing feeling of distress while attempting a decision

Objective

Questioning personal values and beliefs while attempting a decision

Related Factors

Interference with decision making
Interference with support system

Lack of experience with decision making
Lack of relevant information
Lack of support system
Multiple or divergent sources of information
Perceived threat to value system
Unclear personal values/beliefs

Suggestions for Use

None

Suggested Alternative Diagnoses

Parental Role Conflict
Therapeutic Regimen Management, Ineffective Individual

Patient Outcomes and Evaluation Criteria

Include patient-specific target date, evaluation and documentation intervals, and any other patient-specific outcomes.

The patient will:

- Acknowledge the advantages/disadvantages of available choices.
- Evaluate available choices in relation to personal values.
- Decide on course of action.
- Report a decrease in tension or distress.

NIC Priority Interventions

Decision-Making Support: Providing information and support for a patient who is making a decision regarding health care.

Nursing Actions

Target actions to problem etiologies. Individualize actions to meet the unique needs of each patient.

Ongoing Assessments

- Assess patient's understanding of available choices.
- Evaluate patient's level of tension or distress.

Patient Teaching

- Provide accurate information about choices.

Collaborative Activities

- Use resources as appropriate.

Other

- Assist patient in identifying a course of action and adapt as necessary.
- Encourage patient to discuss decision and process with the health care team, family, and significant others.
- Explore with patient the advantages and disadvantages of each choice.
- Help patient decide the importance of each advantage and disadvantage through discussion, "weighing," prioritizing, and eliminating obviously unacceptable choices.

Denial, Ineffective (5.1.1.1.3) (Y02.3)

Definition: The state of a conscious or unconscious attempt to disavow the knowledge or meaning of an event to reduce anxiety/fear to the detriment of health (NANDA).

Defining Characteristics

Major

Objective

Delay in seeking or refusal of health care attention to the detriment of health

Failure to perceive personal relevance of symptoms or danger

Minor

Subjective

Displacing fear of impact of the condition

Displacing source of symptoms to other organs

Failure to admit fear of death or invalidism

Inability to admit impact of disease in life pattern

Inappropriate affect
Minimizing symptoms

Objective

Making dismissive gestures or comments when speaking of distressing events

Related Factors

Specific to patient

Suggestions for Use

None

Suggested Alternative Diagnoses

Coping, Defensive
Coping, Ineffective Family: Compromised
Coping, Ineffective Family: Disabling
Coping, Ineffective Individual
Grieving, Dysfunctional
Noncompliance (specify)
Rape-Trauma Syndrome: Silent Reaction
Therapeutic Regimen Management, Ineffective Individual

Patient Outcomes and Evaluation Criteria

Include patient-specific target date, evaluation and documentation intervals, and any other patient-specific outcomes.

The patient will:

- Begin to acknowledge symptoms.
- Recognize significance of symptoms.
- Report significant symptoms.

NIC Priority Interventions

Anxiety Reduction: Minimizing apprehension, dread, foreboding, or uneasiness related to an unidentified source of anticipated danger.

Counseling: Use of an interactive helping process focusing on the needs, problems, or feelings of the patient and significant others to enhance or support coping, problem solving, and interpersonal relationships.

Nursing Actions

Target actions to problem etiologies. Individualize actions to meet the unique needs of each patient.

Ongoing Assessments

- Assess patient's understanding of symptoms/illness.

Patient Teaching

- Teach recognition of symptoms and desired patient responses.

Other

- Establish a therapeutic relationship with patient that will allow exploration of denial.
- Engage patient in discussion about anxiety, fears, symptoms, and impact of illness.
- Include patient/family in a multidisciplinary conference to develop a plan of action. Plan may include:

  Arranging for follow-up support after discharge.
  Meeting with patients in similar situations to learn new ways to cope and to decrease anxiety and fear.
  Using every opportunity to reinforce consequences of patient's actions.

Diarrhea (1.3.1.2) (Y20.3)

Definition: A state in which an individual experiences a change in normal bowel habits characterized by the frequent passage of loose, fluid, unformed stools (NANDA).

Defining Characteristics

Major

Subjective

Abdominal cramping

Abdominal pain
Urgency to defecate

Objective

Change in usual consistency, frequency, and volume of stool
Loose/liquid stool

Minor

Objective

Change in color of stool

Related Factors

Dietary changes
Excessive alcohol intake
Food intolerance
Impaction
Increased intestinal motility secondary to ____
Medications (specify)
Stress

Suggestions for Use

None

Suggested Alternative Diagnosis

Bowel Incontinence

Patient Outcomes and Evaluation Criteria

The patient will:

- Describe dietary requirements to maintain usual bowel pattern.
- Gain weight.
- Pass stool of usual consistency.
- Pass stool with decreasing frequency.
- Report presence of optimal bowel pattern.
- Practice hygiene adequate to prevent skin breakdown.

NIC Priority Interventions

Diarrhea Management: Prevention and alleviation of diarrhea.

Nursing Actions

Target actions to problem etiologies. Individualize actions to meet the unique needs of each patient.

Ongoing Assessments

- Assess and document:

  Condition of perianal skin q ____.
  Frequency, color, and consistency of stool q ____.
  Impaction q ____.
  Skin turgor and condition of oral mucosa as indicators of dehydration q ____.
- Guaiac stools q ____.
- Have patient identify usual bowel pattern. Document.
- Help patient to identify stressors that may contribute to diarrhea. Document.
- Monitor laboratory values (electrolytes, CBC), and report abnormalities.
- Weigh patient daily.

Patient Teaching

- Inform patient of possibility of medication-induced diarrhea.
- Instruct patient in diet and use of antidiarrheal medications to promote optimal bowel pattern at home.

Collaborative Activities

- Consult with dietitian for adjustment of dietary fiber.
- Consult with pediatrician for alternative type of feeding.
- Request order from physician for antidiarrheal, antispasmodic, and/or topical medications.

Other

- Provide care in an accepting, nonjudgmental manner.
- Provide fluids of patient's choice ___ (specify).
- Provide privacy and safety for patient during bowel elimination.

Disuse Syndrome: Risk for (1.6.1.5) (Y23.1)

Definition: A state in which an individual is at risk for deterioration of body systems as the result of prescribed or unavoidable inactivity (NANDA).

Defining Characteristics

Presence of risk factors, such as the following:

Objective

Altered level of consciousness
Mechanical immobilization
Paralysis
Prescribed immobilization
Severe pain

Risk Factors

See defining characteristics.

Suggestions for Use

This label describes potential complications of immobility. It is a "syndrome diagnosis" under which a number of actual and potential problems are clustered. When the risk factor is immobility, it is not necessary to write separate risk diagnoses such as Risk for Impaired Skin Integrity or Risk for Activity Intolerance. These more specific labels should be used only if an actual (rather than a potential) problem develops or if the risk factor is something other than immobility. Furthermore, this diagnosis should not be written with an etiology. As a syndrome diagnosis, the etiology (disuse) is contained in the label itself (Carpenito 1993).

Suggested Alternative Diagnoses

If an actual problem occurs as a result of immobility or if the etiology of a potential (risk) problem is something other than immobility, consider using a more restricted physiologic nursing diagnosis, such as one of the following:

Infection: Risk for
Injury: Risk for
Peripheral Neurovascular Dysfunction: Risk for

Actual or Risk for

Activity Intolerance
Body Image Disturbance
Breathing Pattern, Ineffective
Constipation
Mobility, Impaired Physical
Powerlessness
Sensory/Perceptual Alterations: All (specify)
Sexuality Patterns, Altered
Skin Integrity, Impaired
Swallowing, Impaired
Tissue Perfusion, Altered: Peripheral
Urinary Retention

Patient Outcomes and Evaluation Criteria

Include patient-specific target date, evaluation and documentation intervals, and any other patient-specific outcomes.

Goals of care for this label are broad. They focus on preventing complications of immobility for all body systems. For example, the patient will:

- Be oriented to time, place, and person.
- Have adequate peripheral circulation.
- Maintain normal urinary function.
- Maintain optimal respiratory function.
- Maintain satisfactory body image.
- Not develop bone demineralization, constipation, contractures, or pressure ulcers.

NIC Priority Interventions

Energy Management: Regulating energy use to treat or prevent fatigue and optimize function.

Nursing Actions

The outcomes and interventions selected are determined by the patient's affected body system and the degree of disuse. For patient outcomes and nursing actions specific to each body system, see the labels listed under suggested alternative diagnoses.

Diversional Activity Deficit (6.3.1.1) (Y50.2)

Definition: The state in which an individual experiences decreased stimulation from or decreased interest/engagement in recreational leisure activities (NANDA).

Defining Characteristics

Subjective

Complaining of inability to initiate or continue with usual activity

Expressing apathy, boredom

Objective

Anger, hostility

Disruptive behavior

Flat affect

Increase in daytime sleep periods

Restlessness

Withdrawn behavior

Related Factors

Deficit in social skills

Disturbance in motivation

Forced inactivity

Frequent/lengthy medical treatments

Impaired perception of reality

Long-term hospitalization

Prolonged bed rest

Suggestions for Use

None

Suggested Alternative Diagnoses

Adjustment, Impaired
Social Interaction, Impaired

Patient Outcomes and Evaluation Criteria

Include patient-specific target date, evaluation and documentation intervals, and any other patient-specific outcomes.

The patient will:

- Demonstrate socially acceptable behaviors during activities.
- Help identify activity alternatives that may provide stimulation.
- Verbalize acceptance of limitations that interfere with usual leisure activities.

NIC Priority Interventions

Recreation Therapy: Purposeful use of recreation to promote relaxation and enhancement of social skills.

Self-Responsibility Facilitation: Encouraging a patient to assume more responsibility for own behavior.

Nursing Actions

Target actions to problem etiologies. Individualize actions to meet the unique needs of each patient.

Ongoing Assessments

- Observe and record:

  Efforts to participate in activities.
  Interests expressed by patient.

Collaborative Activities

- Identify resources, such as volunteers and occupational therapists, that could assist patient in recreational/leisure activities.

Other

- Alternate patient care routines, involving patient in plans.
- Encourage family, friends, and significant persons to visit.
- Encourage patient to participate in activities of interest that can be provided during hospitalization. Specify ____.
- Encourage patient to verbalize feelings and concerns regarding limitations.
- Introduce and encourage new or alternative leisure-time activities. Specify.
- Introduce patient to other patients who have successfully dealt with similar situations.
- Provide appropriate stimuli, such as music, games, visitors, and relaxation therapy, to vary monotonous routines and stimulate thought.
- Provide compatible roommate, if possible.

Dysfunctional Ventilatory Weaning Response (DVWR) (1.5.1.3.2) (None)

Definition: A state in which a patient cannot adjust to lowered levels of mechanical ventilator support, which interrupts and prolongs the weaning process (NANDA).

Defining Characteristics

Nurses have defined three levels of DVWR, in which these defining characteristics occur in response to weaning (Logan & Jenny 1990).

Mild DVWR

Major

Objective

Restlessness

Slight increased respiratory rate from baseline

Minor

Subjective

Responds to lowered levels of mechanical ventilator support with:

- Expressed feelings of increased need for oxygen, breathing discomfort, fatigue, warmth
- Queries about possible machine malfunction

Objective

Responds to lowered levels of mechanical ventilator support with increased concentration on breathing

Moderate DVWR

Major

Objective

Responds to lowered levels of mechanical ventilator support with:

- Baseline increase in respiratory rate < 5 breaths/minute
- Slight increase from baseline blood pressure < 20mm Hg
- Slight increase from baseline heart rate < 20 beats/minute

Minor

Subjective

Apprehension

Objective

Color changes; pale, slight cyanosis
Decreased air entry on auscultation
Diaphoresis
Eye widening ("wide-eyed" look)
Hypervigilance to activities
Inability to cooperate
Inability to respond to coaching
Slight respiratory accessory muscle use

Severe DVWR

Major

Objective

Responds to lowered levels of mechanical ventilatory support with:

Agitation
Deterioration in arterial blood gases from current baseline
Increase from baseline blood pressure > 20 mm Hg
Increase from baseline heart rate > 20 beats/minute
Respiratory rate increases significantly from baseline

Minor

Objective

Adventitious breath sounds, audible airway secretions
Cyanosis
Decreased level of consciousness
Discoordinated breathing with the ventilator
Full respiratory accessory muscle use
Paradoxical abdominal breathing
Profuse diaphoresis
Shallow, gasping breaths

Related Factors

Physical

Inadequate nutrition
Ineffective airway clearance
Sleep pattern disturbance
Uncontrolled pain or discomfort

Situational

Adverse environment (noisy, active environment, negative events in the room, low nurse-patient ratio, extended nurse absence from bedside, unfamiliar nursing staff)
History of multiple unsuccessful weaning attempts.
History of ventilator dependence > 1 week
Inadequate social support
Inappropriate pacing of diminished ventilator support
Uncontrolled episodic energy demands or problems

Psychological

Anxiety: moderate, severe
Decreased motivation
Decreased self-esteem
Fear
Hopelessness

Insufficient trust in the nurse
Knowledge deficit of the weaning process
Patient perceived inefficacy about the ability to wean
Patient role
Powerlessness

Suggestions for Use

DVWR is concerned specifically with patient responses to separation from the mechanical ventilator. Other respiratory diagnoses may also occur during weaning, for example, Ineffective Airway Clearance, Ineffective Breathing Pattern, and Impaired Gas Exchange. This diagnostic label does not include the reasons for the weaning problems. If you do not know the etiology of the DVWR, use "unknown etiology."

Suggested Alternative Diagnoses

Airway Clearance, Ineffective
Breathing Pattern, Ineffective
Gas Exchange, Impaired
Respiratory Function, Altered (Risk for)

Patient Outcomes and Evaluation Criteria

Include patient-specific target date, evaluation and documentation intervals, and any other patient-specific outcomes.

The patient will:

- Achieve established weaning goals.
- Be physiologically stable for weaning process.
- Be psychologically and emotionally ready for weaning process.
- Demonstrate necessary physical and emotional resources to achieve weaning goals.
- Demonstrate understanding of the weaning process and his/her role in achieving weaning process goals.
- Participate in goal setting for weaning process.

NIC Priority Interventions

Mechanical Ventilation: Use of an artificial device to assist a patient to breathe.

Mechanical Ventilatory Weaning: Assisting the patient to breathe without the aid of a mechanical ventilator.

Nursing Actions

Target actions to problem etiologies. Individualize actions to meet the unique needs of each patient.

Ongoing Assessments

- Assess patient's readiness to wean by considering the following respiratory indicators:

  Arterial blood gases stable with $PaO_2 > 60$ on 40–60% oxygen.
  Cough effectively enough to handle secretions.
  Length of time on ventilator.
  Maximum inspiratory force > –25 cm H_2O (normal –80 to –1000) so independent respiration can be initiated.
  Stable spontaneous respiratory rate < 35 breaths/minute (BPM).
  Unassisted tidal volume > 5 ml/kg ideal body weight.
  Vital capacity > 13 ml/kg ideal body weight.

- Assess patient's readiness to wean by considering the following nonrespiratory indicators:

  Absence of constipation, diarrhea, or ileus.
  Absence of fever and/or infection.
  Adequate nutritional status as evidenced by acceptable serum albumin, transferrin, midarm muscle circumference > 15 percentile.
  Adequate rest and sleep.
  Electrolytes within normal limits for patient.
  Hemoglobin and hematocrit within normal limits for patient.
  Improving body strength and endurance.
  Normal blood pressure for patient.
  Psychological/emotional readiness.

Stable heart rate and rhythm.
Tolerable pain or discomfort level.

- Monitor patient's response to current medications and correlate with weaning goals.

Patient Teaching

- Instruct patient/family in weaning process and goals, which should include:

How patient may feel as process evolves.
Participation of family.
Participation required by patient.
What patient can expect from nurse.
Why weaning is necessary.

Collaborative Activities

- Discuss weaning process and goals with physician and respiratory care practitioner, including patient's present and preexisting medical condition(s).
- Reevaluate appropriateness of weaning process with physician if weaning goals are not attainable.

Other

- Document in nursing care plan those strategies that promote success with weaning process to ensure consistency (eg, communication method with patient, family participation, coaching methods, and so on).
- Encourage self-care to increase sense of control and participation in own care. Normalize ADLs to patient's tolerance.
- Establish a trusting relationship that instills patient's confidence in nurse to assist patient with weaning process.
- Establish effective methods of communication between patient and others (eg, writing, blinking eyes, squeezing hand, and so on).
- Initiate weaning process by:

Checking equipment to make sure it is attached to oxygen.
Checking for presence of bilateral breath sounds.
Checking that settings are as ordered.
Checking tubing for kinks and excessive moisture.

Checking vital signs and patient for indicators of nontolerance or fatigue q5–15 minutes. Reconnect patient to ventilator at preweaning settings if indicators of nontolerance occur.

Documenting weaning process and patient's tolerance in nurses notes or flow sheet.

Explaining procedure to patient and family.

Measuring and recording baseline respiratory rate, heart rate, blood pressure, EKG rhythm, lung sounds, vital capacity, tidal volume, inspiratory force, saturated oxygen via pulse oxymeter.

Preoxygenating, hyperinflating, suctioning, reoxygenating patient prior to weaning.

Providing a quiet environment during weaning time.

Providing diversions such as television or radio.

Sitting patient in an upright position to decrease abdominal pressure on the diaphragm, allowing for better lung expansion.

Starting the weaning time when patient has rested and is awake and alert.

Staying with patient during weaning time to provide coaching and reassurance.

Understanding the rationale for weaning orders [use of CPAP (Continuous Positive Airway Pressure); SIMV (Synchronized Intermittent Mandatory Ventilation); PSV (Pressure Support Ventilation); MMV (Mandatory Minute Ventilation)]; or T-piece.

Dysreflexia (Actual/Risk for) (1.2.3.1) (Y25.0)

Definition: The state in which an individual with a spinal cord injury at T7 or above experiences a life-threatening, uninhibited sympathetic response of the nervous system to a noxious stimulus (NANDA).

Defining Characteristics

Major

Subjective

Pounding diffuse headache

Objective

Bradycardia

Diaphoresis above injury

Pallor below injury

Paroxysmal hypertension (sudden periodic elevation of blood pressure, where systolic is > 140 and diastolic is > 90)

Red splotches on skin

Tachycardia

Minor

Subjective

Blurred vision

Chest pain

Metallic taste in mouth

Paresthesia

Objective

Chills

Conjunctival congestion

Goose bumps

Horner's syndrome (contraction of pupil, partial ptosis of eyelid, enophthalmos, absence of sweating over affected side of face)

Nasal congestion

Related Factors

Bladder distention in spinal cord injury

Bowel distention in spinal cord injury

Skin irritation or skin lesion in spinal cord injury

Suggestions for Use

Dysreflexia is a potential problem for the patient with high spinal cord injury. Dysreflexia cannot continue as an actual nursing diagnosis. If it occurs as an actual problem and independent nursing actions do not resolve it, medical treatment is necessary. In that event, the collaborative problem, Potential Complication of High Spinal Cord Injury: Dysreflexia, should be used.

As a rule, Risk for Dysreflexia is a more useful label than Actual Dysreflexia because the patient is in a potential state most of the time (Carpenito 1993, p. 303). The suggested alternative diagnoses represent noxious stimuli that can trigger a sympathetic response in the patient with spinal cord injury. They may be used as actual problems or as the etiology of Dysreflexia or Risk for Dysreflexia.

Suggested Alternative Diagnoses

Constipation (Fecal Impaction)
Skin Integrity, Impaired
Urinary Retention

Patient Outcomes and Evaluation Criteria

Include patient-specific target date, evaluation and documentation intervals, and any other patient-specific outcomes.

The patient will:

- Demonstrate ability to maintain bowel and bladder routine.
- Identify early signs and symptoms of dysreflexia.
- Maintain blood pressure at ____ or less.

NIC Priority Interventions

Dysreflexia Management: Prevention and elimination of stimuli which cause hyperactive reflexes and inappropriate autonomic responses in a patient with a cervical or high thoracic cord lesion.

Nursing Actions

Target actions to problem etiologies. Individualize actions to meet the unique needs of each patient.

Ongoing Assessments

- Assess for bladder distention q4 hours.
- Assess for bowel elimination q day.
- Assess patient's knowledge of condition, including history of previous episodes, early signs and symptoms, and bowel and bladder regimen.
- Assess skin condition at least daily, noting any reddened areas above level of spinal cord injury.
- Obtain baseline temperature, blood pressure, and pulse. Baseline temperature, blood pressure, and pulse are ____.

Patient Teaching

- Ask patient to report any early signs and symptoms of condition that occur.
- Instruct patient in early signs and symptoms of condition: pounding headache, flushing diaphoresis of face and thorax.
- Review with caretaker needed interventions during onset of crisis.

Other

During onset of crisis, carry out management plan as follows:

- Administer antihypertensive medications as ordered.
- Decrease blood pressure by elevating head of bed or putting patient in sitting position.
- Monitor blood pressure q3–5 minutes.
- Stop activity, and have someone notify physician.
- Quickly eliminate noxious stimulus in the following order:

  Bladder: Check catheter for patency, or catheterize patient.

  Bowel: If distended, apply anesthetic ointment to rectal area, and disimpact. Consider enema or flatus tube.

  Body temperature: Maintain normal body temperature.

Family Processes, Altered (3.2.2) (Y70)

Definition: The state in which a family that normally functions effectively experiences dysfunction (NANDA).

Defining Characteristics

Subjective

Differing expectations expressed by family members
Verbal hostility between family members/patient/staff

Objective

Absence of family interaction
Entry of new family member into home (eg, elder, newborn)
Failure to accomplish current developmental tasks
Family hindrance of nursing/medical care
Inability of family system to meet physical, emotional, security, and spiritual needs of its members
Inability to accept/express wide range of feelings
Inability to accept/receive help appropriately
Inability to deal with traumatic event constructively
Inability to express/accept feelings of members
Inappropriate level and direction of energy
Lack of family involvement in community activities
Lack of respect for individuality and autonomy of family members
Parents do not demonstrate respect for each other's views on child-rearing practices
Poorly communicated family rules, rituals, or symbols
Rigidity in function and roles

Related Factors

Change in family roles
Change in family structure
Developmental transition and/or crisis
Hospitalization/change in environment
Illness/disability of family member

Lack of adequate support system
Separation of family members
Situational transitions or crises
Unmet expectations for child
Unmet expectations for childbirth
Unmet expectations for pregnancy

Suggestions for Use

This label describes a family that normally functions effectively but is experiencing a stressor that alters its functioning. The stressors causing Altered Family Processes tend to be situational or developmental transitions and crises such as the following:

Death of a family member
Divorce
Infidelity
Loss of job
Serious illness of a family member

This label is different from Ineffective Family Coping: Compromised, in which the stressor is withdrawal of support by a significant other, and the family coping problem is caused by a change in the relationship between the family members—not necessarily by an external stressor such as death or divorce. Compromised Family Coping may involve the patient and only one significant other, whereas Altered Family Processes involves the entire family.

Altered Family Processes describes a family that has the resources for effectively coping with stressors, in contrast with Ineffective Family Coping: Disabling, which describes a family that demonstrates destructive behaviors. If stressors are not effectively resolved, Altered Family Processes can progress to Ineffective Family Coping.

To differentiate among the suggested alternative diagnoses, carefully examine the defining characteristics and related factors of each.

Suggested Alternative Diagnoses

Caregiver Role Strain (Actual/Risk for)
Coping, Ineffective Family: Compromised
Coping, Ineffective Family: Disabling
Grieving, Dysfunctional
Parental Role Conflict
Parenting, Altered

Family Outcomes and Evaluation Criteria

Include patient-specific target date, evaluation and documentation intervals, and any other patient-specific outcomes.

Family members will:

- Acknowledge change in family roles.
- Identify coping patterns.
- Participate in decision-making processes regarding post-hospital care.

NIC Priority Interventions

Family Integrity Promotion: Promotion of family cohesion.
Family Process Maintenance: Minimization of family process disruption effects.

Nursing Actions

Target actions to problem etiologies. Individualize actions to meet the unique needs of each patient.

Ongoing Assessments

- Assess interaction between patient and family, being alert for potential destructive behaviors.

Patient Teaching

- Teach the family those skills required for care of patient. Specify ____.

Collaborative Activities

- Explore available hospital and community resources with family.

- Initiate a multidisciplinary patient care conference, involving the patient/family in problem solving and facilitation of communication.
- Provide continuity of care by maintaining effective communication between staff members through nurse report, patient care conferences, and care planning.
- Refer family to a financial counselor.
- Request social service consultation to help the family determine posthospitalization needs and identify sources of community support.

Other

- Assist family in identifying behaviors that may be hindering prescribed treatment.
- Assist family in identifying personal strengths.
- Discuss with family appropriate ways to demonstrate feelings.
- Encourage family to express concerns and to help plan posthospital care.
- Encourage family to participate in patient's care.
- Encourage family to verbalize feelings.
- Encourage family to visit patient whenever possible. Provide privacy to facilitate family interactions.
- Promote an open, trusting relationship with family.
- Provide positive reinforcement for effective use of coping mechanisms.

Fatigue (6.1.1.2.1) (Y50.3)

Definition: An overwhelming, sustained sense of exhaustion and decreased capacity for physical and mental work (NANDA).

Defining Characteristics

Major

Subjective

Verbalization of unremitting and overwhelming lack of energy

Objective

Inability to maintain usual routines

Minor

Subjective

Decreased libido

Increased physical complaints

Objective

Accident-proneness

Decreased performance

Disinterest in surroundings

Emotional lability

Inability to concentrate

Irritability

Lethargy, listlessness

Related Factors

Altered body chemistry (eg, medications, drug withdrawal, chemotherapy)

Decreased/increased metabolic energy production

Excessive social and/or role demands

Increased energy requirements to perform activities of daily living

Overwhelming psychologic or emotional demands

States of discomfort

Suggestions for Use

Do not use this label to describe temporary tiredness resulting from lack of sleep. Fatigue describes a chronic condition; the patient's previous energy levels and capabilities cannot be restored. Discriminate carefully between Fatigue and Activity Intolerance. The energy deficit in Fatigue is overwhelming, and may exist even when the patient has not performed any activities.

Fatigue may be the etiology of other nursing diagnoses, such as Self-Care Deficit and Impaired Home Maintenance Management. Conversely, other labels, such as Decreased Cardiac Output, may be the etiology of Fatigue.

Suggested Alternative Diagnoses

Activity Intolerance
Cardiac Output, Decreased
Self-Care Deficit
Sleep Pattern Disturbance

Patient Outcomes and Evaluation Criteria

Include patient-specific target date, evaluation and documentation intervals, and any other patient-specific outcomes.

The patient will:

- Acknowledge disease process/condition that exacerbates symptoms of fatigue.
- Demonstrate ability to maintain usual activity level and social interaction.
- Demonstrate increasing ability to concentrate.
- Differentiate psychologic from physical factors that may cause fatigue.
- Identify measures that modify environment to reduce fatigue.

NIC Priority Interventions

Energy Management: Regulating energy use to treat or prevent fatigue and optimize function.

Nursing Actions

Target actions to problem etiologies. Individualize actions to meet the unique needs of each patient.

Ongoing Assessments

- Assess and document patient's level of fatigue q ____.

Patient Teaching

- Instruct patient in the relationship of fatigue to disease process/condition.

Other

- Assist patient in identifying measures that increase concentration. Consider:

Completing simple tasks.
Initiating tasks after pain medication.
Initiating tasks after rest periods.
Prioritizing necessary tasks.
Reducing surrounding distractions (noise, people, television).

- Discuss with patient/family ways to modify home environment to maintain usual activity level/social interaction and to minimize fatigue.
- Encourage patient to:

Identify measures that prevent or modify fatigue.
Report activities that increase fatigue.
Report onset of pain that may produce fatigue (severity, location, precipitating factors). Document.

- Plan activities with patient/family that minimize fatigue. Plan may include:

Assisting with ADLs as needed. Specify assistance needed.
Including family in plan to minimize fatigue as appropriate. Specify.
Providing positive reinforcement for increase in activity.
Providing rest periods during activities.
Setting small, realistic, attainable goals for patient that decrease fatigue. Specify goals ____.

- Plan activities to allow time for adequate rest:

Avoid unnecessary procedures during resting period
Limit visitation during resting period.

Fear (9.3.2) (Y32)

Definition: Feeling of dread related to an identifiable source which the person validates (NANDA).

Defining Characteristics

Ability to identify object of fear

Related Factors

Environmental stressor/hospitalization
Implications for future pregnancies
Powerlessness
Real or imagined threat to child
Real or imagined threat to own well-being

Suggestions for Use

See suggestions for use for the Anxiety diagnosis.

Suggested Alternative Diagnoses

Anxiety
Post-Trauma Response
Rape-Trauma Syndrome

Patient Outcomes and Evaluation Criteria

Include patient-specific target date, evaluation and documentation intervals, and any other patient-specific outcomes.

The patient will:

- Demonstrate behaviors that may reduce fear.
- Name known sources of fear.
- Report reasonable comfort.

NIC Priority Interventions

Anxiety Reduction: Minimizing apprehension, dread, foreboding, or uneasiness related to an unidentified source of anticipated danger.

Coping Enhancement: Assisting a patient to adapt to perceived stressors, changes, or threats which interfere with meeting life demands and roles.

Security Enhancement: Intensifying a patient's sense of physical and psychological safety.

Nursing Actions

Target actions to problem etiologies. Individualize actions to meet the unique needs of each patient.

Patient Teaching

- Provide patient with information/interaction regarding procedures and hospital routine.

Collaborative Activities

- Assess need for social service and/or psychiatric intervention.
- Encourage a patient/physician discussion of the patient's fear.
- Initiate a multidisciplinary patient care conference to develop a plan of care. Specify plan.

Other

- Convey acceptance of the patient's perception of fear to encourage open communication regarding the source of the fear.
- Encourage and help patient to express the contributing factors that have produced fear.
- Encourage patient to differentiate real from imagined threat to well-being by discussing the sources of fear.
- Provide continuity of patient care through patient assignment and use of care plan.
- Provide frequent verbal and nonverbal reassurances that may assist in reducing the patient's fear state. Avoid clichés.
- Provide frequent, positive reinforcement when patient demonstrates behaviors that may reduce or eliminate fear.
- Remove the source of the patient's fear whenever possible.

Fluid Volume Deficit (1.4.1.2.2.1) (Y22.0)

Definition: The state in which an individual experiences vascular, cellular, or intracellular dehydration (NANDA).

Defining Characteristics

Major

Objective

Change in serum sodium
Change in urine concentration
Change in urine output
Decreased venous filling
Hemoconcentration
Sudden weight loss or gain

Minor

Subjective

Thirst

Objective

Change in mental state
Decreased pulse volume/pressure
Decreased skin turgor
Dry mucous membrane
Dry skin
Hypotension
Increased body temperature
Increased pulse rate
Weakness

Related Factors

Abnormal blood loss (specify)
Abnormal fluid loss (specify)
Excessive continuous consumption of alcohol
Failure of regulatory mechanisms (as in diabetes insipidus, hyperaldosteronism)
Inadequate fluid intake secondary to ____

Suggestions for Use

Use this label for patients experiencing vascular, cellular, or intracellular dehydration. Use the label cautiously, because many fluid balance problems require nurse-physician collaboration. Do not use this label routinely, even as a potential problem, for patients who have a medical order of "NPO." Independent nursing treatments for Fluid Volume Deficit are meant to prevent fluid loss (eg, diaphoresis) and encourage oral fluid intake. For a diagnosis such as Risk for Fluid Volume Deficit related to NPO order, there are no independent nursing actions to prevent or treat either side of the diagnostic statement. The treatment of Fluid Volume Deficit related to NPO status, for example, requires a medical order for intravenous therapy.

Do not use Fluid Volume Deficit (either Actual or Risk) to describe patients who are hemorrhaging or in hypovolemic shock. These situations usually represent collaborative problems.

Incorrect: Risk for Fluid Volume Deficit related to postpartum hemorrhage

Correct: Potential Complication of Childbirth: Postpartum Hemorrhage

Correct: Risk for Postpartum Hemorrhage related to uterine atony

The most appropriate use of the Fluid Volume Deficit label is as a diagnosis (either actual or potential) for patients who are not drinking sufficient amounts of oral fluids. An actual Fluid Volume Deficit may also be the etiology of other nursing diagnoses, such as Altered Oral Mucous Membrane.

Suggested Alternative Diagnoses

Fluid Volume Deficit: Risk for
Oral Mucous Membrane, Altered
Tissue Perfusion, Altered: Renal

Patient Outcomes and Evaluation Criteria

Include patient-specific target date, evaluation and documentation intervals, and any other patient-specific outcomes.

The patient will:

- Be oriented to person, place, and time.
- Have moist mucous membranes.

- Have less concentrated urine. (Specify baseline specific gravity.)
- Report no thirst.
- Report no weakness.

Vital signs will be within normal limits for patient. Specify normal limits.

Serum electrolytes, hemoglobin, and hematocrit will be within normal range for patient. (State normal range.)

NIC Priority Interventions

Electrolyte Management: Promotion of electrolyte balance and prevention of complications resulting from abnormal or undesired serum electrolyte levels (eg, serum calcium, potassium, magnesium, sodium, and phosphate).

Fluid Management: Promotion of fluid balance and prevention of complications resulting from abnormal or undesired fluid levels.

Fluid Monitoring: Collection and analysis of patient data to regulate fluid balance.

Hypovolemia Management: Expansion of intravascular fluid volume in a patient who is volume depleted.

Intravenous (IV) Therapy: Administration and monitoring of intravenous fluids and medications.

Shock Management, Volume: Promotion of adequate tissue perfusion for a patient with severely compromised intravascular volume.

Nursing Actions

Target actions to problem etiologies. Individualize actions to meet the unique needs of each patient. Note that some of these actions are specific for patients who are hemorrhaging—refer to suggestions for use before including those activities in your plan of care.

Ongoing Assessments

- Assess and document:

  Active bleeding. Specify location.

Color, amount, and frequency of emesis, diarrhea, and other drainage.

Dressing changes to evaluate fluid loss from wounds.

Intake and output.

Orientation to person, place, and time q ____.

Skin temperature, dryness, and color.

Skin turgor and mucous membranes q ____.

Specific gravity and color of urine q ____.

Vital signs q ____.

- Evaluate presence of weakness during activity.
- Identify contributing factors that may aggravate dehydration, such as medications, fever, stress, medical orders.
- Review electrolytes, especially Na^+, K^+, chloride, BUN, creatinine, hemoglobin, and hematocrit.
- Weigh patient q ____.

Patient Teaching

- Instruct patient to inform nurse of thirst.

Collaborative Activities

- Confer with physician regarding need for parenteral electrolyte replacement therapy.
- Report and document output over ____ cc.
- Report and document output under ____ cc.
- Report electrolyte abnormalities, especially Na^+, K^+, chloride, BUN, creatinine, hemoglobin, and hematocrit.

Other

- Encourage oral fluid intake. Specify amount to be ingested in 24 hours, quantifying desired intake during the day, evening, and night shifts.
- Limit activity to reduce active bleeding. Specify limitation.
- Offer fluid of patient's choice at bedside.
- Pace activity according to patient's tolerance.

Fluid Volume Deficit: Risk for (1.4.1.2.2.2) (Y22.1)

Definition: The state in which an individual is at risk of experiencing vascular, cellular, or intracellular dehydration (NANDA).

Defining Characteristics

Presence of risk factors such as:

Objective

Deviations affecting access to or intake or absorption of fluids (eg, physical immobility)
Excessive losses through normal routes (eg, diarrhea)
Extremes of age
Extremes of weight
Factors influencing fluid needs (eg, hypermetabolic state)
Knowledge deficit related to fluid volume
Loss of fluid through abnormal routes (eg, indwelling tubes)
Medications (eg, diuretics)

Risk Factors

See defining characteristics.

Suggestions for Use

Do not use routinely for patients who are NPO. Refer to Suggestions for Use for the Fluid Volume Deficit label.

Suggested Alternative Diagnosis

Fluid Volume Deficit

Patient Outcomes and Evaluation Criteria

Include patient-specific target date, evaluation and documentation intervals, and any other patient-specific outcomes.

The patient will:

- Be oriented to person, place, and time.
- Have moist mucous membranes.
- Have less concentrated urine. (Specify baseline specific gravity.)
- Report no thirst.
- Report no weakness.
- Have serum electrolytes, hemoglobin, and hematocrit within normal range. (State normal range.)
- Have vital signs within normal limits for patient. (Specify normal limits.)

NIC Priority Interventions

Electrolyte Management: Promotion of electrolyte balance and prevention of complications resulting from abnormal or undesired serum electrolyte levels (eg, serum calcium, potassium, magnesium, sodium, and phosphate).

Fluid Management: Promotion of fluid balance and prevention of complications resulting from abnormal or undesired fluid levels.

Fluid Monitoring: Collection and analysis of patient data to regulate fluid balance.

Hypovolemia Management: Expansion of intravascular fluid volume in a patient who is volume depleted.

Intravenous (IV) Therapy: Administration and monitoring of intravenous fluids and medications.

Shock Management, Volume: Promotion of adequate tissue perfusion for a patient with severely compromised intravascular volume.

Nursing Actions

Target actions to problem etiologies. Individualize actions to meet the unique needs of each patient. Note that some of these actions are specific for patients who are hemorrhaging—refer to Suggestions for Use for the label Fluid Volume Deficit before including those activities in your plan of care.

Ongoing Assessments

- Assess color, amount, and frequency of emesis, diarrhea, and other drainage.
- Document for active bleeding. Specify location.
- Document intake and output.
- Evaluate fluid loss from wounds during dressing changes.
- Identify contributing factors that may aggravate dehydration, such as medications, fever, stress, medical orders.
- Orient to person, place, and time q ____.
- Review electrolytes, especially Na^+, K^+, chloride, BUN, creatinine, hemoglobin, and hematocrit.
- Assess skin temperature, dryness, and color.
- Assess skin turgor and mucous membranes q ____.
- Specify gravity and color of urine q ____.
- Assess vital signs q ____.
- Weigh patient q ____. Baseline weight is ____.

Patient Teaching

- Instruct patient to inform nurse of thirst.

Collaborative Activities

- Report any electrolyte abnormalities, especially Na^+, K^+, chloride, BUN, creatinine, hemoglobin, and hematocrit, to physician.

Other

- Encourage oral fluid intake. Specify amount to be ingested in 24 hours, quantifying desired intake during the day, evening, and night shifts.
- Limit activity to reduce active bleeding. Specify limitation.
- Offer fluid of patient's choice at bedside.

Fluid Volume Excess (1.4.1.2.1) (Y22.2)

Definition: The state in which an individual experiences increased fluid retention and edema (NANDA).

Defining Characteristics

Subjective

Shortness of breath

Objective

Abnormal breath sounds

Abnormal laboratory values (hematocrit, hemoglobin, sodium, chloride, protein)

Agitation, restlessness

Anasarca

Blood pressure change

Change in mental status

Change in respiratory pattern

Decrease in urine specific gravity

Decreased urine output

Edema

Effusion

Increase in central venous pressure, pulmonary artery pressure, pulmonary wedge pressure

Increased abdominal girth

Intake greater than output

Neck vein distention

Oliguria

Orthopnea

Pleural friction rub

Presence of S_3 heart sound

Rales

Taut, shiny skin

Uremia

Weight gain

Related Factors

Decreased urine output secondary to renal dysfunction, heart failure, sodium retention, immobility, and so on

Increased fluid intake secondary to excess sodium, hyperglycemia, medications, compulsive water drinking, and so on

Insufficient protein secondary to decreased intake or increased losses

Suggestions for Use

Do not use this label for conditions that nurses cannot prevent or treat. The main type of Fluid Volume Excess that nurses can treat independently is peripheral, dependent edema, which can be symptomatically relieved by elevating the patient's affected limbs. Edema (Fluid Volume Excess) is an important risk factor for Impaired Skin Integrity.

If the patient requires medical intervention to resolve the fluid excess, use a collaborative problem such as Potential Complication of Renal Failure: Generalized Edema. Fluid Volume Excess can also be the cause of complications such as Potential Complication of Fluid Volume Excess: Pulmonary Edema.

Examples:

Incorrect: Fluid Volume Excess related to decreased cardiac output

Correct: Potential Complication of Decreased Cardiac Output: Fluid Volume Excess

Correct: Potential Complication of Heart Failure: Pulmonary Edema

Correct: Risk for Impaired Skin Integrity related to fluid volume excess, as manifested by generalized edema

Suggested Alternative Diagnoses

Cardiac Output, Decreased

Skin Integrity, Impaired: Risk for

Patient Outcomes and Evaluation Criteria

Include patient-specific target date, evaluation and documentation intervals, and any other patient-specific outcomes.

Patient will verbalize:

- Understanding of fluid and dietary restrictions.
- Understanding of prescribed medications.

Patient will:

- Achieve target weight. (Specify target weight.)
- Have decreased edema toward normal limits for patient. (Specify normal limits for patient.)
- Maintain skin integrity.
- Maintain vital signs within normal limits for patient. (Specify normal limits.)

NIC Priority Interventions

Fluid Management: Promotion of fluid balance and prevention of complications resulting from abnormal or undesired fluid levels.

Fluid Monitoring: Collection and analysis of patient data to regulate fluid balance.

Nursing Actions

Target actions to problem etiologies. Individualize actions to meet the unique needs of each patient.

Ongoing Assessments

- Measure abdominal girth q ____.
- Assess edematous extremity or body part for impaired circulation and skin integrity, and document q ____.
- Assess effects of medications on edema (such as steroids, diuretics, lithium).
- Assess intake and output q ____.
- Monitor electrolytes.
- Weigh q ____.

- Assess for presence of edema (peripheral, sacral, periorbital). Specify location and degree of edema on scale from 1+ to 4+.
- Assess for pulmonary and/or cardiovascular complications as indicated by increased respiratory distress, increased pulse rate, increased blood pressure, abnormal heart sounds, and/or abnormal lung sounds.
- Assess vital signs q ____.

Patient Teaching

- Instruct patient regarding:

  Causes and resolutions of edema.
  Dietary restrictions.
  Use, dosage, and side-effects of prescribed medication.

Collaborative Activities

- Monitor electrolytes, and report abnormalities to physician.

Other

- Change position q ____.
- Elevate extremities to increase venous return.
- Maintain patient's fluid restriction.

Gas Exchange, Impaired (1.5.1.1) (Y26.2)

Definition: The state in which the individual experiences a decreased passage of oxygen and/or carbon dioxide between the alveoli of the lungs and the vascular system (NANDA).

Defining Characteristics

Objective

Confusion
Hypercapnia
Hypoxia

Inability to move secretions
Irritability
Restlessness
Somnolence

Related Factors

Decreased functional lung tissue secondary to chronic lung disease, pneumonia, thoracotomy, atelectasis, respiratory distress syndrome, mass, diaphragmatic hernia
Decreased pulmonary blood supply secondary to pulmonary hypertension, pulmonary embolus, congestive heart failure, respiratory distress syndrome, anemia
Ventilation-perfusion imbalance

Suggestions for Use

Use of this label is not recommended. Decreased passage of gases between the alveoli of the lungs and the vascular system can be discovered only by means of a medically prescribed diagnostic test: blood gas analysis. A patient might easily have most of the defining characteristics without actually having impaired alveolar gas exchange. Because nurses can neither diagnose nor treat this condition, you should use a diagnostic statement that describes oxygen-related problems that *can* be treated independently (eg, Activity Intolerance). If the patient is *at risk* for Impaired Gas Exchange, write the appropriate collaborative problem, eg, Potential Complication of Thrombophlebitis: Pulmonary Embolus.

See suggestions for use for Ineffective Airway Clearance, Ineffective Breathing Pattern, and Dysfunctional Ventilatory Weaning Response (DVWR).

Suggested Alternative Diagnoses

Activity Intolerance
Airway Clearance, Ineffective
Breathing Pattern, Ineffective
Dysfunctional Ventilatory Weaning Response (DVWR)

Patient Outcomes and Evaluation Criteria

Include patient-specific target date, evaluation and documentation intervals, and any other patient-specific outcomes.

Arterial blood gases are within normal limits for patient.

Pulmonary function is within normal limits for patient.

Patient is able to describe plan for care at home.

NIC Priority Interventions

Acid-Base Management: Promotion of acid-base balance and prevention of complications resulting from acid-base imbalance.

Airway Management: Facilitation of patency of air passages.

Nursing Actions

Target actions to problem etiologies. Individualize actions to meet the unique needs of each patient.

Ongoing Assessments

- Assess patient's lung sounds, respiratory rate, and production of sputum as indicators of effective use of supportive equipment.
- Correlate all assessment data (patient sensorium, breath sounds, respiratory pattern, ABGs, sputum, effect of medications). Document.
- Increase frequency of monitoring when patient appears somnolent.

Patient Teaching

- Explain proper use of supportive equipment (oxygen, suction, spirometer, IPPB).
- Explain to patient and family the reasons for low-flow oxygen by nasal cannula or mask when oxygen is required.
- Inform patient and family that smoking is prohibited.
- Instruct patient and family in plan for care at home (medications, activity, supportive equipment, reportable signs and symptoms, community resources).
- Instruct patient in breathing and relaxation techniques to improve breathing pattern.

Collaborative Activities

- Consult with physician regarding future need for ABG test and use of supportive equipment as indicated by a change in the patient's condition.
- Report changes in correlated assessment data (patient sensorium, breath sounds, respiratory pattern, ABGs, sputum, effect of medications).

Other

- Inform patient before beginning intended procedures, to lower anxiety and increase sense of control.
- Pace activities, to minimize fatigue and shortness of breath.
- Reassure patient during periods of respiratory distress and/or anxiety.
- Reduce potential for increased oxygen consumption by reducing fever, decreasing pain, lessening anxiety, and pacing activity.
- A suggested plan of care for a patient on a ventilator may include:

  Ensuring adequate oxygen delivery by reporting abnormal ABGs, having ambu bag attached to oxygen source at bedside, and hyperoxygenating prior to suctioning.

  Ensuring effective breathing pattern by assessing for synchronization and possible need for sedation.

  Maintaining patent airway by suctioning patient and keeping an ET tube or trach replacement at bedside.

  Monitoring for complications (pneumothorax, unilateral aeration).

  Verifying correct placement of ET tube.

Grieving, Anticipatory (9.2.1.2) (Y33.0)

Definition: A state in which an individual grieves before an actual loss (NANDA).

Defining Characteristics

Subjective

Anger
Disbelief
Guilt
Hope that loss can be prevented
Sense of unreality

Objective

Altered activity level
Altered communication patterns
Altered libido
Altered sleep pattern
Denial
Normal grieving initiated on anticipation of a significant loss
Physiologic symptoms, eg, exhaustion, sighing, choking sensation, tightness in throat, changes in eating habits
Shock
Sorrow, weeping

Related Factors

Impending death of self
Potential loss of body parts or functions
Potential loss of significant person, animal, or possession
Potential loss of social role

Suggestions for Use

Anticipatory Grieving may be a normal, not necessarily maladaptive, response. If it requires no intervention, do not include it in the patient care plan. Anticipatory Grieving occurs *before* the loss. It shares some defining characteristics with Dysfunctional Grieving; however, the following symptoms of Dysfunctional Grieving would *rule out* a diagnosis of Anticipatory Grieving:

Exaggerated and prolonged feelings of guilt
Interference with life functioning
Prolonged anger or hostility
Suicidal thoughts

Suggested Alternative Diagnosis

Grieving, Dysfunctional

Patient Outcomes and Evaluation Criteria

Include patient-specific target date, evaluation and documentation intervals, and any other patient-specific outcomes.

The Patient/family will:

- Demonstrate ability to make mutual decisions regarding anticipated loss.
- Express thoughts and feelings regarding anticipated loss.
- Participate in grief work.
- Use appropriate resources.

NIC Priority Interventions

Grief Work Facilitation: Assistance with the resolution of a significant loss.

Nursing Actions

Target actions to problem etiologies. Individualize actions to meet the unique needs of each patient.

Ongoing Assessments

- Assess past experience of patient/family with loss, existing support systems, current grief work.

Patient Teaching

- Discuss phases of the grieving process with patient/family.

Collaborative Activities

- Refer to appropriate resources. Consider support groups, legal assistance, financial assistance, social services, religious/spiritual assistance.

Other

- Assist patient/family to verbalize fears/concerns of potential loss.
- Discuss with patient/family the impact of anticipated loss on the family unit and its functioning.

- Help patient/family to share mutual fears, plans, concerns, and hopes with each other.
- Respect culture, religion, race, and values of patient/family as patient/family expresses grief.

Grieving, Dysfunctional (9.2.1.1) (Y33.1)

Definition: A state in which an individual reacts to an actual, anticipated, or perceived loss of a significant person, ideal, status, object, or body part with an absent, delayed, exaggerated, or prolonged response.

Defining Characteristics

Subjective

Alteration in dream patterns
Alteration in libido
Anger
Denial of loss
Expressing distress at loss
Expressing guilt
Expressing unresolved issues
Sadness

Objective

Alteration in activity level
Alteration in eating habits
Alteration in sleep patterns
Crying
Developmental regression
Difficulty in expressing loss
Idealization of lost object
Interference with life functioning
Labile affect
Reliving past experiences

Related Factors

Actual loss (specify)
Anticipated loss (specify)
Chronic illness
Perceived loss (specify; objects may include people, possessions, a job, status, home, ideals, parts and processes of the body)
Terminal illness

Suggestions for Use

Most of the defining characteristics may also be present in the normal or anticipatory grief process. Grieving is dysfunctional only if it is prolonged (perhaps for more than a year after the loss) or if the symptoms are unusually numerous or severe. See Suggestions for Use for Anticipatory Grieving.

Suggested Alternative Diagnoses

Adjustment, Impaired
Grieving, Anticipatory
Thought Processes, Altered

Patient Outcomes and Evaluation Criteria

Include patient-specific target date, evaluation and documentation intervals, and any other patient-specific outcomes.

The patient will:

- Demonstrate independence in activities of daily living.
- Participate actively in decision-making process.
- Share grief with significant person.
- Use available support systems.
- Verbalize grief.
- Verbalize meaning of loss.

NIC Priority Interventions

Grief Work Facilitation: Assistance with the resolution of a significant loss.

Nursing Actions

Target actions to problem etiologies. Individualize actions to meet the unique needs of each patient.

Ongoing Assessments

- Assess and document the presence and source of patient's grief.

Patient Teaching

- Discuss the phases of the grieving process with patient.
- Provide patient/family with information about hospital and community resources, such as self-help groups.

Collaborative Activities

- Initiate a patient care conference to review patient/family needs related to their state of the grieving process and to establish a plan of care. Support provided by ____.
- Seek support among peers and others to provide patient care as needed.

Other

- Acknowledge patient's and family's grief reactions while continuing necessary care activities.
- Allow for flexibility in schedule of activities.
- Avoid confrontation of denial, and at the same time do not reinforce denial.
- Balance any misperceptions with reality.
- Demonstrate respect for patient's culture, religion, race, and values as patient expresses grief.
- Discuss with patient/family the impact of the loss on the family unit and its functioning.
- Encourage independence in performance of self-care, assisting patient only as necessary.
- Encourage patient to express grief.
- Establish a schedule for contact with patient. Interact with patient q ____. Document contact.
- Establish a trusting relationship with patient and family.
- Evaluate verbal and nonverbal communication as they relate to grieving process.

- Help patient/family to participate actively in decision-making process.
- Provide a safe, secure, and private environment to facilitate patient/family grieving process.
- Recognize and reinforce the strength of each family member.

Growth and Development, Altered (6.6) (Y54)

Definition: The state in which an individual demonstrates deviations in norms from his/her age group (NANDA).

Defining Characteristics

Major

Objective

Altered physical growth

Delay or difficulty in performing skills (motor, social, or expressive) typical of age group

Inability to perform self-care or self-control activities appropriate for age

Minor

Objective

Decreased responses

Flat affect

Infant irritability

Listlessness

Related Factors

Abuse

Changes in family system

Congenital anomaly

Effects of physical disability

Environment and stimulation deficiencies

Fetal distress during or after birth/delivery

Inadequate bonding

Inadequate caretaking
Inadequate prenatal care
Inconsistent responsiveness
Indifference
Lack of stimulation in environment
Loss
Maternal acute/chronic disease
Maternal age
Multiple caretaking
Neonatal disease
Poverty
Prematurity
Prescribed dependence
Rapid growth
Separation from significant others
Serious illness/injury
Traumatic separation
Unhealthy maternal life-style during pregnancy

Suggestions for Use

Use of this label is not recommended. It is too broad to suggest nursing actions. There are many nursing diagnoses that could be considered "alterations in growth and development" or that could be caused by altered growth and development (eg, Self-Care Deficit, Urinary Incontinence, Impaired Verbal Communication, and Altered Parenting). When possible, use the more specific labels.

Because growth and development are routinely assessed in nursing care of children, a diagnostic statement is usually not required for that application—such assessment is usually included in pediatric standards of care.

This label is not appropriate for a mentally impaired child (eg, Altered Growth and Development related to Down syndrome). Diagnose the specific functional task that the child is unable to perform (eg, Feeding Self-Care Deficit). Likewise, this label is probably not appropriate for a child with failure to thrive. That condition may be described better by one of the family functioning diagnoses or by a diagnosis of Altered Nutrition: Less Than Body Requirements. Altered Growth and Development is most appropriately used for a child who is having difficulty achieving age-specific developmental tasks.

Suggested Alternative Diagnoses

Bowel Incontinence
Communication, Impaired: Verbal
Coping, Ineffective Family: Compromised
Coping, Ineffective Family: Disabling
Coping, ineffective Individual
Parenting, Altered
Self-Care Deficit (specify)
Urinary Incontinence

Patient Outcomes and Evaluation Criteria

Include patient-specific target date, evaluation and documentation intervals, and any other patient-specific outcomes.

Patient will achieve the highest level of wellness, development, and independence possible, given patient's illness/disability.

NIC Priority Interventions

Nutritional Monitoring: Collection and analysis of patient data to prevent or minimize malnourishment.

Nutrition Therapy: Administration of food and fluids to support metabolic processes of a patient who is malnourished or at high risk for becoming malnourished.

Self-Responsibility Facilitation: Encouraging a patient to assume more responsibility for own behavior.

Nursing Actions

Target actions to problem etiologies. Individualize actions to meet the unique needs of each patient.

Ongoing Assessments

- Assess the caretakers' knowledge, resources, support system, coping skills, and level of commitment to develop a plan of care.
- Conduct a thorough health assessment (eg, child's history, temperament, culture, family environment, developmental screening) to determine functional level.
- Identify potential related physical problems (eg, dehydration, falls, URI, skin breakdown), and initiate plans to prevent them.

Collaborative Activities

- Act as case manager to assure comprehensive care by coordinating medical, school, rehabilitation, and social services.

Other

- Assist caretakers to develop a plan of care. (For possible care plans/interventions, refer to Coping, Ineffective Family: Compromised; and Coping, Ineffective Family: Disabling.)
- Assist patient in achieving next level of growth and development through appropriate mastery of tasks specific to his/her level.
- Create an environment where ADLs can be performed with maximum independence.
- Establish a therapeutic and trusting relationship with caretakers.
- Help the family develop a strategy to integrate the patient as an accepted member of the family and community.

Health Maintenance, Altered (6.4.2) (Y.55)

Definition: A state in which an individual is unable to identify, manage, and/or seek out help to maintain health (NANDA).

Defining Characteristics

Subjective

Expressed desire to improve health behaviors

Objective

Demonstrated lack of knowledge regarding basic health practices

History of lack of health-seeking behavior

History of untreated, chronic symptoms of disease process

Inability to take responsibility for meeting basic health practices

Lack of finances, equipment, and/or social resources

Limited use of health care agencies and personnel

Limited use of preventive health measures

Need to adhere to cultural/religious beliefs

Unwillingness to improve health behaviors

Related Factors

Cultural beliefs

Disabling spiritual distress

Dysfunctional grieving

Ineffective family coping

Ineffective individual coping

Lack of ability to make deliberate and thoughtful judgments

Lack of material resources

Lack of or significant alteration in communication skills

Lack of social supports

Motor impairment

Perceptual/cognitive impairment (complete/partial lack of gross and/or fine motor skills)

Religious beliefs

Unachieved developmental tasks

Suggestions for Use

Use this diagnosis for patients who *wish* to change an unhealthy life-style or who *lack knowledge* of their disease or condition. Do not use it to describe patients who are not motivated to change or learn.

Suggested Alternative Diagnoses

Adjustment, Impaired
Denial, Ineffective
Health-Seeking Behaviors
Noncompliance (specify)
Therapeutic Regimen Management, Ineffective Individual

Patient Outcomes and Evaluation Criteria

Include patient-specific target date, evaluation and documentation intervals, and any other patient-specific outcomes.

The patient will:

- Acknowledge adverse effects of health beliefs.
- Acknowledge need for assistance after discharge.
- Verbalize willingness to follow nursing/medical regimen.
- Verbalize knowledge of preventive health measures.

NIC Treatments of Choice

Health System Guidance: Facilitating a patient's location and use of appropriate health services.

Nursing Actions

Target actions to problem etiologies. Individualize actions to meet the unique needs of each patient.

Ongoing Assessments

- Identify beliefs that interfere with health maintenance.
- Identify deficits that interfere with health maintenance.

Collaborative Activities

- Consult with social services to plan for health maintenance needs on discharge.
- Initiate a multidisciplinary patient care conference to plan health maintenance program with patient and family. Plan is ____ (specify).
- Offer information on community resources specific to health maintenance needs of patient/family.

Other

- Encourage discussion of preventive health measures specific to patient needs, such as dietary changes, cessation of smoking, stress reduction, and implementation of exercise program.
- Provide a nonjudgmental environment in which patient/family can share beliefs.

Health-Seeking Behaviors (specify) (5.4) (Y01.0–9)

Definition: A state in which a patient in *stable health is actively seeking ways to alter personal health habits and/or the environment in order to move toward a higher level of health (NANDA).

Defining Characteristics

Major

Subjective

Expressed desire to seek a higher level of wellness

Objective

Observed desire to seek a higher level of wellness

Minor

Subjective

Expressed concern about current environmental conditions on health status

Expressed desire for increased control of health practice

Stated unfamiliarity with wellness community resources

*Stable health status is defined as age-appropriate illness prevention measures achieved, patient reports good or excellent health, and signs and symptoms of disease, if present, are controlled.

Objective

Demonstrated or observed lack of knowledge of health-promoting behaviors
Observed desire for increased control of health practice
Observed unfamiliarity with wellness community resources

Related Factors

Specific to patient.

Suggestions for Use

Use this label for well patients who wish information about disease prevention or health promotion.

Suggested Alternative Diagnoses

Breast-Feeding, Effective (Potential for Enhanced)
Coping, Family: Potential for Growth
Health Maintenance, Altered

Patient Outcomes and Evaluation Criteria

Include patient-specific target date, evaluation and documentation intervals, and any other patient-specific outcomes.

The patient will:

- Describe health-seeking/health-promoting behaviors.
- Describe ways of attaining a higher level of health.
- Utilize wellness community resources.

NIC Priority Interventions

Self-Modification Assistance: Reinforcement of self-directed change initiated by the patient to achieve personally important goals.

Nursing Actions

Target actions to problem etiologies. Individualize actions to meet the unique needs of each patient.

Ongoing Assessments

- Assess patient/family level of knowledge about:

Measures for preventing illness.

Signs and symptoms of disease condition and controllable aspects of the disease.

Patient Teaching

- Provide patient/family with information about available wellness community resources.

Collaborative Activities

- Consult with community services as a primary step toward health promotion for patient/family. Involve patient/family in consultation.

Other

- Assist patient/family in developing a plan for increased health-promoting activities.
- Discuss with patient/family personal health habits, and determine which behaviors may be changed to achieve optimal health (diet, smoking cessation, stress reduction, exercise program).
- Reinforce positive health-seeking behaviors.

Home Maintenance Management, Impaired (6.4.1.1) (Y56)

Definition: A state in which an individual, family, or household member is unable to independently maintain a safe, growth-promoting immediate environment (NANDA).

Defining Characteristics

Major

Subjective

Family/household members describing financial crises or outstanding debts

Family/household members expressing inability to maintain home in a comfortable fashion

Family/household members requesting assistance with home maintenance

Objective

Accumulation of dirt, food wastes, or hygienic wastes
Overtaxed (eg, exhausted, anxious) family members
Repeated hygienic disorders, infestations, or infections
Unwashed or unavailable cooking equipment, clothes, linen

Minor

Objective

Disorderly surroundings
Inappropriate household temperature
Offensive odors
Presence of vermin or rodents

Related Factors

Developmental disability
Home environment obstacles
Impaired cognitive or emotional functioning
Inadequate support system
Individual/family member disease or injury
Insufficient family organization or planning
Insufficient finances
Lack of familiarity with community resources
Lack of knowledge (specify)
Lack of role modeling
Physical impairment of family member other than patient
Psychologic impairment (specify)

Suggestions for Use

This diagnosis emphasizes inability to manage the home environment, for example, laundry, cleaning, and cooking. If the difficulty is with managing medications or treatments, use Ineffective Management of Therapeutic Regimen. If it is primarily a difficulty in managing self-care, such as bathing and dressing, use Self-Care Deficit (specify). Differentiate also between this label and Caregiver Role Strain.

Suggested Alternative Diagnoses

Caregiver Role Strain
Injury: Risk for (Trauma, Falls)
Self-Care Deficit (specify)
Therapeutic Regimen Management, Ineffective Individual

Patient Outcomes and Evaluation Criteria

Include patient-specific target date, evaluation and documentation intervals, and any other patient-specific outcomes.

Patient/family/household member will:

- Describe plan to correct obstacles/hazards in home.
- Follow specific plan for home maintenance.
- Identify options to overcome financial constraints.
- Verbalize awareness of constraints on home situation due to illness of family member.
- Verbalize knowledge of available resources.

NIC Priority Interventions

Home Maintenance Assistance: Helping the patient/family to maintain the home as a clean, safe, and pleasant place to live.

Nursing Actions

Target actions to problem etiologies. Individualize actions to meet the unique needs of each patient.

Ongoing Assessments

- Assess and document need for postdischarge follow-through with public health nurse.

Patient Teaching

- Provide patient/family/household member with written material regarding home maintenance.

Collaborative Activities

- Contact discharge planning/social worker to establish realistic plan for home maintenance.

Other

- Accept and support without judgment the realities of the home situation.
- Help patient/family/household member identify obstacles/hazards in home that may impede home maintenance.
- Help patient/family/household member identify strengths in family unit as well as support systems that will assist in home maintenance.
- Initiate discussion with patient/family about health status of all family members, as illness of other family members may affect home maintenance management.
- Involve patient/family/household member in all planning activities.

Hopelessness (7.3.1) (Y60.0)

Definition: A subjective state in which an individual sees no alternatives or personal choices available and cannot mobilize energy on own behalf (NANDA).

Defining Characteristics

Major

Subjective

Verbal cues such as "I can't," "I don't care," sighing

Objective

Decreased affect

Decreased verbalization

Passivity

Minor

Objective

Alteration in sleep patterns

Avoidance of eye contact

Closing eyes

Decrease in appetite
Decreased response to stimuli
Lack of initiative
Lack of involvement in care/passive allowance of care
Shrugging in response to speaker

Related Factors

Abandonment
Failing or deteriorating physical condition
Lack of social supports
Long-term stress
Lost spiritual belief
Prolonged activity restrictions creating isolation

Suggestions for Use

Differentiate between this label and Powerlessness. Hopelessness implies that the person believes there *is* no solution to his/her problem ("no way out"). In Powerlessness, the person may know of a solution to the problem, but believes it is beyond his/her control to achieve the solution. Long-term feelings of Powerlessness may lead to Hopelessness. Although both diagnoses share some defining characteristics, the following are specific only to Powerlessness: Irritability, resentment, anger, guilt, and fear of alienation from caregivers. For some patients, Hopelessness may be a risk factor for suicide.

Suggested Alternative Diagnoses

Coping, Ineffective Individual
Grieving, Dysfunctional (may be an etiology of Hopelessness)
Powerlessness
Violence, Self-Directed: Risk for

Patient Outcomes and Evaluation Criteria

Include patient-specific target date, evaluation and documentation intervals, and any other patient-specific outcomes.

The patient will:

- Identify personal strengths.
- Initiate behaviors that may reduce feelings of hopelessness.

NIC Priority Interventions

Hope Instillation: Facilitation of the development of a positive outlook in a given situation.

Nursing Actions

Target actions to problem etiologies. Individualize actions to meet the unique needs of each patient.

Ongoing Assessments

- Assess and document potential for suicide.

Patient Teaching

- Provide information on community resources, such as community agencies, social agencies, self-improvement classes, stress-reduction classes, counseling. Specify.

Collaborative Activities

- Obtain psychiatric consultation.

Other

- Encourage active participation in group activities to provide opportunity for social supports and problem solving.
- Explore with patient factors that contribute to feelings of hopelessness.
- Involve family/significant person in treatment plan.
- Provide opportunities for patient to initiate interactions and activities.
- Provide positive reinforcement for behaviors that demonstrate initiative, such as eye contact, self-disclosure, reduction in amount of sleep time, self-care, increased appetite.
- Spend time with patient to provide opportunity to explore alternative coping measures. Schedule q ____.

Hyperthermia (1.2.2.3) (Y25.1)

Definition: A state in which an individual's body temperature is elevated above his/her normal range (NANDA).

Defining Characteristics

Major

Objective

Increase in body temperature above normal range

Minor

Subjective

Nausea

Objective

Confusion
Flushed skin
Increased respiratory rate
Light-headedness
Seizures/convulsions
Skin warm to touch
Tachycardia

Related Factors

Dehydration
Excessive clothing
Illness or trauma
Inability or decreased ability to perspire
Increased metabolic rate
Medication/anesthesia
Prolonged exposure to hot environment
Vigorous activity

Suggestions for Use

Severe Hyperthermia is a life-threatening condition requiring both medical and nursing intervention; as such it would be best described by a collaborative diagnosis. For many patients, an elevated temperature is not a problem, but merely a symptom of a disease process, which is treated by a medication such as acetaminophen or aspirin. Many Hyperthermias (maybe most) require no independent nursing treatment. One of the suggested alternative diagnoses may be more useful.

Suggested Alternative Diagnoses

Body Temperature, Altered: Risk for
Hyperthermia: Risk for
Thermoregulation, Ineffective

Patient Outcomes and Evaluation Criteria

Include patient-specific target date, evaluation and documentation intervals, and any other patient-specific outcomes.

Patient's temperature will be restored to normal.

Patient/family will:

- Demonstrate proper method of taking temperature.
- Describe measures to prevent/minimize increase in body temperature.
- Report early signs and symptoms of hyperthermia.

NIC Treatment of Choice

Fever Treatment: Management of a patient with hyperpyrexia caused by nonenvironmental factors.

Temperature Regulation: Attaining and/or maintaining body temperature within a normal range.

Vital Signs Monitoring: Collection and analysis of cardiovascular, respiratory, and body temperature data to determine and prevent complications.

Nursing Actions

Target actions to problem etiologies. Individualize actions to meet the unique needs of each patient.

Ongoing Assessments

- Monitor temperature q ____.

Patient Teaching

- Instruct patient/family in measures for prevention and early recognition of hyperthermia.

Collaborative Activities

- Administer antipyretics per doctor's order.

Other

- Encourage intake of oral fluids.
- Remove excess clothing, and cover patient with only a sheet.
- Use cooling measures: submerge in tepid bath; apply cool washcloths to axillae, groin, forehead, and nape of neck; use a circulating fan in patient's room; use a cooling blanket.

(See nursing actions for Body Temperature, Altered: Risk for on page 25.)

Hypothermia (1.2.2.2) (Y25.2)

Definition: The state in which an individual's body temperature is reduced below normal range (NANDA).

Defining Characteristics[1]

Mild

Amnesia
Apathy
Cold skin
Confusion
Disorientation
Hypertension

[1]Matz, R.: Hypothermia: Measures and countermeasures, *Hospital Practice* 1986, 21 (1A): 45–71.

Pallor
Piloerection (goose bumps)
Shivering
Slurred speech
Tachycardia

Moderate

Bradycardia
Cardiac arrhythmias
Dilated pupils
Cyanosis
Shivering

Severe

Absent reflexes
Cardiac arrhythmias
Decreased urine output
Muscular rigidity
Respirations 5/min

Related Factors

Aging
Consumption of alcohol
Damage to hypothalamus
Decreased basal metabolic rate
Hypothyroidism
Immaturity of newborn's temperature regulatory system
Inability or decreased ability to shiver
Inactivity
Inadequate clothing
Loss of subcutaneous fat
Low birth weight (infant)
Malnutrition
Medications causing vasodilation
Prolonged exposure to cool or cold environment
Trauma

Suggestions for Use

Because severe Hypothermia (rectal temperature below 35C or 95F) may cause complications such as impaired myocardial or respiratory function, such low readings should be reported to the physician.

Suggested Alternative Diagnoses

Body Temperature, Altered: Risk for
Hypothermia: Risk for

Patient Outcomes and Evaluation Criteria

Include patient-specific target date, evaluation and documentation intervals, and any other patient-specific outcomes.

Patient's temperature is restored to normal.

Patient/family will:

- Describe measures to prevent/minimize decrease in body temperature.
- Verbalize early signs and symptoms of hypothermia.

NIC Priority Interventions

Hypothermia Treatment: Rewarming and surveillance of a patient whose core body temperature is below 35C.

Temperature Regulation: Attaining and/or maintaining body temperature within a normal range.

Vital Signs Monitoring: Collection and analysis of cardiovascular, respiratory, and body temperature data to determine and prevent complications.

Nursing Actions

Target actions to problem etiologies. Individualize actions to meet the unique needs of each patient.

Ongoing Assessments

- Place patient on cardiac monitor.
- Record baseline vital signs.
- Take patient's temperature with a low-range thermometer.

Patient Teaching

- Instruct patient/family in measures for prevention and early recognition of hypothermia.

Collaborative Activities

- For severe hypothermia, assist physician with core-warming techniques (eg, hemodialysis, peritoneal dialysis, colonic irrigation, intragastric balloon, inhalation re-warming).[2]

Other

- Provide warmth: dry clothing, heated blankets, mechanical heating devices, adjusted room temperature, hot water bottles, submersion in warm water, warm oral fluids as tolerated.

(See nursing actions for Body Temperature, Altered: Risk for on page 25.)

Infant Feeding Pattern, Ineffective (6.5.1.4) (Y53)

Definition: A state in which an infant demonstrates an impaired ability to suck or coordinate the suck-swallow response (NANDA).

Defining Characteristics

Objective

Inability to coordinate sucking, swallowing, breathing
Inability to initiate or sustain an effective suck

Related Factors

Anatomical abnormalities
Neurological impairment/delay
Oral hypersensitivity
Prematurity
Prolonged NPO

[2]Reuler, J.: Hypothermia: Pathophysiology, clinical settings, and management, *Annals of Internal Medicine* 1978, 89: 519–527.

Suggestions for Use

This label describes a baby with sucking or swallowing difficulties. It focuses on the nutritional needs of the infant. The goal of nursing activities is to prevent weight loss or promote weight gain. Use the following defining characteristics to discriminate among this label and the suggested alternative diagnoses.

	Key Defining Characteristics
Ineffective Breast-Feeding	Dissatisfaction with feeding process
Ineffective Infant Feeding Pattern	Inability of infant to suck or poorly coordinated suck-swallow response
Interrupted Breast-Feeding	Mother wishes to maintain lactation; unable to put baby to breast for some feedings (eg, because of working)

Suggested Alternative Diagnoses

Breast-Feeding, Ineffective
Breast-Feeding, Interrupted
Nutrition, Altered: Less Than Body Requirements

Patient Outcomes and Evaluation Criteria

Include patient-specific target date, evaluation and documentation intervals, and any other patient-specific outcomes.

Infant will:

- Coordinate suck-swallow with respirations while maintaining heart rate and color.
- Maintain steady and acceptable weight gain.

NIC Priority Interventions

Enteral Tube Feeding: Delivering nutrients and water through an intestinal tube.

Nonnutritive Sucking: Provision of sucking opportunities for infant who is gavage fed or who can receive nothing by mouth.

Nursing Actions

Target actions to problem etiologies. Individualize actions to meet the unique needs of each patient.

Ongoing Assessments

- Assess infant's readiness for nipple feeding:

  Coordination of sucking, swallowing, and breathing (34 weeks).
  Gag reflex (32 weeks).
  Mature sucking reflex (32–34 weeks).
  Neonatal Oral Motor Assessment Scale (NOMAS).
  Presence of rooting reflex (28–36 weeks).

- At each feeding, assess infant's nipple feeding skills by evaluating if infant:

  Actively initiates swallow in coordination with suck.
  Actively sucks liquid from bottle.
  Completes feeding in acceptable time.
  Coordinates sucking, swallowing, and breathing.
  Loses minimal liquid from mouth.

- At each feeding, assess respiratory function and behavioral state and monitor infant for problems such as regurgitation, abdominal distention, and increased residuals.
- Daily assess whether the infant is ready to advance. Consider a feeding flow sheet to facilitate assessment; document infant's state, oxygen needs, preferred nipple, position, formula type/temperature, amount of feeding taken in first 10 minutes, total feeding, total feeding time, daily weight, and stool pattern.
- Prior to discharge, assess mother's readiness to feed infant; teach feeding techniques, and support her during feeding.

Patient Teaching

To increase success with nipple feeding:

- Avoid techniques that interrupt infant's learning by allowing passive flow of liquid without infant's active participation (twisting or jiggling bottle, moving nipple up and down, moving nipple in and out of infant's mouth, moving infant's jaw up and down).

- Burp the infant frequently.
- Choose most appropriate nipple (size, shape, firmness, size of hole).
- Consider varying formula (thickness, taste, temperature).
- Establish regular respiration by calming the infant prior to feeding; during feeding remove nipple at first sign of respiratory or state changes.
- Feed the premature infant when fully alert and eager.
- Overfill bottle above amount of scheduled feeding to make sucking easier and to minimize sucking of air.
- Position the infant in a semiupright position with head slightly forward and chin tilting down.
- Provide consistent caregivers to better read infant's cues and facilitate infant learning; involve mother at earliest opportunity.
- Reduce light and noise levels.
- Remain relaxed and patient during feeding; allow brief rest periods; pace the infant to complete feeding in appropriate time (too quickly may compromise safety, too slowly may increase fatigue and calorie expenditure).
- Use facilitation techniques (prior to feeding, increase oral sensitivity by stroking the infant's lips, cheeks, and tongue; during feeding, place your fingers on each cheek and under the jaw midway between the chin and throat to provide inward and forward support of the cheeks and tongue).

Collaborative Activities

- Establish support network to ensure that mother has help with day-to-day lactation/breast-feeding problems as they occur.
- Refer to a physical or occupational therapist any infant who is not progressing with feeding or has structural or oral motor defects.

Other

- Arrange for home visit within 72 hours of discharge.

- Determine most appropriate feeding method (nipple feeding, intermittent gavage, continuous feeding with NG tube, jejunal tube, or gastrostomy).

Infection: Risk for (1.2.1.1) (Y25.3)

Definition: The state in which an individual is at increased risk for being invaded by pathogenic organisms (NANDA).

Defining Characteristics

Presence of risk factors, such as:

Altered peristalsis
Broken skin
Change in pH secretions
Chronic disease
Decrease in ciliary action
Decreased hemoglobin
Immunosuppression
Inadequate acquired immunity
Insufficient knowledge to avoid exposure to pathogens
Invasive procedures
Leukopenia
Malnutrition
Pharmaceutical agents
Rupture of amniotic membranes
Stasis of body fluids
Suppressed inflammatory response
Tissue destruction and increased environmental exposure
Trauma
Traumatized tissue

Risk Factors

See defining characteristics.

Suggestions for Use

Do not use this label routinely for patients with surgical incisions. For the normal surgical population, maintaining routine standards of care will prevent incision infection. Likewise, do not use Risk for Infection routinely for patients who have an indwelling catheter. Aseptic technique is expected. Everyone is, in a sense, at risk for infection. Therefore, use this nursing diagnosis only for those patients who are at higher than "usual" risk—for example, those with nutritional deficits or compromised immune systems. For patients with actual Infection, use the collaborative problem, Potential Complication: Sepsis.

Suggested Alternative Diagnoses

Nutrition, Altered: Less Than Body Requirements
Protection, Altered
Skin Integrity, Impaired

Patient Outcomes and Evaluation Criteria

Include patient-specific target date, evaluation and documentation intervals, and any other patient-specific outcomes.

Patient will:

- Be free of signs and symptoms of infection.
- Demonstrate adequate personal hygiene.

Patient/family will:

- Identify factors that may increase the risk of infection.
- Identify signs and symptoms of infection.
- Verbalize willingness to alter life-style to decrease risk of infection.

NIC Priority Interventions

Immunization/Vaccination Administration: Provision of immunizations for prevention of communicable disease.

Infection Control: Minimizing the acquisition and transmission of infectious agents.

Infection Protection: Prevention and early detection of infection in a patient at risk.

Nursing Actions

Target actions to problem etiologies. Individualize actions to meet the unique needs of each patient.

Ongoing Assessments

- Evaluate patient's risk for urinary, pulmonary, fungal, or viral infections.
- Monitor patient for signs and symptoms of infection (consider temperature, pulse rate, drainage, appearance of wound, secretions, appearance of urine, skin temperature, skin lesions).
- Monitor laboratory values (consider CBC, cultures, serum protein, and albumin).
- Observe performance of personal hygiene practices to protect against infection.

Patient Teaching

- Explain to patient/family why illness and/or therapy increases the risk for infection.
- Instruct in performance of personal hygiene practices to protect against infection.
- Instruct patient/family in signs and symptoms of infection, including elevated temperature, warm skin, wound warmth/redness/tenderness, unexpected drainage from wound site, generalized pain/discomfort, increased heart rate, localized swelling/redness/pain.

Collaborative Activities

- Refer patient/family to social services and/or community resources to assist patient/family in managing home, hygiene, nutrition.
- Report suspicious findings (eg, laboratory values) to physician.

Other

- Assist patient/family in beginning to make needed life-style changes, using whatever resources seem appropriate. Specify plan.
- Help patient/family identify factors in their environment, life-style, or health practices that increase risk of infection.
- Protect patient from cross-contamination by not assigning same nurse to another patient with an infection, not rooming patient with an infected patient, limiting visitors as indicated, and providing protective isolation when indicated.

Injury: Risk for (1.6.1) (Y23)

Definition: A state in which the individual is at risk of injury as a result of environmental conditions interacting with the individual's adaptive and defensive resources (NANDA).

Defining Characteristics

Presence of risk factors, such as:

Internal

Biochemical Regulatory Function

Abnormal blood profile
Decreased hemoglobin
Effector dysfunction
Immune-autoimmune disorder
Integrative dysfunction
Leukocytosis/leukopenia
Malnutrition
Sensory dysfunction
Sickle cell
Thalassemia
Tissue hypoxia

Physical

Altered mobility
Broken skin

Developmental Age

Physiological

Psychosocial factors

Psychologic

Affective

Orientation

External

Biological

Immunization level of community

Microorganisms

Chemical

Drugs (pharmaceutical agents, alcohol, caffeine, nicotine, preservatives, cosmetics, and dyes)

Nutrients (vitamins, food types)

Poisons

Pollutants

Physical

Cognitive, affective, and psychomotor factors

Design, structure, and arrangement of community, building, or equipment

Mode of transport

Nosocomial agents

People/provider

Staffing patterns

Risk Factors

See defining characteristics.

Suggestions for Use

This is a broad label that includes internal risk factors such as altered clotting factors and decreased hemoglobin. NANDA has not identified any critical defining characteristics for this title, so it is important to identify only those patients who are at unusually high risk for this problem. Everyone has at least some risk for accidents and injury, but the label should be used only for those who require nursing intervention to prevent injury.

This label consists of five subcategories that describe *injury* more specifically: Risk for Suffocation, Poisoning, Trauma, Aspiration, and Disuse Syndrome. When possible, use these more specific labels instead of Risk for Injury because they provide clearer direction for nursing care. None of the subcategories needs further specification except for Risk for Trauma, which includes wounds, burns, and fractures, as well as an unlimited number of other risk factors.

Note that it may be useful to use the label Sensory/Perceptual Alterations as an etiology for Risk for Injury.

Suggested Alternative Diagnoses

Aspiration: Risk for
Home Maintenance Management, Impaired
Infection, Risk for
Poisoning: Risk for
Protection, Altered
Sensory/Perceptual Alterations: Visual, Auditory, Kinesthetic, Gustatory, Tactile, Olfactory (specify)
Suffocation: Risk for
Thought Processes, Altered
Trauma: Risk for
Violence, Risk for: Self-Directed

Patient Outcomes and Evaluation Criteria

Include patient-specific target date, evaluation and documentation intervals, and any other patient-specific outcomes.

Patient/family will:

- Identify appropriate safety factors that protect individual/child from injury.
- Identify risks that increase susceptibility to injury.

The patient will:

- Avoid physical injury.
- Verbalize strategies that prevent injury.

NIC Priority Interventions

Fall Prevention: Instituting special precautions with patient at risk for injury from falling.

Surveillance, Safety: Purposeful and ongoing collection and analysis of information about the patient and the environment for use in promoting and maintaining patient safety.

Nursing Actions

Ongoing Assessments

- Assess high-risk areas that may lead to injury to patient/family.
- Check patient for presence of constrictive clothing, cuts, burns, bruises.
- To determine safety needs of patient, assess and document:

  Changes in mental status.
  Degree of intoxication.
  Maturational age.
  Patient's motor and/or sensory deficit.

Patient Teaching

- Instruct patient/family in techniques to prevent injury at home (specify).
- Instruct patient to use caution in use of heat therapy devices.
- Provide educational materials related to strategies and countermeasures to prevent injury.
- Provide information on environmental hazards and characteristics (eg, stairs, windows, cupboard locks, swimming pools, streets, gates).

Collaborative Activities

- Refer to educational classes in the community.

Other

- Do not support patient's hallucinations or otherwise contribute to disorientation.
- Encourage patient to request assistance with activities.

- Explore strategies to prevent injury.
- Reorient patient to reality and immediate environment when necessary.
- Use heating devices with caution to prevent burns in patients with sensory deficit.

Knowledge Deficit (specify) (8.1.1) (Y40.0–9)

Definition: A state in which the individual/family does not comprehend, learn, or demonstrate knowledge of health care measures necessary to maintain or improve health.

Defining Characteristics

Subjective

Verbalization of limited knowledge/understanding of health care measures

Objective

Inaccurate follow-through of instruction

Inaccurate performance on tests

Inappropriate or exaggerated behaviors (eg, hysteria, hostility, agitation, or apathy)

Related Factors

Cognitive limitation

Information misinterpretation

Lack of interest in learning

Lack of motivation

Lack of recall

Limited exposure to information (specify)

Limited practice of skill (specify)

Unfamiliarity with information resources

Unreadiness to learn

Suggestions for Use

Knowledge Deficit is not recommended as a problem label for the following reasons:

1. Knowledge Deficit is not truly a *human response.* "Response" suggests a behavior or action; Knowledge Deficit is simply a state of being.
2. Knowledge Deficit does not necessarily describe a health state.
3. Knowledge Deficit does not necessarily describe a *problem.* Nursing diagnoses should reflect altered functioning; but Knowledge Deficit simply means the person lacks some knowledge, not that her/his functioning is changed as a result of that lack.

Knowledge Deficit can contribute to a number of problem responses, including Anxiety, Altered Parenting, Self-Care Deficit, or Ineffective Coping. Therefore, it may be used effectively as the etiology of a nursing diagnosis. For example: Risk for Injury (Trauma) related to lack of knowledge of proper application of seat-belts when pregnant; or Anxiety related to lack of knowledge of procedures involved in bone marrow aspiration.

If Knowledge Deficit is used as the problem side of a nursing diagnosis, one goal must be "Patient will acquire knowledge about . . ." This causes the nurse to focus on giving information rather than on the behaviors caused by the patient's lack of knowledge, reinforcing the belief that giving information will change behavior and solve problems. On the other hand, when Knowledge Deficit is used as an etiology, it focuses attention on behaviors that indicate self-doubt, decisional conflict, anxiety, and so on. Note the difference in nursing care suggested by these diagnostic statements:

Knowledge Deficit (Bone Marrow Aspiration) related to lack of prior experience

Anxiety related to Knowledge Deficit (bone marrow aspiration)

Patient teaching is an important intervention for most patients and for all nursing diagnoses (eg, Constipation, Ineffective Breast-Feeding, Altered Nutrition). It is not necessary, or even desirable, to have a Knowledge Deficit diagnosis on every patient's care plan. You should simply include teaching as one of the nursing interventions for the other diagnoses you make.

Some patients, such as a newly diagnosed diabetic, require a great deal of teaching in order to acquire necessary self-care skills. Such *special* teaching plans should be a part of the routine care on standardized care plans for these patients, and should not require an individualized diagnosis. However, if the agency does not have a standardized plan or protocol, it will be necessary to write an individualized teaching plan. Even then, Knowledge Deficit should be used as the etiology of a response, for example:

Risk for Altered Health Maintenance (Diabetes Management) related to Knowledge Deficit (medication, diet, exercise, and skin care) secondary to new diagnosis.

If used at all, Knowledge Deficit should describe conditions in which the patient needs new or additional knowledge. It should not be used for problems involving the patient's *ability* to learn (as in Knowledge Deficit related to severe anxiety about outcome of surgery). Rakel and Bulechek (1990) propose a diagnosis of "Situational Learning Disability: Impaired Ability to Learn" or "Situational Learning Disability: Lack of Motivation to Learn" for such conditions. However, these are not NANDA labels.

Knowledge Deficit is under review by NANDA and may eventually be dropped from the taxonomy of nursing diagnoses. To date, NANDA has not developed a definition or critical defining characteristics for it. At least two studies show that Knowledge Deficit is one of the diagnoses most frequently used (misused) by nurses (Gordon 1985; Lambert and Jones 1989). This may be due in part to premature diagnosing: it is easy to recognize a knowledge deficit, label it as a problem, and not look beyond that to the *human response* to the lack of knowledge. Misuse of this diagnosis also occurs because of the mistaken belief that information giving is effective in changing human behavior.

Suggested Alternative Diagnoses

Adjustment, Impaired
Coping, Ineffective Individual
Denial, Ineffective
Health Maintenance, Altered
Noncompliance (specify)

Patient Outcomes and Evaluation Criteria

Include patient-specific target date, evaluation and documentation intervals, and any other patient-specific outcomes.

Patient/family will:

- Identify need for additional information regarding prescribed treatment.
- Verbalize understanding of need for support services to ensure completion of learning.
- Demonstrate ability to follow necessary health care measures.
- Demonstrate ability to ____ (specify skill).

NIC Priority Interventions

Health System Guidance: Facilitating a patient's location and use of appropriate health services.

Teaching, Disease Process: Assisting the patient to understand information related to a specific disease process.

Teaching, Individual: Planning, implementation, and evaluation of a teaching program designed to address a patient's particular needs.

Teaching, Infant Care: Instruction on nurturing and physical care needed during the first year of life.

Teaching, Preoperative: Assisting a patient to understand and mentally prepare for surgery and the postoperative recovery period.

Teaching, Prescribed Activity/Exercise: Preparing a patient to achieve and/or maintain a prescribed level of activity.

Teaching, Prescribed Diet: Preparing a patient to correctly follow a prescribed diet.

Teaching, Prescribed Medication: Preparing a patient to safely take prescribed medications and monitor for their effects.

Teaching, Procedure/Treatment: Preparing a patient to understand and mentally prepare for a prescribed procedure or treatment.

Teaching, Psychomotor Skill: Preparing a patient to perform a psychomotor skill.

Teaching, Safe Sex: Providing instruction concerning sexual protection during sexual activity.

Nursing Actions

Target actions to problem etiologies. Individualize actions to meet the unique needs of each patient.

Ongoing Assessments

- Assess and document:

  Patient's level of understanding of prescribed treatment.
  Patient's readiness to learn treatment regimen.

- Check for accurate feedback to ensure that patient understands prescribed treatment.

Patient Teaching

- Provide literature specific to patient's learning needs.
- Provide teaching at patient's level of understanding, repeating information as necessary. Be realistic.
- Reinforce teaching as necessary, using multiple teaching approaches, return demonstrations, and verbal and written feedback.
- Provide information on community resources that will help patient maintain treatment regimen.
- Involve support person/family in teaching process.

Collaborative Activities

- Develop a coordinated multidisciplinary teaching plan. Plan is ____ (specify).
- Plan with patient and physician adjustment in treatment to facilitate patient's ability to follow prescribed treatment.

Other

- Interact with patient in a nonjudgmental manner to facilitate learning.
- Document patient's progress in nurse's notes.

Mobility, Impaired Physical (6.1.1.1) (Y50.4)

Definition: A state in which the individual experiences a limitation of ability for independent physical movement (NANDA).

Level I: Independently uses equipment or device

Level II: Requires help from another person for assistance, supervision, or teaching

Level III: Requires help from another person and equipment/device

Level IV: Is dependent and does not participate in activity[1]

Specify level ___.

Defining Characteristics

Objective

Decreased muscle strength, control, and/or mass

Impaired motor coordination

Inability to move purposefully within the physical environment, including bed mobility, transfer, and ambulation

Limited range of motion

Reluctance to attempt movement

[1]Adapted from Jones, E., et al: *Patient Classification for Long-Term Care: User's Manual* (HEW Publication No. HRA-74-3107, November 1974).

Related Factors

Decreased strength and endurance secondary to ____
Depression/severe anxiety
Medically prescribed limitations
Musculoskeletal impairment
Neuromuscular impairment
Pain/discomfort
Perceptual/cognitive impairment

Suggestions for Use

Use Impaired Mobility to describe individuals with limited ability for independent physical movement, such as decreased ability to move arms or legs or generalized muscle weakness, or when nursing interventions will focus on restoring mobility and function or preventing further deterioration. For example:

Impaired Physical Mobility related to ineffective management of chronic pain secondary to rheumatoid arthritis

Do not use this label to describe temporary immobility that cannot be changed by the nurse (eg, traction, prescribed bedrest), or permanent paralysis. In these and many other instances, Impaired Mobility can be used effectively as the etiology of a problem. For example:

Impaired Tissue Integrity (Decubitus Ulcer) related to Impaired Physical Mobility +4

Suggested Alternative Diagnoses

Disuse Syndrome: Risk for
Injury: Risk for
Self-Care Deficit

Patient Outcomes and Evaluation Criteria

Include patient-specific target date, evaluation and documentation intervals, and any other patient-specific outcomes.

Patient will:

- Verbalize acceptance of limitations.
- Demonstrate correct use of assistive devices with supervision.
- Use assistive devices correctly and independently.
- Request assistance with mobilization activities.
- Perform mobilization activities with assistance.

NIC Priority Interventions

Exercise Therapy, Ambulation: Promotion and assistance with walking to maintain or restore autonomic and voluntary body functions during treatment and recovery from illness or injury.

Exercise Therapy, Joint Mobility: Use of active or passive body movement to maintain or restore joint flexibility.

Positioning: Moving the patient or a body part to provide comfort, reduce the risk of skin breakdown, promote skin integrity, and/or promote healing.

Nursing Actions

Ongoing Assessments

Assessment and documentation is an ongoing process to determine at which performance level patient's mobility is impaired.

Level I Nursing Actions

- Assistive device is ____ (specify).
- Document patient's safe performance of activities with assistive devices.
- Develop and document a plan for maintaining/increasing mobility. Plan is ____ (specify).
- Provide positive reinforcement during activities.
- Assess need for assistance from home health agency and need for durable medical equipment.

Level II Nursing Actions

- Assess patient's learning needs regarding ____ (specify).
- Assess need for assistance from home health agency and need for durable medical equipment.

- Instruct patient in use of assistive device ____ (specify).
- Instruct and encourage patient in active/passive range-of-motion exercises to maintain or develop muscle strength and endurance.
- Instruct the patient in safe transfer from bed to wheelchair or commode.
- Instruct patient regarding weight-bearing status.
- Instruct patient regarding correct body alignment.
- Instruct and encourage patient to use a trapeze and/or weights to enhance and maintain strength of upper extremities.
- Provide positive reinforcement during activities.
- Assist patient with mobility as necessary. Specify.
- Supervise all mobilization attempts.
- Document patient's safe performance of activities.
- Develop and document a plan for maintaining/increasing mobility. (Use OT/PT as resource in planning patient care activities.) Plan is ____ (specify).

Levels III and IV Nursing Actions

- Provide patient/family the opportunity to share feelings and concerns.
- Encourage patient/family to view limitations realistically.
- Provide positive reinforcement during activities.
- Develop a plan to include the following:

  Active and passive range-of-motion exercises.
  Type of assistive device.
  Positioning of patient in bed/chair.
  Ways to transferelated tourn patient.
  The number of personnel needed to mobilize patient.
  Necessary elimination equipment (bedpan/urinal/fracture pan).
  Schedule of activities.
  Maximization of patient's mobility, given necessary constraints.

- Document patient's responses to plan.
- Use OT/PT as resource in planning patient care activities.

Noncompliance (specify) (5.2.1.1) (Y02.4)

Definition: (1) A person's informed decision not to adhere to a therapeutic recommendation (NANDA). (2) Failure to adhere to a therapeutic recommendation after having made an informed decision *to* do so, and after expressing intention to do so (Gordon 1987).

Defining Characteristics

Subjective

*Patient/family report of patient's noncompliance with treatment regimen

Objective

*Direct observation of failure to adhere to treatment regimen
Failure to progress
Failure to keep appointments
Abnormal diagnostic test results
Evidence of exacerbation of symptoms

*Critical

Related Factors

Cultural beliefs
Denial of illness
Dysfunctional relationship between patient and provider
Negative consequence of treatment regimen
Negative perception of treatment regimen
Perceived benefits of continued illness
Spiritual beliefs

Suggestions for Use

According to NANDA, Noncompliance should be diagnosed when a patient makes an informed decision *not* to adhere to a therapeutic recommendation: for instance, when a patient decides to stop taking a medication with unpleasant side-effects. Nursing intervention might then be directed at convincing the patient of the value of continuing with the therapy, but the nurse should balance this with respect for the patient's autonomy when a truly informed decision has been made. Remember that a decision to refuse therapy can be as rational as a decision to have therapy.

Gordon's (1987) definition (see Definition) is more useful. If the patient is informed and *intends* to follow instructions, then nursing intervention can be directed at finding and removing the factors that keep him from doing so. For example, a patient may state, "My husband doesn't need to lose weight, and he loves fried food and pastries. He just won't eat the diet foods, and I really don't have time to cook one meal for myself and one for the rest of the family." This client would like to comply with her diet, but situational factors are making it difficult. You could write a nursing diagnosis of Noncompliance with Low-Calorie Diet related to inconvenience of preparing special foods and lack of family support. That diagnosis does suggest independent nursing interventions.

Following is a comparison of the NANDA and Gordon definitions of Noncompliance.

NANDA Definition of Noncompliance	*Gordon's Definition of Noncompliance*
Patient has the necessary information	Patient has the necessary information
Patient makes informed choice not to comply with treatment	Patient has said he wants and intends to comply with treatment
	Patient does not comply

Noncompliance should not be used for patients who are unable to follow instructions (eg, too weak, cognitive disability) or who lack necessary information. If those factors are contributing to Noncompliance, then it is better to use the diagnosis Altered Health Maintenance.

Some nurses believe that Noncompliance has a negative connotation. When using this label, be sure to express the etiology in neutral, nonjudgmental terms. Geissler (1991) has suggested the term *nonadherence,* although it is not yet a NANDA label.

Suggested Alternative Diagnoses

Denial, Ineffective
Health Maintenance, Altered
Therapeutic Regimen Management, Ineffective Individual

Patient Outcomes and Evaluation Criteria

Include patient-specific target date, evaluation and documentation intervals, and any other patient-specific outcomes.

Patient will:

- Acknowledge consequences of continued noncompliant behavior.
- Not abuse health care providers physically or verbally.
- Participate in the development of plan of care.
- Follow agreed-on plan of care.

NIC Priority Interventions

Health System Guidance: Facilitating a patient's location and use of appropriate health services.

Self-Modification Assistance: Reinforcement of self-directed change initiated by the patient to achieve personally important goals.

Nursing Actions

Target actions to problem etiologics. Individualize interventions to meet the unique needs of each patient.

Ongoing Assessments

- Identify probable cause of patient's noncompliant behavior.

Patient Teaching

- Help patient/family to understand the need for following prescribed treatment and the consequences of noncompliance.

Collaborative Activities

- Initiate patient care conference to establish plan for consistent approach to patient. Plan is ____ (specify).
- Evaluate patient's need for emotional support from hospital resources/social worker.
- Consult with physician about possible alteration in medical regimen to encourage patient's compliance.

Other

- Encourage the patient to express feelings and concerns about hospitalization and relationship with health care providers.
- Involve the patient in determining what behavior constitutes compliance.
- Give positive reinforcement for compliance to encourage ongoing positive behaviors.
- Develop a written contract with the patient, and evaluate compliant behaviors on a continuing basis. Contract is ____ (specify).
- Inform patient that physical/verbal abuse is not acceptable and will not be tolerated.
- Discuss with patient/family those factors that may have precipitated noncompliance with treatment regimen.
- Provide emotional support to family members to help them maintain a positive relationship with patient.

Nutrition, Altered: Less Than Body Requirements (1.1.2.2) (Y24.0)

Definition: The state in which an individual experiences an intake of nutrients insufficient to meet metabolic needs (NANDA).

Defining Characteristics

NANDA does not specify critical defining characteristics for this label. The author recommends using this label only if one of the starred cues is present.

Subjective

Abdominal pain
Alteration in taste sensation
Indigestion/stomach cramps
Perceived inability to ingest food
Reported lack of food
Satiety immediately after ingesting food

Objective

*Body weight 20% or more under ideal for height and frame
*Food intake less than metabolic needs—either total calories or specific nutrients
*Inadequate food intake of less than recommended daily allowance—either total calories or specific nutrients
*Weight loss with adequate food intake
Aversion to eating
Capillary fragility
Diarrhea and/or steatorrhea
Difficulty in swallowing/chewing
Evidence of lack of food
Excessive loss of hair
Hyperactive/hypoactive bowel sounds
Lack of information, misinformation

Lack of interest in food
Misconceptions
Pale conjunctival and mucous membranes
Poor muscle tone
Refusal to eat
Ulcerated oral mucosa
Weakness of muscles required for swallowing or mastication

Related Factors

Chemical dependence (specify)
Chronic illness (specify)
Difficulty in chewing
Difficulty in swallowing
Economic factors
Food intolerance
High metabolic needs
Inadequate sucking reflex in the infant
Lack of basic nutritional knowledge
Limited access to food
Loss of appetite
Nausea/vomiting
Parental neglect
Psychologic impairment (specify)

Suggestions for Use

Use this label for patients who are able to eat, but unable ingest, digest, or absorb nutrients adequate to meet metabolic needs. Inadequate ingestion might occur because of decreased appetite, nausea, being too poor to buy food, or any number of situations. Examples of patients unable to digest food or absorb particular nutrients are those with allergies, diarrhea, lactose intolerance, or poorly fitting dentures.

Do not use this label routinely for persons who are NPO (nothing by mouth) or for those completely unable to ingest food for other reasons (eg, unconscious patients). Nurses cannot prescribe independent nursing interventions for a diagnosis such as Altered Nutrition: Less Than Body Requirements related to NPO. They cannot give the missing nutrients and they cannot change the NPO order. Additionally, the patient is often NPO for only a short time before and after surgery; thus, any lack of nutrients is temporary and is resolved without nursing intervention. Long-term NPO status is a risk factor for other nursing diagnoses, such as Risk for Altered Oral Mucous Membrane, and for collaborative problems such as Potential Electrolyte Imbalance.

The patient might have a total nutritional deficit, or perhaps be deficient in only one nutrient. When the deficit is other than total, it should be specified, as follows:

Altered Nutrition: Less Than Body Requirements *for Protein* related to lack of knowledge of nutritious foods and limited budget for food

Suggested Alternative Diagnoses

Breast-Feeding, Ineffective
Swallowing, Impaired

Patient Outcomes and Evaluation Criteria

Include patient-specific target date, evaluation and documentation intervals, and any other patient-specific outcomes.

Patient will:

- Maintain weight at ____ kg.
- Describe components of nutritionally adequate diet.
- Verbalize willingness to follow diet.
- Abstain from nonprescribed medication/substances.
- Tolerate prescribed diet.
- Gain ____ kg.

NIC Priority Interventions

Eating Disorders Management: Prevention and treatment of severe diet restriction and overexercising or binging and purging of food and fluids.

Nutrition Management: Assisting with or providing a balanced dietary intake of foods and fluids.

Weight Gain Assistance: Facilitating gain of body weight.

Nursing Actions

Target actions to problem etiologies. Individualize interventions to meet the unique needs of each patient.

General Interventions for All Altered Nutrition

Ongoing Assessments

- Monitor and document food intake.
- Assess and document bowel sounds and abdominal distention q ____.
- Monitor laboratory values, especially transferrin, albumin, and electrolytes.
- Weigh patient q ____.

Collaborative Activities

- Confer with dietitian to establish caloric requirements, especially for patients with high energy needs, such as those with burns, trauma, fever, and wounds, as well as postoperative patients.
- Confer with dietitian to establish protein requirements for patients with inadequate protein intake or experiencing protein losses, such as patients with anorexia nervosa or glomerular disease/peritoneal dialysis.
- Confer with physician regarding need for appetite stimulant, supplemental feedings, nutritional tube feedings, or TPN so that adequate caloric intake is maintained.

Other

- Develop meal plan with patient to include schedule of meals, eating environment, patient likes/dislikes, food temperature.
- Encourage family member to bring food of patient's preference from home.

Difficulty in Chewing/Swallowing

Ongoing Assessments

- Assess and document degree of swallowing difficulty.

Collaborative Activities

- Request occupational therapy consultation.

Other

- Reassure patient, and provide calm atmosphere during meals.
- Have suction catheters available at bedside, and suction during meals as needed.
- Place patient in semi-Fowler's or high-Fowler's position to facilitate swallowing; have patient remain in this position for 30 minutes following meals to prevent aspiration.
- Place food on unaffected side of mouth to facilitate swallowing.
- When feeding patient, use syringe, if necessary, to facilitate swallowing.

Nausea/Vomiting

Ongoing Assessments

- Identify factors precipitating nausea and vomiting.
- Document color, amount, and frequency of emesis.

Patient Teaching

- Instruct patient in slow, deep breathing and voluntary swallowing to decrease nausea and/or vomiting.

Collaborative Activities

- Administer antiemetics on a set schedule to prevent nausea. Schedule is ____ (specify).

Other

- Minimize factors that may precipitate nausea and vomiting. Specify.
- Offer cool, wet washcloth to be placed on forehead or back of neck.
- Ask patient to notify nurse of nausea.
- Offer oral hygiene q ____.

Loss of Appetite

Ongoing Assessments

- Identify factors that may contribute to patient's loss of appetite (such as medications, emotional concerns).

Other

- Give positive feedback to patient who shows increased appetite.

Infant Feeding

Ongoing Assessments

- Assess mother's feeding techniques.
- Monitor baby's intake.

Patient Teaching

- Instruct mother in feeding techniques that may increase baby's intake.

Collaborative Activities

- Confer with pediatrician regarding change in formula, change in schedule, supplemental feedings, and/or gavage feedings as appropriate.

Other

- Use ____ nipples.
- Feed baby on demand.
- Provide privacy for mother and baby during feedings.
- Feed baby q ____.

Nutrition, Altered: More Than Body Requirements (1.1.2.1) (Y24.1)

Definition (Actual): The state in which an individual is experiencing an intake of nutrients that exceeds metabolic needs (NANDA).

Defining Characteristics

Subjective

Reports little or no exercise

Objective

*Triceps skinfold greater than 15mm in men and 25mm in women

*Weight 20% over ideal for height and frame

Concentrating food intake at end of day

Conforming to cultural norms

Dysfunctional eating patterns

Eating in response to external cues, such as time of day or social situation

Eating in response to internal cues, such as anxiety, anger, depression, boredom, stress, loneliness

Little or no exercise

Medications that stimulate appetite

Pairing food with other activities

Selecting foods that do not meet daily requirements

Substituting sweets for addiction

*Critical

Related Factors

Chemical dependence

Concentrating food intake at end of day

Decreased metabolic requirements

Dysfunctional eating patterns

Eating in response to external cues, eg, time of day or social situation

Eating in response to internal cues other than hunger, eg, anxiety

Ethnic/cultural norms

Excessive intake in relation to metabolic needs

Increased appetite

Lack of basic nutritional knowledge

Lack of physical exercise

Observed use of food as reward or comfort measure

Pairing food with other activities

Rapid transition across growth percentiles in infants or children

Reported or observed higher baseline weight at beginning of each pregnancy

Reported or observed obesity in one or both parents

Reported use of solid food as major food source before 5 months of age

Suggestions for Use

This diagnosis is most appropriate for patients who are motivated to lose weight (eg, a woman who has gained weight after pregnancy). It is not appropriate for patients who are overweight but not motivated to participate in a weight loss program. Consider Altered Health Maintenance instead. Note that Altered Nutrition: More Than Body Requirements focuses attention on nutrition instead of on life-style changes necessary for weight loss (eg, exercise). Eating in response to stressors might be described as Ineffective Individual Coping.

Although some of the nursing actions and one of the NIC interventions specify "eating disorders management" as an intervention for this diagnosis, the focus of nursing for a patient who is binging and purging is much more complex than excess calorie intake; this diagnosis has limited use in that situation.

Suggested Alternative Diagnoses

Coping, Ineffective Individual

Health Maintenance, Altered

Therapeutic Regimen Management, Ineffective Individual

Patient Outcomes and Evaluation Criteria

Include patient-specific target date, evaluation and documentation intervals, and any other patient-specific outcomes.

Patient will:

- Acknowledge weight problem.
- Verbalize desire to lose weight.

- Participate in a structured weight-loss program.
- Participate in a regular exercise program.
- Approach ideal weight (specify ____)
- Refrain from binge eating.

NIC Priority Interventions

Eating Disorders Management: Prevention and treatment of severe diet restriction and overexercising or binging and purging of food and fluids.

Nutrition Management: Assisting with or providing a balanced dietary intake of foods and fluids.

Weight Reduction Assistance: Facilitating loss of weight and/or body fat.

Nursing Actions

Target actions to problem etiologies. Individualize interventions to meet the unique needs of each patient.

Ongoing Assessments

- Monitor laboratory values that may be indicative of malnutrition (eg, serum albumin, serum protein, transferrin).

Patient Teaching

- Instruct patient/family in food selection, preparation, and portions.
- Provide information regarding available community resources, such as weight-loss groups, dietary counseling, exercise programs, self-help groups.

Collaborative Activities

- Confer with dietitian to implement weight-loss/eating disorder program that includes dietary management and activity expenditure.

Other

- Explore with patient/family factors that may be contributing to obesity.
- Help patient to identify physical problems that may be related to obesity/eating disorder.
- Develop a weight-loss plan to include:

Two-week food and daily activity diary (amount, time, location, mood, social setting).

Target weight loss.

Self-monitoring.

Education, eg, causes of obesity, nutritional information, energy expenditure.

Positive reinforcement.

Behavior substitution.

Exercise regimen.

Planning for social/business situations that include food.

Group support.

Strategies for control/avoidance of stimulus to eating.

- Develop a plan for managing eating disorders to include:

Frequency of meals and snacks.

Diet of complex carbohydrates, protein.

Avoidance of simple sugars, fast food, caffeine, soft drinks.

Discussion of emotions that stimulate eating.

Recognition of high-risk situations (types of foods, social situations, interpersonal stresses, unmet personal expectations, eating in secret/private).

Behavior substitution.

Group support.

- Provide frequent positive reinforcement for weight loss, maintenance of dietary regimen, improved eating behaviors, exercise.

Nutrition, Altered: More Than Body Requirements (Potential for) (1.1.2.3) (Y24.2)

Definition (Potential for): The state in which an individual is at risk of experiencing an intake of nutrients that exceeds metabolic needs (NANDA).

Defining Characteristics

Presence of risk factors such as the following:

Subjective

Increased appetite

Eating in response to internal cues other than hunger, eg, anxiety

Reported use of solid food as major food source before 5 months of age

Objective

*Obesity in one or both parents

*Rapid transition across growth percentiles in infants or children

Chemical dependence

Concentrating food intake at end of day

Decreased metabolic requirements

Dysfunctional eating patterns

Eating in response to external cues, eg, time of day or social situation

Ethnic/cultural norms

Excessive intake in relation to metabolic needs

Lack of basic nutritional knowledge

Lack of physical exercise

Observed use of food as reward or comfort measure

Pairing food with other activities

Reported or observed higher baseline weight at beginning of each pregnancy

*Critical

Risk Factors

See defining characteristics.

Suggestions for Use

See Altered Nutrition: More Than Body Requirements.

Suggested Alternative Diagnoses

Coping, Ineffective Individual
Health Maintenance, Altered
Therapeutic Regimen Management, Ineffective Individual

Patient Outcomes and Evaluation Criteria

Include patient-specific target date, evaluation and documentation intervals, and any other patient-specific outcomes.

Patient will:

- Acknowledge presence of risk factors.
- Participate in a regular exercise program.
- Maintain ideal weight ____ (specify).
- Eat a balanced diet.

NIC Priority Interventions

Nutrition Management: Assisting with or providing a balanced dietary intake of foods and fluids.

Weight Reduction Assistance: Facilitating loss of weight and/or body fat.

Nursing Actions

Target actions to problem etiologies. Individualize interventions to meet the unique needs of each patient.

Ongoing Assessments

- Monitor weight.
- Monitor presence of risk factors.

Patient Teaching

- Instruct patient/family in food selection, preparation, and portions.
- Provide information regarding available community resources, such as dietary counseling, exercise programs, self-help groups.

Other

- Explore with patient/family factors that may contribute to obesity.

- Develop a weight-management plan to include:

  Two-week food and daily activity diary (amount, time, location, mood, social setting).
  Ideal weight.
  Self-monitoring.
  Education, eg, causes of obesity, nutritional information, energy expenditure.
  Positive reinforcement.
  Behavior substitution.
  Exercise regimen.
  Anticipatory planning for social/business situations that include food.
  Strategies for control/avoidance of stimulus to eating.

- Develop a plan for management of eating to include:

  Frequency of meals and snacks.
  Diet of complex carbohydrates, protein.
  Avoidance of simple sugars, fast food, caffeine, soft drinks.
  Discussion of emotions that stimulate eating.
  Recognition of high-risk situations (types of foods, social situations, interpersonal stresses, unmet personal expectations, eating in secret/private).

- Provide frequent positive reinforcement for good nutrition and exercise.

Oral Mucous Membrane, Altered (1.6.2.1.1) (Y27.0)

Definition: The state in which an individual experiences disruptions in the tissue layers of the oral cavity (NANDA).

Defining Characteristics

Subjective

Discomfort with hot or cold foods
Oral pain/discomfort

Objective

Bad breath
Coated tongue
Dental caries
Dry mouth
Dry, cracked lips
Edema
Hemorrhagic gingivitis
Hyperemia
Irritation, inflammation, or ulceration of oral mucosa
Lack of or decreased salivation
Leukoplakia
Oral lesions or ulcers
Oral plaque
Stomatitis
Vesicles

Related Factors

Chemotherapy
Dehydration
Inadequate oral hygiene
Infection
Lack of or decreased salivation
Malnutrition
Medication
Mouth breathing
NPO for more than 24 hours
Radiation to head and neck
Trauma (*chemical,* eg, acidic foods, drugs, noxious agents, alcohol; *mechanical,* eg, ill-fitting dentures, braces, nasogastric or endotracheal tubes, surgery in oral cavity)

Suggestions for Use

None

Suggested Alternative Diagnosis

Tissue Integrity, Impaired

Patient Outcomes and Evaluation Criteria

Include patient-specific target date, evaluation and documentation intervals, and any other patient-specific outcomes.

Patient will:

- Ingest foods and fluids with increasing comfort.
- Perform essential oral hygiene according to prescribed instruction.
- Have no increase in mucosal irritation, ulceration, or inflammation.
- Have restored integrity of mucosa.

NIC Priority Interventions

Oral Health Restoration: Promotion of healing for a patient who has an oral mucosa or dental lesion.

Nursing Actions

Target actions to problem etiologies. Individualize interventions to meet the unique needs of each patient.

Ongoing Assessments

- Assess patient's oral mucosa for irritation, ulceration, and inflammation.
- Identify substances that irritate oral mucosa, such as tobacco, alcohol, food, medication, extremes in food temperature, seasonings. Specify irritants.
- Assess and document patient's understanding of need for oral care and ability to perform oral care.
- Monitor oral intake.

Patient Teaching

- Instruct patient/family in routine for oral care.

Collaborative Activities

- Confer with physician regarding an order for antifungal mouthwash or oral topical anesthetic as adjunct to oral hygiene if fungal infection exists.

Other

- Plan meals with patient and dietitian to ensure optimal nutrition and hydration.
- Plan for oral care is ____ (specify). (Consider use of toothettes or soft child's toothbrush, bulb syringe, suction catheter, high-strength peroxide, and saline mouthwash.)
- Avoid use of commercial mouthwash, sugared candies, and gum.
- Provide mouth care prior to meals and q ____ hours to ensure optimal oral hygiene and adequate nutrition.
- Assist patient during meals as needed.
- Clean dentures after each meal.

Pain [Acute] (9.1.1) (Y31.0)

Definition: A state in which an individual reports discomfort or an uncomfortable sensation (adapted from NANDA).

Defining Characteristics

Subjective

Communication of pain descriptors, eg, pain, discomfort, nausea, night sweats, muscle cramps, itching skin, numbness, tingling of extremities

Objective

Alteration in muscle tone
Crying
Diaphoresis, pallor
Facial mask of pain
Grimacing
Guarding, protective behavior
Increased respiratory rate
Increased/decreased pulse rate
Limited attention span

Moaning
Pacing
Restlessness
Withdrawal/focus on self

Related Factors

Injury
Noxious stimulus (eg, biological, chemical, physical, psychological injury agents; specify)
Recent surgery

Suggestions for Use

NANDA has not developed critical defining characteristics for Pain, but it can be diagnosed on the patient's report alone, because that is sometimes the only sign of pain. None of the other defining characteristics, taken alone, would be sufficient to diagnose Pain. The related factors indicate that a patient can suffer both physical and psychological pain. Qualifier words should be added to this diagnosis to indicate the severity, location, and nature of the pain. For example:

Severe, stabbing chest pain related to fractured ribs
Mild frontal headache related to sinus congestion

It is important to differentiate between Acute and Chronic Pain because the nursing focus is different for each. Acute Pain (eg, postoperative incision pain) is usually a collaborative problem managed primarily by administering narcotic analgesics. There are a few independent nursing interventions, such as teaching the patient to splint the incision while moving about, but these alone would not provide adequate pain relief. The nurse takes a more active role in teaching patients self-management of Chronic Pain. When Pain is acute or caused by a stressor not amenable to nursing intervention (eg, surgical incision), it may be an etiology rather than a problem. For example:

Ineffective Airway Clearance related to weak cough related to Pain secondary to chest incision

Sexual Dysfunction related to partner's Severe Chronic Pain secondary to arthritis

In differentiating between Acute and Chronic Pain, the following comparison may be helpful:

	Acute Pain	*Chronic Pain*
Defining Characteristics	Duration less than 6 months	Duration longer than 6 months
	Autonomic responses such as pallor, increase in vital signs, and diaphoresis	Personality changes Weight loss

Suggested Alternative Diagnosis

Pain, Chronic

Patient Outcomes and Evaluation Criteria

Include patient-specific target date, evaluation and documentation intervals, and any other patient-specific outcomes.

Patient will:

- Report a decrease in pain.
- Report reasonable comfort.
- Demonstrate individualized relaxation techniques that are effective for achieving comfort.

Patient's level of pain is maintained at ____ or less (scale of 0–10).

NIC Priority Interventions

Analgesic Administration: Use of pharmacologic agents to reduce or eliminate pain.

Epidural Analgesia Administration: Preparation and delivery of narcotic analgesics into the epidural space.

Pain Management: Alleviation of pain or a reduction in pain to a level of comfort that is acceptable to the patient.

Patient-Controlled Analgesia (PCA) Assistance: Facilitating patient control of analgesic administration and regulation.

Nursing Actions

Target actions to problem etiologies. Individualize interventions to meet the unique needs of each patient.

Ongoing Assessments

- Ask patient to rate pain/discomfort on a scale of 0–10 (0 = no pain/discomfort, 10 = worst pain). Document intensity of pain/discomfort.
- Assess nonverbal cues regarding level of pain/discomfort.
- Complete initial pain assessment questionnaire.
- Consider the impact of religion, culture, beliefs, and circumstances on patient's perception of pain/discomfort.
- If patient is preverbal or cognitively impaired, use family members for information.
- In assessing patient's pain, use words that are consistent with patient's age and developmental level.[1]
- Use pain flow sheet to monitor pain relief of analgesics and possible side-effects.
- Use self-report as first choice to obtain assessment information.

Patient Teaching

- Explain reason for pain/comfort medication. Instruct patient to ask for pain/comfort medication before pain/discomfort becomes too severe.
- Instruct patient to inform nurse if pain relief is not achieved.
- Explain pain-management regimen to patient/family.
- Inform patient of procedures that may increase pain, and offer suggestions for coping.
- Instruct patient in use of sitz bath to increase comfort.

[1]Acute Pain Management Guideline Panel. Acute pain management: Operative or medical procedure and trauma. *Clinical Practice Guideline.* AHCPR Pub. No. 92-0032. Rockville, MD: Agency for Health-Care Policy and Research, Public Health Service, U.S. Department of Health and Human Services, February, 1992.

- Include in discharge instruction: specific drug to be taken; frequency of drug administration; potential side-effects; potential drug interaction; specific precautions to follow when taking the medication (eg, physical activity limitations, dietary restrictions); name of person to notify about pain problem.

Collaborative Activities

- Confer with physician on pain management, and assess need for change in pain medication order and use of nonpharmacologic interventions such as TENS and ice/heat application.

Other

- Help patient identify comfort measures that have worked in the past, such as analgesics, distraction, relaxation, and application of heat/cold.
- Explore feelings about fear of addiction. To reassure patient, ask, "If you didn't have this pain, would you still want to take this drug?" Document the pain-management plan.
- Convey acceptance of patient's report of discomfort by a willingness to provide comfort measures.
- Adjust frequency of dosage as indicated by pain assessment and side-effects.
- Note that the elderly have increased sensitivity to analgesic effects of opiates, with higher peak effect and longer duration of pain relief.
- Be alert to possible drug–drug and drug–disease interactions in the elderly, who often have multiple chronic, painful illnesses and take multiple medications.
- Administer pain medication prior to activities/procedures.
- Manage immediate post-operative pain with scheduled opiate (eg, q4 hours for 36 hours) or patient-controlled analgesia (PCA).
- Offer position change, back rubs, and relaxation techniques as supplements/alternative to medications for pain relief.
- Change bed linen prn.
- Encourage patient to maintain optimal activity level.
- Provide care in an unhurried, supportive manner.

- Involve patient in decisions regarding care activities.
- Help patient focus on activities rather than on pain/discomfort by providing diversion through television, radio, tapes, and visitors.

Pain, Chronic (9.1.1.1) (Y31.1)

Definition: A state in which an individual experiences pain that continues for more than 6 months in duration (NANDA).

Defining Characteristics

Major

Subjective

Verbal report or observed evidence of pain existing more than 6 months

Minor

Subjective

Fear of drug addiction
Fear of drug tolerance
Fear of reinjury
Frustration
Nausea

Objective

Altered ability to continue previous activities
Changes in sleep pattern
Depression
Facial mask
Guarded movements
Weight changes
Withdrawal, physical and social

Related Factors

Altered body function (specify)

Chronic physical-psychosocial disability
Metastatic cancer
Neurologic injury

Suggestions for Use

See Pain [Acute] suggestions for use.

In differentiating between Acute and Chronic Pain, the following comparison may be helpful:

	Acute Pain	*Chronic Pain*
Defining Characteristics	Duration less than 6 months	Duration longer than 6 months (may be continuous or intermittent)
	Autonomic responses such as pallor, increase in vital signs, and diaphoresis	Personality changes Weight loss

Suggested Alternative Diagnosis

Pain [Acute]

Patient Outcomes and Evaluation Criteria

Include patient-specific target date, evaluation and documentation intervals, and any other patient-specific outcomes.

Patient will:

- Report reasonable comfort.
- Report increasing ability to cope with pain.
- Verbalize knowledge of alternative measures for pain relief.

Patient's level of pain is maintained at ____ or less (scale 0–10).

NIC Priority Interventions

Analgesic Administration: Use of pharmacologic agents to reduce or eliminate pain.

Pain Management: Alleviation of pain or a reduction in pain to a level of comfort that is acceptable to the patient.

Patient-Controlled Analgesia (PCA) Assistance: Facilitating patient control of analgesic administration and regulation.

Nursing Actions

Target actions to problem etiologies. Individualize interventions to meet the unique needs of each patient.

Ongoing Assessments

- Ask patient to rate pain on a scale of 0–10 (0 = no pain and 10 = worst pain). Document patient's report of pain intensity.
- Assess and document effects of long-term medication use.
- Assess and document patient's response to pain-relief measures.
- Be alert to verbal and nonverbal cues regarding level of pain experienced by the patient.
- Complete initial pain assessment questionnaire.
- Use pain flow sheet to monitor pain relief and side effects.
- Use self-report as first choice to obtain assessment information. If patient is preverbal or cognitively impaired, use family members for information.

Patient Teaching

- Convey to patient that total pain relief may not be achievable.
- Explain home pain-management regimen to patient/family.
- Include in discharge instruction: specific drug to be taken; frequency of drug administration; potential side-effects; potential drug interaction; specific precautions to follow when taking the medication (eg, physical activity limitations, dietary restrictions); name of person to notify about pain problem.

- Instruct patient to inform nurse if desired pain relief is not achieved.
- Instruct patient/family in use of alternative pain-relief measures.

Collaborative Activities

- Consult with physician for orders regarding alternative pain-relief measures, such as TENS, biofeedback, ice/heat application.
- Initiate a multidisciplinary patient care conference to develop a plan to manage discomfort. Plan should include identification and treatment of each symptom and its cause.

Other

- Assist patient in identifying reasonable and acceptable level of pain.
- Convey acceptance of patient's report of discomfort by a willingness to provide comfort measures.
- Incorporate patient's methods of pain relief in care.
- Offer patient pain-relief measures to supplement pain medication, such as biofeedback, relaxation techniques, back rub, and guided imagery.
- Provide care in an unhurried, supportive manner, allowing for sufficient rest periods.

Parental Role Conflict (3.2.3.1) (None)

Definition: The state in which a parent(s) who normally functions effectively experiences role confusion and conflict in response to crisis (adapted from NANDA).

Defining Characteristics

Major

Subjective

Expressed concern about perceived/actual loss of control over decisions relating to child

Expressed concern/feelings of inadequacy to provide for child's physical and emotional needs during hospitalization or in the home

Expressed concerns about changes in parental role, family functioning, family communication, family health

Objective

Demonstration of disruption in caretaking routines

Minor

Subjective

Verbalization, demonstration of feelings of guilt, anger, fear, anxiety, and/or frustrations about effect of child's illness on family process

Objective

Reluctance to participate in usual caretaking activities, even with encouragement and support

Related Factors

Change in marital status, career, roles

Financial crisis

Interruptions in family life due to home care regimen (treatments, caregivers, lack of respite)

Intimidation with invasive or restrictive modality (ie, isolation, intubation), specialized care centers or policies (eg, apnea monitoring, postural drainage, hyperalimentation)

Legal crisis

Relocation

Separation from child due to chronic illness

Suggestions for Use

Use this label when a situation causes unsatisfactory role performance by previously effective parents.

Suggested Alternative Diagnoses

Caregiver Role Strain (Actual/Risk for)
Family Processes, Altered
Parenting, Altered
Parenting, Altered: Risk for

Parent Outcomes

Include patient-specific target date, evaluation and documentation intervals, and any other patient-specific outcomes.

Parent(s) will:

- Verbalize desired parenting role.
- Demonstrate ability to modify parenting role in response to crisis.
- Express a sense of adequacy in providing for child's needs.

NIC Priority Interventions

Crisis Intervention: Use of short-term counseling to help the patient cope with a crisis and resume a state of functioning comparable to or better than the precrisis state.

Family Process Maintenance: Minimization of family process disruption effects.

Role Enhancement: Assisting a patient, significant other, and/or family to improve relationships by clarifying and supplementing specific role behaviors.

Nursing Actions

Target actions to problem etiologies. Individualize interventions to meet the unique needs of each patient.

Assessment

- Ask parents to describe how they want to be involved in the care of their hospitalized child.

Patient Teaching

- Explain rationale for treatments, and encourage questions to minimize misunderstandings and maximize participation.

Collaborative Activities

- Refer to community resources, support groups, social services.

Other

- Confront parents with their ineffective parenting behaviors (during this crisis), and discuss alternatives.
- Develop a plan of care involving parents. Consistently implement plan.
- Discuss with parent(s) a strategy for meeting personal/family's current needs.
- Give positive reinforcement for constructive parental actions.

Parenting, Altered (3.2.1.1.1) (None)

Definition: The state in which a nurturing figure experiences an inability to create an environment which promotes the optimum growth and development of another human being (NANDA).

Defining Characteristics

Subjective

Expressed disappointment with child
Verbalization of resentment toward child
Verbalization of role inadequacy
Verbalized disgust at body functions of child
Verbalized inability to control child

Objective

*Inattentiveness to child's needs
*Reluctant/inappropriate caretaking behaviors (toilet training, sleep/rest, feeding, discipline)
*Reported history of child abuse or abandonment by primary caretaker

Abandonment or runaway
Avoidance of contact with child
Child out of control
Child receiving care from multiple caretakers without consideration of needs of the infant/child
Compulsive seeking of role approval from others
Evidence of physical and/or psychologic trauma to child
Frequent accidents/illnesses
Growth and development lag
Inappropriate or inconsistent discipline practices
Inappropriate visual, tactile, auditory stimulation
Lack of parental attachment behaviors
Negative identification and attachment of meanings to child's characteristics
Noncompliance with health appointments for child

*Critical

Related Factors

Absent or ineffective role model
Dysfunctional relationship between parents/nurturing figures
Interruption in bonding process
Lack of cognitive functioning
Lack of knowledge/skill (specify)
Lack of or inappropriate response of child to parent
Lack of support for nurturing figure(s)
Physical/emotional abuse of parent
Psychologic impairment (specify)
Significant stress (specify)
Substance abuse (specify)
Unmet maturational needs of parent
Unrealistic expectations of self, infant, partner

Suggestions for Use

This label represents a less healthy level of functioning than Parental Role Conflict.

Suggested Alternative Diagnoses

Caregiver Role Strain (Actual/Risk for)
Coping, Ineffective Family: Disabling
Family Processes, Altered
Parental Role Conflict
Parenting, Altered: Risk for
Role Performance, Altered

Parent Outcomes

Include patient-specific target date, evaluation and documentation intervals, and any other patient-specific outcomes.

Parent(s) will:

- Report increasing confidence in care of child.
- Report increasing confidence in parenting role.
- Demonstrate nurturing behaviors toward child, including constructive discipline.
- Identify effective ways to express anger/frustration that are not harmful to child.
- Identify community resources that assist with home care.
- Actively participate in counseling.
- Participate in parenting classes.

NIC Priority Interventions

Attachment Promotion: Facilitation of the development of the parent-infant relationship.

Family Integrity Promotion: Promotion of family cohesion and unity.

Nursing Actions

Target actions to problem etiologies. Individualize interventions to meet the unique needs of each patient.

Collaborative Activities

- Develop a plan for meeting needs of parent. Plan may include counseling, support groups, and hot lines.
- Offer to make initial telephone call to appropriate community resources.

- Report actual or suspected child abuse to appropriate authority.
- Request social service consultation to help the family identify sources of community support.

Other

- Acknowledge and reinforce parenting strengths and skills.
- Encourage expression of feelings (guilt, anger, ambivalence) regarding parenting role.
- Help parent identify deficits/alterations in parenting skills.
- Initiate a plan to assist parent in developing/adapting parenting skills. Consider:

  Frequent opportunities for parent/child interaction.
  Role modeling of parenting skills of nurse.
  Identifying realistic expectations of parenting role.

- Explore available resources with parent.

Parenting, Altered: Risk for (3.2.1.1.2) (None)

Definition: Possibility of changes in ability of nurturing figure(s) to create an environment which promotes the optimum growth and development of another human being (NANDA).

Defining Characteristics

Presence of risk factors such as:

Subjective

Negative identification of or attachment of meanings to child's characteristics

Verbalizes desire to have child call parent by first name instead of traditional cultural tendencies

Verbalizes resentment towards the child

Objective

*History of child abuse or abandonment by primary caretaker
*Inappropriate caretaking behaviors (toilet training, sleep/rest feeding)
*Inattentive to child's needs
Child receives care from multiple caretakers without consideration for the needs of the child
Compulsively seeking role approval from others
Growth and development lag in the child
Inappropriate or inconsistent discipline practices
Inappropriate visual, tactile, auditory stimulation
Lack of parental attachment behaviors
Noncompliance with health appointments for self and/or child

*Critical

Risk Factors

Absent or ineffective role model
Absent or ineffective support system
Adult children of alcoholics
History of child abuse or abandonment of parent
Lack of knowledge regarding effective parenting
Lack of or inappropriate response of child to parent
Mental or physical illness/disability
Perceived threat to parent's physical or emotional survival
Poverty/homelessness
Presence of significant stress
Unmet maturational needs of parent

Suggestions for Use

The critical defining characteristics NANDA lists for this diagnosis are the same as those for actual Altered Parenting. If they are present, use Altered Parenting instead of this diagnosis.

NANDA states that, in general, adjustment to parenting is a normal maturational process that calls for nursing interventions to prevent potential problems and promote health.

Suggested Alternative Diagnoses

Caregiver Role Strain: Risk for
Coping, Ineffective Family
Family Processes, Altered
Parental Role Conflict

Parent Outcomes

Include patient-specific target date, evaluation and documentation intervals, and any other patient-specific outcomes.

Parent(s) will:

- Identify own risk factors that may lead to ineffective parenting.
- Identify high-risk situations that may lead to ineffective parenting.
- Use identified resources to maintain/learn/improve parenting skills.
- Maintain satisfactory parenting role.

NIC Priority Interventions

Attachment Promotion: Facilitation of the development of the parent-infant relationship.

Family Integrity Promotion: Promotion of family cohesion and unity.

Nursing Actions

Target actions to problem etiologies. Individualize interventions to meet the unique needs of each patient.

Patient/Parent Teaching

- Provide reading material as appropriate.

Collaborative Activities

- Refer to community support/educational programs to assist with development of parenting skills and provide anticipatory guidance.

Other

- Help parent(s) identify high-risk situations/factors that may hinder effective parenting.

- Help parent(s) to develop strategies to maintain/learn/ improve parenting skills.
- Acknowledge and reinforce parenting strengths and skills.

Peripheral Neurovascular Dysfunction: Risk for (6.1.1.1.1) (None)

Definition: A state in which an individual is at risk of experiencing a disruption in circulation, sensation, or motion of an extremity (NANDA).

Defining Characteristics

Presence of risk factors such as:

Objective

Burns

Fractures

Immobilization

Mechanical compression, eg, tourniquet, cast, brace, dressing, or restraint

Orthopedic surgery

Trauma

Vascular obstruction

Risk Factors

See defining characteristics.

Suggestions for Use

Use this label for situations nurses can prevent by reducing or eliminating causative factors (eg, Risk for Peripheral Neurovascular Dysfunction related to compression from restraints). For situations requiring medical treatment (eg, thrombophle-bitis), use a collaborative problem such as Potential Complication of Thrombophlebitis in Left Leg: Peripheral Neurovascular Dysfunction.

Suggested Alternative Diagnoses

None

Patient Outcomes and Evaluation Criteria

Include patient-specific target date, evaluation and documentation intervals, and any other patient-specific outcomes.

Patient/family will:

- Verbalize signs and symptoms of peripheral neurovascular dysfunction.
- Describe measures to prevent development of neurovascular dysfunction.

Patient will:

- Remain free of injury from compression devices or restraints.
- Demonstrate optimal healing and adaptation to cast, traction, or dressing.

NIC Priority Interventions

Circulatory Care: Promotion of arterial and venous circulation.

Exercise Therapy: Joint Mobility: Use of active or passive body movement to maintain or restore joint flexibility.

Peripheral Sensation Management: Prevention or minimization of injury or discomfort in the patient with altered sensation.

Nursing Actions

Ongoing Assessments

Perform the following neurovascular assessments every hour for the first 24 hours following casting, injury, traction, or restraints. Then, if stable, q4 hours:

- Assess and document circulation (color, temperature, capillary refill, edema, and distal pulses) to involved extremity.
- Assess for and report increasing and progressive pain that is present on passive movement and not relieved by narcotics, which may be first sign of compartment syndrome.

- Assess motor function, movement, and strength of the involved peripheral nerve.
- Conduct systematic evaluation of the sensory function of the involved peripheral nerve (interview patient for subjective symptoms, pinprick, paresthesias).

Patient Teaching

- Emphasize importance of keeping follow-up appointments with physician.
- Teach patient/family routine cast care and measures to prevent complications.
- Teach patient/family signs and symptoms of peripheral nerve injury and importance of immediate medical attention (pain not relieved by medication, paresthesia of involved body part).

Other

- Avoid tight dressings and appliances to prevent ischemia.
- Elevate involved extremity to increase venous return and minimize edema.
- Institute immediate treatment if compartment syndrome is suspected: keep involved extremity at heart level, notify physician, and anticipate removal of anterior cast, occlusive bandages, and surgical intervention.
- Listen to patient's expressed complaints of pain, burning, and changes in sensation.
- Recognize that restlessness, fussiness, and crying may be nonverbal cues of physical distress in infants, children, or adults with impaired verbal communication.

Personal Identity Disturbance (7.1.3) (Y61.1)

Definition: Alteration in one's ability to distinguish between the self (ego) and nonself (adapted from NANDA).

Defining Characteristics

Objective

Change in social involvement

Extension of body boundary to incorporate environmental objects

Grandiose behavior

Related Factors

Chronic illness

Chronic pain

Congenital defects

Psychologic impairment (specify)

Situational crisis (specify)

Suggestions for Use

None

Suggested Alternative Diagnosis

Thought Processes, Altered

Patient Outcomes and Evaluation Criteria

Include patient-specific target date, evaluation and documentation intervals, and any other patient-specific outcomes.

Patient will:

- Acknowledge impact of situation on existing personal relationships/life-style/role performance.
- Express willingness to use suggested resources on discharge.
- Identify personal strengths.
- Maintain close personal relationships.
- Verbalize willingness to consider life-style change.

NIC Priority Interventions

Decision-Making Support: Providing information and support for a patient who is making a decision regarding health care.

Self-Esteem Enhancement: Assisting a patient to increase his/her personal judgment of self-worth.

Nursing Actions

Target actions to problem etiologies. Individualize interventions to meet the unique needs of each patient.

Ongoing Assessments

- Assess need for assistance from social services department for planning care with patient/family.

Collaborative Activities

- Offer to make initial phone call to appropriate community resources for patient/family.
- Request psychiatric consultation.

Other

- Actively listen to patient/family, and acknowledge reality of concerns about treatments, progress, and prognosis.
- Assist patient to identify personal strengths.
- Develop a plan of care with patient/family that identifies coping mechanisms and personal strengths and acknowledges limitations. Specify plan.
- Encourage patient to verbalize concerns about close personal relationships.
- Encourage patient to verbalize consequences of physical and emotional changes that have influenced self-concept.
- Encourage patient/family to air feelings and to grieve.
- Help patient identify alternative behaviors that are congruent with a change in personal relationships, life-style, and/or role performance.
- Provide care in a nonjudgmental manner, maintaining the patient's privacy and dignity.

Poisoning: Risk for (1.6.1.2) (Y23.2)

Definition: Accentuated risk of accidental exposure to or ingestion of drugs or dangerous products in doses sufficient to cause poisoning (NANDA).

Defining Characteristics

Presence of risk factors, such as:

Internal (individual)

Cognitive or emotional difficulties

Insufficient finances

Lack of proper precautions

Lack of safety or drug education

Reduced vision

Verbalization of occupational setting without adequate safeguards

External (environmental)

Availability of illicit drugs potentially contaminated by poisonous additives

Chemical contamination of food and water

Dangerous products placed or stored within the reach of children or confused persons

Flaking, peeling paint or plaster in presence of young children

Large supplies of drugs in house

Medicines stored in unlocked cabinets accessible to children or confused persons

Paint, lacquer, and so on in poorly ventilated areas or without effective protection

Presence of atmospheric pollutants

Presence of poisonous vegetation

Unprotected contact with heavy metals or chemicals

Risk Factors

See defining characteristics.

Suggestions for Use

Use the most specific label for which defining characteristics are present.

Suggested Alternative Diagnoses

Home Maintenance Management, Impaired
Injury, Risk for
Parenting, Altered

Patient Outcomes and Evaluation Criteria

Include patient-specific target date, evaluation and documentation intervals, and any other patient-specific outcomes.

Patient/family will:

- Develop strategies to prevent poisoning.
- Identify risks that increase possibility of poisoning.
- Identify and implement appropriate safety measures that protect individual/child from poisoning.
- Use measures to protect self and others from injury.

NIC Priority Interventions

Environmental Management, Safety: Monitoring and manipulation of the physical environment to promote safety.

Surveillance, Safety: Purposeful and ongoing collection and analysis of information about the patient and the environment for use in promoting and maintaining patient safety.

Nursing Actions

Target actions to problem etiologies. Individualize interventions to meet the unique needs of each patient.

Ongoing Assessments

- Assess high-risk areas that may lead to injury to patient/family.

Patient Teaching

- Provide educational materials related to strategies and countermeasures.

- Provide information on environmental hazards and characteristics (eg, stairs, windows, cupboard locks, swimming pools, streets, gates).
- Provide information on Poison Control Center and exposure to medications and household products.

Collaborative Activities

- Refer to community classes (CPR, first aid, swimming classes).

Other

- Explore strategies to prevent injury.

Post-Trauma Response (9.2.3) (Y34)

Definition: The state of an individual experiencing a sustained painful response to unexpected extraordinary life events (NANDA).

Defining Characteristics

Major

Subjective

Excessive verbalization of traumatic event
Guilt about behavior required for survival
Intrusive thoughts
Reliving the event; flashback
Repetitive nightmares or dreams
Verbalization of guilt about the behavior required for survival
Verbalization of survival guilt

Minor

Subjective

Emotional numbness
Reported difficulty with interpersonal relationships
Reported phobia regarding trauma

Reported pronounced changes in sexual behavior

Objective

Amnesia about traumatic event
Irritability
Poor impulse control
Sleep pattern disturbance
Substance abuse
Suicide attempt(s)
Withdrawal from activities and commitments

Related Factors

Accidents
Assault
Catastrophic illness
Disaster
Epidemic
Kidnapping
Participation in combat
Rape
Terrorism
Torture

Suggestions for Use

If the related factor is rape, consider the suggested alternative diagnoses.

Suggested Alternative Diagnoses

Rape-Trauma Syndrome: Compound Reaction
Rape-Trauma Syndrome: Silent Reaction

Patient Outcomes and Evaluation Criteria

Include patient-specific target date, evaluation and documentation intervals, and any other patient-specific outcomes.

Patient will:

- Verbalize feelings related to traumatic event.
- Acknowledge value of counseling.
- Identify community resources for postdischarge care.

NIC Priority Interventions

Counseling: Use of short-term counseling to help the patient cope with a crisis and resume a state of functioning comparable to or better than the precrisis state.

Support System Enhancement: Facilitation of support to patient by family, friends, and community.

Nursing Actions

Target actions to problem etiologies. Individualize interventions to meet the unique needs of each patient.

Ongoing Assessments

- Assess patient's potential for suicide.

Patient Teaching

- Provide information/referral on community resources (rape counselors, clergy, crisis centers, support groups, mental health professionals, social services, Victims' Assistance, Survivors of Trauma).

Collaborative Activities

- Follow hospital/agency policy regarding legal responsibility for reporting to authorities.
- Initiate a multidisciplinary patient care conference to develop a plan of care. Specify.

Other

- Encourage active participation in group activities to provide opportunity for social supports and problem solving.
- Encourage patient to verbalize account of the event.
- Encourage verbalization of concerns by using caregivers who have an established rapport with patient and are knowledgeable about, and comfortable with, exploration of patient concerns.
- Enhance patient's feeling of safety:

  Promote a caring and therapeutic relationship between patient and nurse.

  Monitor/hold phone calls at patient's request.

  Monitor/limit visitation.

- Initiate suicide precautions.
- Involve family/significant person in treatment plan.
- Plan room assignment, considering private vs. semiprivate and choice of roommate.
- Provide opportunities for patient to initiate interactions and activities.
- Support the patient needing an invasive medical procedure (which may precipitate flashbacks):

  Encourage patient to discuss feelings after procedure.
  Explain necessity of procedure.
  Premedicate if needed to minimize distress/discomfort.
  Stay with patient during procedure.

Powerlessness (7.3.2) (Y60.1)

Definition: Perception that one's own action will not significantly affect an outcome; a perceived lack of control over a current situation or immediate happening (NANDA).

Defining Characteristics

Severe

Subjective

Verbal expressions of having no control or influence over situation, self-care, or outcome

Objective

Apathy

Depression over physical deterioration that occurs despite patient compliance with regimens

Moderate

Subjective

Expressions of dissatisfaction and frustration over inability to perform previous tasks and/or activities

Expression of doubt regarding role performance

Fear of alienation from caregivers
Reluctance to express true feelings

Objective

Dependence on others that may result in irritability, resentment, anger, and guilt
Does not defend self-care practices when challenged
Does not monitor progress
Inability to seek information regarding care
Nonparticipation in care or decision making when opportunities are provided
Passivity

Low

Subjective

Expressions of uncertainty about fluctuating energy levels

Objective

Passivity

Related Factors

Chronic illness
Complications threatening pregnancy
Health care environment
Illness-related regimen
Interpersonal interaction
Life-style of helplessness
Terminal illness
Treatment regimen

Suggestions for Use

Differentiate between Powerlessness and Hopelessness. Hopelessness implies that the person believes there *is* no solution to his/her problem ("no way out"). In situations of Powerlessness, patients may know of a solution to their problem, but believe it is beyond their control to achieve the solution.

Suggested Alternative Diagnoses

Disuse Syndrome: Risk for
Grieving, Dysfunctional

Hopelessness
Self-Esteem, Low: Chronic

Patient Outcomes and Evaluation Criteria

Include patient-specific target date, evaluation and documentation intervals, and any other patient-specific outcomes.

Patient will:

- Verbalize feelings of powerlessness.
- Identify actions within his/her control.
- Participate in decision making regarding plan of care.

NIC Priority Interventions

Self-Esteem Enhancement: Assisting a patient to increase his/her personal judgment of self-worth.

Self-Responsibility Facilitation: Encouraging a patient to assume more responsibility for own behavior.

Nursing Actions

Target actions to problem etiologies. Individualize interventions to meet the unique needs of each patient.

Collaborative Activities

- Initiate a multidisciplinary patient care conference to discuss and develop patient care routine. Plan is ____ (specify).

Other

- Allow patient as much control over his/her situation as possible.
- Discuss with patient realistic options in care, providing explanations for these options.
- Explain to patient the rationale for any change in the plan of care.
- Help patient to identify factors that may contribute to powerlessness.
- Involve patient in decision making about care routine.
- Provide flexibility in care regimen as needed by patient.
- Use nurse/patient relationship to assist patient in expressing feelings about his/her situation.

Protection, Altered (1.6.2) (None)

Definition: The state in which an individual experiences a decrease in the ability to guard the self from internal or external threat such as illness or injury (NANDA).

Defining Characteristics

Major

Objective

Altered clotting
Deficient immunity
Impaired healing
Maladaptive stress response
Neurosensory alteration

Minor

Subjective

Cough
Dyspnea
Itching

Objective

Anorexia
Cough
Disorientation
Fatigue
Immobility
Insomnia
Perspiring
Pressure sores
Restlessness
Weakness

Related Factors

Abnormal blood profiles (eg, leukopenia, thrombocytopenia, anemia, coagulation)

Alcohol abuse

Diseases (eg, cancer, immune disorders)

Drug therapies (eg, antineoplastic, corticosteroid, immune, anticoagulant, thrombolytic)

Extremes of age

Inadequate nutrition

Treatments (eg, surgery, radiation)

Suggestions for Use

When possible, use a more specific label such as Risk for Infection, Impaired Skin Integrity, Impaired Tissue Integrity, Altered Oral Mucous Membrane, or Fatigue.

Suggested Alternative Diagnoses

Infection: Risk for

Injury: Risk for

Peripheral Neurovascular Dysfunction: Risk for

Skin Integrity, Impaired: Risk for

Patient Outcomes and Evaluation Criteria

Include patient-specific target date, evaluation and documentation intervals, and any other patient-specific outcomes.

Patient/family will:

- Demonstrate behaviors that decrease risk of injury/infection/bleeding.
- Identify early signs and symptoms of injury/infection/bleeding.
- Report early signs and symptoms of injury/infection/bleeding.
- Verbalize willingness to change behavior to decrease risk of injury/infection/bleeding.

Patient will:

- Be free of signs and symptoms of injury/infection/bleeding.
- Report an increase in his/her ability to manage stress.

NIC Priority Interventions

Environmental Management, Violence Prevention: Monitoring and manipulation of the physical environment to decrease the potential for violent behavior directed toward self, others, or environment.

Infection Control: Minimizing the acquisition and transmission of infectious agents.

Infection Protection: Prevention and early detection of infection in a patient at risk.

Surveillance, Safety: Purposeful and ongoing collection and analysis of information about the patient and the environment for use in promoting and maintaining patient safety.

Nursing Actions

Prevention of Infection

- See nursing actions for Risk for Infection on page 150.

Prevention of Injury

- See nursing actions for Risk for Injury on page 154.

Prevention of Bleeding

Assessment

- Evaluate extent of patient's bleeding risk.

Patient Teaching

- Advise patient to wear medical identification bracelet and to alert dentist, physician.
- Instruct patient to avoid trauma (eg, from contact sports, sharp objects, stiff toothbrush).
- Teach patient signs and symptoms of bleeding and when to report.
- Teach patient first aid for bleeding.

Restoration and Growth

Patient Teaching

- Provide information on community resources/support groups.

Collaborative Activities

- Consult dietitian for suggestions to improve nutrition.
- Confer with social services to identify appropriate referral for counseling.

Other

- Explore with patient ways to enhance sleep/rest.
- Assist patient in achieving optimum sleep, rest, nutrition, activity, and stress management.
- Discuss relaxation techniques with patient/family, and make appropriate referrals.
- Assist patient/family in identifying and planning an appropriate exercise program.

Rape-Trauma Syndrome (9.2.3.1) (Y34.0)

Definition: The stress response pattern that occurs as a result of forcible or attempted forcible sexual penetration against the victim's will and consent. This syndrome includes an acute phase of disorganization of the victim's life-style and a long-term process of reorganization of life-style (adapted from NANDA).*

Defining Characteristics

Acute Phase (Several Weeks)

Emotional Reactions

Anger
Confusion
Embarrassment
Fear of physical violence and death
Fear of pregnancy, sexually transmitted diseases
Humiliation

*This syndrome includes Rape-Trauma, Compound Reaction and Silent Reaction. Each appears as a separate diagnosis in this text.

Inability to make decisions
Memory disturbance
Psychotic states
Revenge
Self-blame
Suicidal/homicidal behavior

Multiple Physical Symptoms

GI irritability (eg, stomach pains, appetite disturbance, nausea)
GU disturbance (eg, vaginal discharge, itching, burning on urination, generalized pain)
Muscle tension (eg, tension headaches and fatigue)
Physical trauma (eg, general soreness, bruises, lesions, trauma to mouth and rectum)
Sleep pattern disturbance (eg, hyperalertness, edginess, nervousness)

Long-Term Phase

Life-Style Changes

Changing residences
Initiating period of celibacy
Seeking out family, friends for support
Taking trips

Recurrent Dreams and Nightmares

Mastery dreams (indicate recovering)
Reliving rape and victimization
Symbolic dreams related to the rape

Emotional Reactions

Body image disturbance
Promiscuity
Psychotic states
Suicidal/homicidal behavior

Fears and Phobias

Fear of being alone
Fear of crowds
Fear of environment (location of rape/attempted rape)
Fear of initiating/continuing relationships that may lead to intimacy
Sexual fears

Related Factors

Patient's biopsychosocial response to event.

Suggestions for Use

None

Suggested Alternative Diagnoses

Rape-Trauma Syndrome: Compound Reaction
Rape-Trauma Syndrome: Silent Reaction

Patient Outcomes and Evaluation Criteria

Include patient-specific target date, evaluation and documentation intervals, and any other patient-specific outcomes.

Patient will:

- Describe a plan that includes safety measures to reduce future risk.
- Experience decreased symptoms of stress response.
- Return to previous level of biopsychosocial functioning.

NIC Priority Interventions

Crisis Intervention: Use of short-term counseling to help the patient cope with a crisis and resume a state of functioning comparable to or better than the precrisis state.

Rape-Trauma Treatment: Provision of emotional and physical support immediately following an alleged rape.

Nursing Actions

Target actions to problem etiologies. Individualize interventions to meet the unique needs of each patient.

Ongoing Assessments

- Assess need for hospitalization for physical or psychologic trauma.

Patient Teaching

- Refer patient/family to rape crisis counseling.

- Support and educate significant others. Encourage expression of feelings, and discuss therapeutic response to victim and changed behaviors.

Collaborative Activities

- Initiate rape protocol specific to health care facility taking into consideration preservation of evidence, physical assessment, specimen collection, reporting to legal authorities, and medical follow-up.

Other

- Allow adequate time for patient to respond to even simple questions.
- Approach patient in a nonjudgmental and supportive manner.
- Assist patient/family to establish support network.
- Counsel immediate family, spouse, or partner to maintain close relationship with victim, with attention to dispelling feelings of blame (self or projected).
- Encourage patient to verbalize feelings.
- Identify with patient/family predictable behaviors in response to rape-trauma event.
- Treat physical injuries.

Rape-Trauma Syndrome: Compound Reaction (9.2.3.1.1) (Y34.1)

Definition: The stress response pattern that occurs as a result of forcible or attempted forcible sexual penetration against the victim's will and consent. It includes an acute phase of disorganization of the victim's life-style and a long-term process of reorganization of life-style. In the compound reaction, previous psychiatric and/or medical conditions are reactivated (adapted from NANDA).

Defining Characteristics

Acute Phase (Several Weeks)

Emotional Reactions

Anger
Confusion
Embarrassment
Fear of physical violence and death
Fear of pregnancy, sexually transmitted diseases
Humiliation
Inability to make decisions
Memory disturbance
Psychotic states
Reliance on alcohol or drugs
Revenge
Self-blame
Signs of previous psychiatric conditions (acute psychosis, mania, major depression, suicidal behaviors, paranoia, delusions)
Suicidal/homicidal behavior

Multiple Physical Symptoms

GI irritability (eg, stomach pains, appetite disturbance, nausea)
GU disturbance (eg, vaginal discharge, itching, burning on urination, generalized pain)
Muscle tension (eg, tension headaches and fatigue)
Physical trauma (eg, general soreness, bruises, lesions, trauma to mouth and rectum)
Signs of previous medical conditions
Sleep pattern disturbance (eg, hyperalertness, edginess, nervousness)

Long-Term Phase

Life-Style Changes

Changing residences
Initiating period of celibacy
Seeking out family, friends for support
Taking trips

Recurrent Dreams and Nightmares

Mastery dreams (indicate recovering)

Reliving rape and victimization

Symbolic dreams related to the rape

Emotional Reactions

Body image disturbance

Promiscuity

Psychotic states

Suicidal/homicidal behavior

Fears and Phobias

Fear of being alone

Fear of crowds

Fear of environment (location of rape/attempted rape)

Fear of initiating/continuing relationships that may lead to intimacy

Sexual fears

Related Factors

Patient's biopsychosocial response to event.

Suggestions for Use

None

Suggested Alternative Diagnoses

Rape-Trauma Syndrome

Rape-Trauma Syndrome: Silent Reaction

Patient Outcomes and Evaluation Criteria

Include patient-specific target date, evaluation and documentation intervals, and any other patient-specific outcomes.

Patient safety will be maintained during reactivation of psychiatric and/or medical conditions.

Patient will:

- Actively participate in rape counseling.
- Discontinue use of alcohol/drugs.

- Identify the existence of a relationship between his/her own psychiatric and/or medical conditions and the rape episode.
- Return to previous level of biopsychosocial functioning.

NIC Priority Interventions

Counseling: Use of an interactive helping process focusing on the needs, problems, or feelings of the patient and significant others to enhance or support coping, problem solving, and interpersonal relationships.

Rape-Trauma Treatment: Provision of emotional and physical support immediately following an alleged rape.

Nursing Actions

Target actions to problem etiologies. Individualize interventions to meet the unique needs of each patient.

Ongoing Assessments

- Assess and document patient's orientation to person, place, time, and situation.
- Assess for suicidal ideation.
- Perform physical assessment based on patient's complaints to determine presenting medical conditions.
- Perform psychosocial assessment that focuses on rape.

Patient Teaching

- Educate significant others. Discuss therapeutic response to victim and changed behaviors.

Collaborative Activities

- Refer patient/family to rape crisis counseling.

Other

- Allow adequate time for patient to respond to even simple questions.
- Approach patient in a nonjudgmental and supportive manner.
- Assist patient/family to establish support network.
- Correlate physical and psychosocial assessment data to determine patient's status.

- Counsel immediate family, spouse, or partner to maintain close relationship with victim, with attention to dispelling feelings of blame (self or projected).
- Encourage patient to verbalize feelings.
- Establish a plan of care to stabilize medical/psychologic condition to proceed with rape-trauma counseling.
- Identify with patient/family predictable behaviors in response to rape-trauma event.
- Provide necessary safety precautions indicated by suicide risk assessment.
- Support significant others. Encourage expression of feelings.

Rape-Trauma Syndrome: Silent Reaction (9.2.3.1.2) (Y34.2)

Definition: The stress response pattern that occurs as a result of forcible or attempted forcible sexual penetration against the victim's will and consent. It includes an acute phase of disorganization of the victim's life-style and a long-term process of reorganization of life-style. In the silent reaction, the rape/attempted rape is not verbalized (adapted from NANDA).

Defining Characteristics

Subjective

Blocking of associations
Frequent, violent nightmares
Long periods of silence
Minor stuttering
No verbalization of the occurrence of rape
Persistently low self-confidence and self-esteem
Physical distress
Severe anxiety during assessment interview

Objective

Avoidance of close relationships
Change in sexual behavior/relationships
Irritability toward gender of perpetrator
Sudden change in relationships
Sudden onset of phobic reactions
Suspiciousness

Related Factors

Patient's biopsychosocial response to event.

Suggestions for Use

None

Suggested Alternative Diagnoses

Rape-Trauma Syndrome
Rape-Trauma Syndrome: Compound Reaction

Patient Outcomes and Evaluation Criteria

Include patient-specific target date, evaluation and documentation intervals, and any other patient-specific outcomes.

Patient will:

- Acknowledge rape/attempted rape.
- Describe a plan that includes safety measures to reduce future risk.
- Experience a decrease in stress response symptoms.
- Return to previous level of biopsychosocial functioning (specify).
- Verbalize details of the rape/attempted rape as a means of catharsis.
- Verbalize feelings associated with rape/attempted rape.

NIC Priority Interventions

Counseling: Use of an interactive helping process focusing on the needs, problems, or feelings of the patient and significant others to enhance or support coping, problem solving, and interpersonal relationships.

Rape-Trauma Treatment: Provision of emotional and physical support immediately following an alleged rape.

Nursing Interventions

Target actions to problem etiologies. Individualize interventions to meet the unique needs of each patient.

Patient Teaching

- Educate significant others. Discuss therapeutic response to victim and changed behaviors.
- Explain to patient a rape victim's expected thoughts, feelings, behaviors.

Collaborative Activities

- Refer patient/family to rape crisis counseling.

Other

- Assist patient/family to establish support network.
- Confirm with patient that a traumatic event recently occurred, and specifically identify it as "rape."
- Encourage patient to ventilate thoughts, feelings, behaviors.
- Establish therapeutic relationship that will allow exploration of silent reaction.
- Support significant others. Encourage expression of feelings.

Relocation Stress Syndrome (6.7) (None)

Definition: Physiological and/or psychosocial disturbances as a result of transfer from one environment to another (NANDA).

Defining Characteristics

Major

Subjective

Anxiety

Apprehension

Increased confusion (elderly population)
Loneliness

Objective

Change in environment/location
Depression

Minor

Subjective

Increased verbalization of needs
Unfavorable comparison of post/pretransfer staff
Verbalization of being concerned/upset about transfer
Verbalization of unwillingness to relocate

Objective

Change in eating habits
Dependency
Gastrointestinal disturbances
Insecurity
Lack of trust
Restlessness
Sad affect
Sleep disturbance
Vigilance
Weight change
Withdrawal

Related Factors

Decreased physical health status.
Feeling of powerlessness
History and types of previous transfers
Impaired psychosocial health status
Lack of adequate support system
Little or no preparation for the impending move
Losses involved with decision to move
Moderate to high degree of environmental change
Past, concurrent, and recent losses

Suggestions for Use

None

Suggested Alternative Diagnoses

None

Patient Outcomes and Evaluation Criteria

Include patient-specific target date, evaluation and documentation intervals, and any other patient-specific outcomes.

Patient will:

- Demonstrate decrease in physiological/psychosocial disturbances.
- Demonstrate ability to adjust to new environment.
- Verbalize acceptance of new environment.

Patient/family will establish a new supportive social network.

NIC Priority Interventions

Coping Enhancement: Assisting a patient to adapt to perceived stressors, changes, or threats which interfere with meeting life demands and roles.

Discharge Planning: Preparation for moving a patient from one level of care to another within or outside the current health care agency.

Hope Instillation: Facilitation of the development of a positive outlook in a given situation.

Self-Responsibility Facilitation: Encouraging a patient to assume more responsibility for own behavior.

Nursing Actions

Target actions to problem etiologies. Individualize interventions to meet the unique needs of each patient.

Ongoing Assessments

- Assess patient's orientation, mood (depressed, angry, anxious), and physiological status on admission and q ____.
- Assess patient's response to past relocations by interviewing patient and family.

Collaborative Activities

- Maintain consistency in caregivers and care routines as much as possible. Consider a case manager.
- Utilize other resources to assist in transition to new environment.

Other

- Allow patient as much control over his/her situation as possible.
- Encourage patient to verbalize thoughts and feelings about relocation.
- Encourage verbalization of concerns, feelings, fears about recent change in environment.
- Establish new environment as close to previous environment as possible to maintain consistency in placement of personal belongings, placement of furniture, pictures, and so on.
- Explore with patient/family methods to expand/develop patient's social network.
- If future transfers are necessary, avoid transfers at night, at change-of-shift, and unplanned or abrupt transfers.
- Involve patient in decision making about care routine.
- Orient patient to new environment q ____.
- To ease the transfer, encourage family to stay with patient, bring familiar objects from home, and provide familiar socialization.

Role Performance, Altered (3.2.1) (None)

Definition: Disruption in the way one perceives one's role performance (NANDA). Alteration in one's ability to perform those functions and activities expected of a particular role in a given society.

Defining Characteristics

Objective

Change in others' perception of role
Change in physical capacity to resume role
Change in self-perception of role
Change in usual patterns of responsibility
Concern about ability to continue role performance
Conflict in roles
Denial of role
Lack of knowledge of role

Related Factors

Assumption of new role
Chronic illness
Chronic pain
Psychologic impairment (specify)
Situational crisis (specify)
Surgery
Treatment side effects
Unmet expectations for childbirth
Unmet expectations for pregnancy

Suggestions for Use

When applicable, use the more specific labels Parental Role Conflict, Sexual Dysfunction, Altered Family Processes, and so forth. Some degree of role conflict and disruption is present for everyone. For a patient having difficulty with role performance, consider using Altered Role Performance as the etiology of another diagnosis that describes the impact on functioning (eg, Self-Concept Disturbance, or Risk for Impaired Home Maintenance Management related to Altered Role Performance).

Suggested Alternative Diagnoses

Caregiver Role Strain (Actual/Risk for)
Family Processes, Altered
Home Maintenance Management, Impaired

Parental Role Conflict
Self-Esteem, Low: Situational
Sexual Dysfunction

Patient Outcomes and Evaluation Criteria

Include patient-specific target date, evaluation and documentation intervals, and any other patient-specific outcomes.

Patient will:

- Acknowledge impact of situation on existing personal relationships/life-style/role performance.
- Demonstrate ability to function within limitations.
- Describe actual change in function.
- Express willingness to use resources on discharge.
- Identify personal strengths.
- Maintain close personal relationships.
- Verbalize willingness to consider life-style change.

NIC Priority Interventions

Role Enhancement: Assisting a patient, significant other, and/or family to improve relationships by clarifying and supplementing specific role behaviors.

Nursing Actions

Target actions to problem etiologies. Individualize interventions to meet the unique needs of each patient.

Ongoing Assessments

- Assess need for assistance from social services department for planning care with patient/family.

Collaborative Activities

- Offer to make initial phone call to appropriate community resources for patient/family.

Other

- Actively listen to patient/family, and acknowledge reality of concerns about treatments, progress, and prognosis.

- Assist patient in identifying personal strengths.
- Develop a plan of care with patient/family that identifies coping mechanisms and personal strengths and acknowledges limitations. Specify plan.
- Discuss with patient/family the impact of patient's change in role performance and the potential change in family members' role functions.
- Encourage patient to verbalize concerns about close personal relationships.
- Encourage patient to verbalize consequences of physical and emotional changes that have influenced self-concept.
- Encourage patient/family to air feelings and to grieve.
- Help patient identify alternative behaviors that are congruent with a change in personal relationships, life-style, and/or role performance.
- Provide care in a nonjudgmental manner, maintaining the patient's privacy and dignity.

Self-Care Deficit (6.5) (None)

This label includes the following specific deficits in self-care: Self-Care Deficit: Bathing/Hygiene, Self-Care Deficit: Dressing/Grooming, Self-Care Deficit: Feeding, Self-Care Deficit: Toileting, and Self-Care Deficit: Total. Because the nursing interventions are different for each, they are presented separately in this text.

Suggestions for Use

Self-Care Deficit describes a state in which a person experiences impaired ability to perform self-care activities such as bathing, dressing, eating, and toileting. If the person is unable to perform any self-care, the situation is described as Total Self-Care Deficit. However, the diagnosis is subdivided into more specific problems, each with its own critical defining characteristics; these problems can exist alone or in various combinations. For example:

Feeding Self-Care Deficit
Feeding and Bathing/Hygiene Self-Care Deficit

Self-Care Deficits are often caused by Activity Intolerance, Impaired Physical Mobility, Pain, Anxiety, or Perceptual or Cognitive Impairment (eg, Feeding Self-Care Deficit +2 related to hyperactivity). As an etiology, Self-Care Deficit can cause Depression, Fear of becoming dependent, and Powerlessness (eg, Fear of becoming totally dependent related to Total Self-Care Deficit +2 secondary to residual weakness from CVA).

Self-Care Deficit should be used to label only those conditions in which the focus is to support or improve the patient's self-care abilities. Outcome and evaluation criteria for this diagnosis must reflect improved functioning. Therefore, if the diagnosis is used for states not amenable to treatment, there is no hope of achieving the stated outcomes. The focus of nursing interventions is twofold: (1) to increase the patient's ability to perform self-care, and (2) to help patients with limitations and perform care the patient cannot do.

Suggested Alternative Diagnoses

Activity Intolerance
Mobility, Impaired Physical
Sensory/Perceptual Alterations
Thought Processes, Altered

Self-Care Deficit: Bathing/ Hygiene (specify level) (6.5.2) (Y51)

Definition: A state in which the individual experiences an impaired ability to perform or complete bathing/hygiene activities for self (NANDA).

Defining Characteristics

Objective

*Inability to wash body or body parts

Inability to regulate water temperature or flow

Inability to obtain or get to water source

*Critical

Related Factors

Decreased strength and endurance

Depression

Developmental disability

Intolerance to activity

Medically imposed restrictions

Musculoskeletal impairment

Neuromuscular impairment

Pain/discomfort

Perceptual or cognitive impairment

Psychologic impairment (specify)

Severe anxiety

Suggestions for Use

See Self-Care Deficit.

In order to promote efforts to restore functioning, the patient's functional level must be classified. NANDA uses the following scale.[1]

0 = Completely independent

1 = Requires use of equipment or device

2 = Requires help from another person for assistance, supervision, or teaching

3 = Requires help from another person and equipment device

4 = Dependent, does not participate in activity

[1]Code adapted from E. Jones, et al. *Patient Classification for Long-Term Care: Users' Manual,* HEW Publication No. HRA-74-3107, November 1974; as it appears in *NANDA Nursing Diagnoses: Definitions and Classification 1994.*

The following definitions and descriptors may be helpful in determining which number to assign to a patient's functional level:

	Totally Dependent (+4)	*Moderately Dependent* (+3)	*Semi-dependent* (+2)
Bathing	Patient needs complete bath; cannot assist at all.	Nurse supplies all equipment; positions patient; washes back, legs, perineum, and all other parts, as needed. Patient can assist.	Nurse provides all equipment; positions patient in bed/ bathroom. Patient completes bath, except for back and feet.
Oral Hygiene	Nurse completes entire procedure.	Nurse prepares brush; rinses patient's mouth; positions patient.	Nurse provides equipment; patient does task.

Suggested Alternative Diagnoses

Activity Intolerance
Mobility, Impaired Physical
Self-Care Deficit
Sensory/Perceptual Alterations
Thought Processes, Altered

Patient Outcomes and Evaluation Criteria

Include patient-specific target date, evaluation and documentation intervals, and any other patient-specific outcomes.

Patient will:

- Accept total care by caregiver, if needed.
- Acknowledge need for assistance or total care.
- Be able to use adaptive devices.

- Participate in bathing and oral hygiene to optimal level.
- Perform independent bathing and oral hygiene.
- Verbalize satisfactory body cleanliness and oral hygiene.

NIC Priority Interventions

Bathing: Cleaning of the body for the purposes of relaxation, cleanliness, and healing.

Self-Care Assistance, Bathing/Hygiene: Assisting patient to perform personal hygiene.

Nursing Actions

Ongoing Assessments

- Assess ability to use assistive devices.
- Assess for improved or deteriorating functional level.
- Assess oral mucous membranes and body cleanliness daily.

Patient Teaching

- Instruct patient in alternative methods for bathing and oral hygiene. Specify method and teaching plan.

Collaborative Activities

- Offer pain medications prior to bathing.
- Refer patient and family to social services.
- Use OT/PT as resource in planning patient care activities.

Other

- Acknowledge and reinforce patient's accomplishments.
- Create opportunities for small successes. Specify.
- Discuss limitations in self-care with patient.
- Encourage independence in bathing and oral hygiene, assisting patient only as necessary.
- Encourage patient to set own pace during self-care.
- Include family in provision of care.
- Include patient in determining care routine.
- Plan for postdischarge care with patient and family.
- Specify functional level and provide bathing and oral hygiene needs as follows: ____.

Self-Care Deficit: Dressing/ Grooming (specify) (6.5.3) (Y52)

Definition: A state in which the individual experiences an impaired ability to perform or complete dressing and grooming activities for self (NANDA).

Defining Characteristics

Objective

*Impaired ability to put on or take off necessary items of clothing

Impaired ability to fasten clothing

Impaired ability to obtain or replace articles of clothing

Subjective

Inability to maintain appearance at a satisfactory level

*Critical

Related Factors

Decreased strength and endurance
Depression
Developmental disability
Intolerance to activity
Musculoskeletal impairment
Neuromuscular impairment
Pain/discomfort
Perceptual or cognitive impairment
Psychologic impairment (specify)
Severe anxiety

Suggestions for Use

See Self-Care Deficit.

NANDA uses the following scale to classify functional level:[1]

0 = Completely independent
1 = Requires use of equipment or device
2 = Requires help from another person for assistance, supervision, or teaching
3 = Requires help from another person and equipment device
4 = Dependent, does not participate in activity

The following definitions and descriptors may be helpful in determining which number to assign to a patient's functional level:

	Totally Dependent (+4)	*Moderately Dependent* (+3)	*Semi-dependent* (+2)
Dressing/ Grooming	Patient needs to be dressed and cannot assist the nurse; nurse combs patient's hair.	Nurse combs patient's hair; assists with dressing; buttons and zips clothing, ties shoes.	Nurse gathers items for patient; may button, zip, or tie clothing. Patient dresses self.

Suggested Alternative Diagnoses

Activity Intolerance
Mobility, Impaired Physical
Self-Care Deficit
Sensory/Perceptual Alterations
Thought Processes, Altered

Patient Outcomes and Evaluation Criteria

Include patient-specific target date, evaluation and documentation intervals, and any other patient-specific outcomes.

[1]Code adapted from E. Jones, et al. *Patient Classification for Long-Term Care: Users' Manual,* HEW Publication No. HRA-74-3107, November 1974; as it appears in *NANDA Nursing Diagnoses: Definitions and Classification 1994.*

Patient will:

- Accept care by caregiver.
- Be able to dress and comb hair independently.
- Be able to use adaptive devices to facilitate dressing.
- Be neatly dressed.
- Express satisfaction with dressing and hair grooming.
- Have clean, neat hair.
- Participate in self-care (dressing, hair care) to optimal level.
- Recognize/acknowledge need for help.

NIC Priority Interventions

Dressing: Choosing, putting on, and removing clothes for a person who cannot do this for self.

Hair Care: Promotion of neat, clean, attractive hair.

Nursing Actions

Ongoing Assessments

- Assess ability to use assistive devices.
- Assess energy level and activity tolerance.
- Assess for improved or deteriorating ability to dress and perform hair care.
- Assess for sensory, cognitive, or physical deficits that may make dressing difficult for the patient.

Patient Teaching

- Demonstrate use of assistive devices and adaptive activities.
- Instruct patient in alternative methods for dressing and hair care. Specify method and teaching plan.

Collaborative Activities

- Offer pain medications prior to dressing and grooming.
- Refer patient and family to social services.
- Use OT/PT as resource in planning patient care activities.

Other

- Accommodate cognitive deficits.
- Acknowledge and reinforce patient's accomplishments.
- Create opportunities for small successes. Specify.
- Discuss limitations in dressing and hair care with patient.
- Encourage independence in dressing/grooming, assisting patient only as necessary.
- Encourage patient to set own pace during dressing/grooming. Allow sufficient time.
- Help patient choose clothing that is loose fitting and easy to put on.
- Include family in provision of care.
- Include patient in determining care routine.
- Keep verbal communication short and simple.
- Lay clothes out for patient in the order they will be needed when dressing.
- Plan for postdischarge care with patient and family.
- Provide assistive devices such as long-handled shoe horn, Velcro fasteners and closures, buttonhooks, zipper pull, and so on.
- Provide for privacy while dressing.
- Provide for safety by keeping environment uncluttered and well lighted.
- Specify functional level and provide basic care (dressing and hair care) as follows: ____. Use nonverbal cues (eg, hand one article of clothing at a time, in the order needed).

Self-Care Deficit: Feeding (specify) (6.5.1) (Y53)

Definition: A state in which the individual experiences an impaired ability to perform or complete feeding activities for self (NANDA).

Defining Characteristics

Objective

*Impaired ability to bring food from a receptacle to the mouth
Excessive dropping or spilling of food
Inability to cut food

Subjective

Expression of frustration with feeding self

*Critical

Related Factors

Decreased strength and endurance
Depression
Developmental disability
Intolerance to activity
Musculoskeletal impairment
Neuromuscular impairment
Pain/discomfort
Perceptual or cognitive impairment
Psychologic impairment (specify)
Severe anxiety

Suggestions for Use

See Self-Care Deficit.

NANDA uses the following scale to classify functional level:[1]

0 = Completely independent
1 = Requires use of equipment or device
2 = Requires help from another person for assistance, supervision, or teaching
3 = Requires help from another person and equipment device
4 = Dependent, does not participate in activity

[1]Code adapted from E. Jones, et al. *Patient Classification for Long-Term Care: Users' Manual,* HEW Publication No. HRA-74-3107, November 1974; as it appears in *NANDA Nursing Diagnoses: Definitions and Classification 1994.*

The following definitions and descriptors may be helpful in determining which number to assign to a patient's functional level:

	Totally Dependent (+4)	*Moderately Dependent* (+3)	*Semi-dependent* (+2)
Feeding	Patient needs to be fed, totally.	Nurse cuts food; opens containers; positions patient; monitors and encourages eating.	Nurse positions patient; gathers supplies; monitors eating.

Suggested Alternative Diagnoses

Activity Intolerance
Mobility, Impaired Physical
Self-Care Deficit
Sensory/Perceptual Alterations
Thought Processes, Altered

Patient Outcomes and Evaluation Criteria

Include patient-specific target date, evaluation and documentation intervals, and any other patient-specific outcomes.

Patient will:

- Accept feeding by caregiver.
- Be able to feed self independently.
- Be able to use adaptive devices to eat.
- Express satisfaction with eating.
- Have adequate intake of food and fluids.
- Improve ability to feed self.
- Recognize/acknowledge need for help with eating.
- Report increased satisfaction with ability to feed self.

NIC Priority Interventions

Feeding: Providing nutritional intake for patient who is unable to feed self.

Nursing Actions

Ongoing Assessments

- Assess ability to use assistive devices.
- Assess energy level and activity tolerance.
- Assess for improved or deteriorating ability to feed self.
- Assess for sensory, cognitive, or physical deficits that may make self-feeding difficult.

Patient Teaching

- Demonstrate use of assistive devices and adaptive activities.
- Instruct patient in alternative methods for eating/drinking. Specify method and teaching plan.

Collaborative Activities

- Offer pain medications prior to eating.
- Refer patient and family to social services.
- Use OT/PT as resource in planning patient care activities.

Other

- Accommodate cognitive deficits:

  Avoid using sharp eating utensils (eg, steak knives).
  Check for food in cheeks.
  Have meals in quiet environment to limit distraction from task.
  Keep verbal communication short and simple.
  Serve one food at a time, in small amounts.

- Acknowledge and reinforce patient's accomplishments.
- Assist with setting up tray and cutting food, opening packages, buttering bread, and so forth, as needed.
- Create opportunities for small successes. Specify.
- Discuss with patient limitations in ability to feed self.
- Encourage independence in eating and drinking, assisting patient only as necessary.
- Encourage patient to set own pace during meals. Allow sufficient time.
- Encourage patient to wear dentures and eyeglasses.
- Include family in feeding patient.
- Include patient in determining care routine.

- Plan for postdischarge care with patient and family.
- Provide assistive devices such as plate guards, padded handles on utensils, and suction cups to stabilize plates.
- Provide for privacy while eating, if patient is embarrassed.
- Provide oral hygiene before and after meals.
- Serve "finger foods" (eg, fruit, bread) to promote independence.
- Specify functional level and provide basic care (feeding) as follows: ____.

Self-Care Deficit: Toileting (specify level) (6.5.4) (Y57)

Definition: A state in which the individual experiences an impaired ability to perform or complete toileting activities for self (NANDA).

Defining Characteristics

Objective

*Unable to get to toilet or commode

*Unable to sit on or rise from toilet or commode

*Unable to manipulate clothing for toileting

*Unable to carry out proper toilet hygiene

Unable to flush toilet or commode

*Critical

Related Factors

Decreased strength and endurance

Depression

Developmental disability

Intolerance to activity

Medically imposed restrictions

Musculoskeletal impairment

Neuromuscular impairment

Pain/discomfort

Perceptual or cognitive impairment
Psychologic impairment (specify)
Severe anxiety

Suggestions for Use

See Self-Care Deficit.

NANDA uses the following scale to classify functional levels:[1]

0 = Completely independent
1 = Requires use of equipment or device
2 = Requires help from another person for assistance, supervision, or teaching
3 = Requires help from another person and equipment device
4 = Dependent, does not participate in activity

The following definitions and descriptors may be helpful in determining which number to assign to a patient's functional level:

	Totally Dependent	*Moderately Dependent*	*Semi-dependent*
	(+4)	(+3)	(+2)
Toileting	Patient is incontinent; nurse places patient on bedpan or commode.	Nurse provides bedpan; positions patient on or off bedpan; places patient on commode.	Patient can walk to bathroom/commode with assistance; nurse helps with clothing.

Suggested Alternative Diagnoses

Activity Intolerance
Mobility, Impaired Physical
Self-Care Deficit

[1]Code adapted from E. Jones, et al. *Patient Classification for Long-Term Care: Users' Manual,* HEW Publication No. HRA-74-3107, November 1974; as it appears in *NANDA Nursing Diagnoses: Definitions and Classification 1994.*

Sensory/Perceptual Alterations
Thought Processes, Altered

Patient Outcomes and Evaluation Criteria

Include patient-specific target date, evaluation and documentation intervals, and any other patient-specific outcomes.

Patient will:

- Accept help from caregiver.
- Be able to toilet self.
- Have increased ability to toilet self.
- Recognize/acknowledge need for help with toileting.

NIC Priority Interventions

Environmental Management: Manipulation of the patient's surroundings for therapeutic benefit.

Self-Care Assistance, Toileting: Assisting another with elimination.

Nursing Actions

Ongoing Assessments

- Assess ability to ambulate independently and safely.
- Assess ability to use assistive devices (walkers, canes, and so on).
- Assess energy level and activity tolerance.
- Assess for improved or deteriorating ability to feed self.
- Assess for sensory, cognitive, or physical deficits that may limit self-toileting.

Patient Teaching

- Demonstrate use of assistive equipment and adaptive activities.
- Instruct patient and family in transfer and ambulation techniques. Specify method and teaching plan.

Collaborative Activities

- Offer pain medications prior to toileting.
- Refer patient and family to social services.

- Use OT/PT as resource in planning patient care activities and obtaining necessary equipment.

Other

- Accommodate cognitive deficits:

  Encourage patient to wear regular clothing instead of pajamas or gowns to help maintain continence.

  Keep verbal communication short and simple.

  Offer bedpan/commode every 2 hours, after meals, and at bedtime.

- Acknowledge and reinforce patient's accomplishments.
- Allow sufficient time for toileting to avoid fatigue and frustration.
- Avoid use of indwelling catheters and condom catheters if possible.
- Create opportunities for small successes. Specify.
- Discuss with patient specific limitations in ability to toilet self (ambulating, hygiene, and so on).
- Encourage independence in toileting, assisting patient only as necessary for hygiene and safety.
- Encourage patient to wear clothes that are easy to manage.
- Encourage patient to wear eyeglasses.
- Include family in assisting patient.
- Keep bedpan or urinal within patient's reach.
- Keep call bell within reach; answer call bell promptly.
- Maintain a safe environment, including good lighting and a clear pathway to the toilet area.
- Plan for postdischarge care with patient and family.
- Provide assistive devices such as plate guards, padded handles on utensils, suction cups to stabilize plates, and so on.
- Provide for privacy: close door, pull curtains around bed, ask visitors to leave.
- Specify functional level and provide basic care (toileting) as follows: ____.

(See Urinary Incontinence for additional interventions for incontinence.)

Self-Esteem Disturbance (7.1.2) (None)

Definition: Negative self-evaluation/feelings about self or self-capabilities, which may be directly or indirectly expressed (NANDA).

Defining Characteristics

Subjective

Describes change in social involvement
Expressions of shame/guilt
Verbalization of negative feelings about self

Objective

Denial of problems obvious to others
Difficulty in accepting positive feedback; exaggeration of negative feedback
Difficulty in making decisions
Evaluation of self as unable to deal with events
Grandiosity
Hesitation to try new things/situations
Hypersensitivity to slight or criticism
Lack of eye contact
Lack of follow-through
Nonparticipation in therapy
Projection of blame/responsibility for problems
Rationalization of personal failures

Related Factors

Assumption of new role
Chronic illness
Chronic pain
Congenital anomalies
Psychologic impairment (specify)
Situational crisis (specify)
Unmet expectations for child

Unmet expectations for childbirth
Unmet expectations for pregnancy

Suggestions for Use

When you have adequate supporting clinical data, use more specific labels such as Chronic or Situational Low Self-Esteem. This label has some defining characteristics in common with Body Image Disturbance; however, the diagnoses can be differentiated by the presence, in Body Image Disturbance, of preoccupation with change in or loss of a body part or function. Body Image Disturbance is very specific, but it may contribute to the broader, more pervasive Self-Esteem Disturbance.

Suggested Alternative Diagnoses

Body Image Disturbance
Hopelessness
Personal Identity Disturbance
Powerlessness
Self-Esteem, Low: Chronic
Self-Esteem, Low: Situational

Patient Outcomes and Evaluation Criteria

Include patient-specific target date, evaluation and documentation intervals, and any other patient-specific outcomes.

Patient will:

- Acknowledge impact of situation on existing personal relationships/life-style/role performance.
- Express willingness to use resources on discharge.
- Identify personal strengths.
- Maintain close personal relationships.
- Verbalize willingness to consider life-style change.

NIC Priority Interventions

Self-Esteem Enhancement: Assisting a patient to increase his/her personal judgment of self-worth.

Nursing Actions

Ongoing Assessments

- Assess need for assistance from social services department for planning care with patient/family.

Collaborative Activities

- Offer to make initial phone call to appropriate community resources for patient/family.

Other

- Actively listen to patient/family, and acknowledge reality of concerns about treatments, progress, and prognosis.
- Assist patient in identifying personal strengths.
- Develop a plan of care with patient/family that identifies coping mechanisms and personal strengths and acknowledges limitations. Specify plan.
- Encourage patient to maintain usual daily grooming routine.
- Encourage patient to verbalize concerns about close personal relationships.
- Encourage patient to verbalize consequences of physical and emotional changes that have influenced self-concept.
- Encourage patient to wear clothing to enhance physical and emotional self-esteem.
- Encourage patient/family to air feelings and to grieve.
- Help patient identify alternative behaviors that are congruent with a change in personal relationships, life-style, and/or role performance.
- Provide care in a nonjudgmental manner, maintaining the patient's privacy and dignity.

Self-Esteem, Low: Chronic (7.1.2.1) (Y61.2)

Definition: Long-standing, negative self-evaluation/feelings about self or self-capabilities (NANDA).

Defining Characteristics

Major

Subjective

Consistent verbalization of negative feelings about self
Consistently expressed feelings of shame/guilt
Expressed inability to deal with events
Rationalization or rejection of positive feedback

Objective

Exaggeration of negative feedback about self
Reluctance to try new states/things/situations

Minor

Subjective

Excessive seeking of reassurance
Excessive positive self-appraisal/bragging

Objective

Excessive passivity
History of acquiescence to the opinion of others
History of lack of success in work or personal life
Indecisiveness
Lack of eye contact
Projection of blame/responsibility for problems
Self-destructive behavior (alcohol, drug abuse)
Self-neglect

Related Factors

Chronic illness
Congenital anomaly
Psychologic impairment (specify)
Repeatedly unmet expectations

Suggestions for Use

Chronic Low Self-Esteem is different from Situational Low Self-Esteem in that the symptoms are long-standing and seem to result from frequent, actual, or perceived lack of success in work or role performance.

Suggested Alternative Diagnoses

Coping, Ineffective Individual
Hopelessness
Powerlessness
Self-Esteem Disturbance
Self-Esteem, Low: Situational

Patient Outcomes and Evaluation Criteria

Include patient-specific target date, evaluation and documentation intervals, and any other patient-specific outcomes.

Patient will:

- Acknowledge personal strengths.
- Decrease verbalization of low self-esteem.
- Express a willingness to seek counseling.
- Participate in making decisions regarding plan of care.
- Practice behaviors that generate self-confidence.
- Verbalize increasing self-confidence.

NIC Priority Interventions

Self-Esteem Enhancement: Assisting a patient to increase his/her personal judgment of self-worth.

Nursing Actions

Target actions to problem etiologies. Individualize interventions to meet the unique needs of each patient.

Patient Teaching

- Provide information about the value of counseling and available community resources.
- Teach positive behavioral skills through role play, role model, discussion, and so on.

Collaborative Activities

- Seek assistance from hospital resources as needed (social workers, psychiatric clinical specialist, pastoral care services).

Other

- Actively involve patient in developing a plan of care. Plan may include:

  Assigning a primary nurse to maintain consistency for patient and to communicate plan to team members.
  Assisting patient to identify personal strengths.
  Giving feedback regarding observed positive behaviors.
  Involving patient in diversional activity.
  Redirecting patient's focus to personal strengths.
  Setting limits about negative verbalization (frequency, content, audience).
  Identifying positive coping behaviors.
  Providing opportunities for skill practice.
  Structuring interactions/activities to minimize potential for failure.

Self-Esteem, Low: Situational (7.1.2.2) (Y61.3)

Definition: Negative self-evaluation/feelings about self which develop in response to a loss or change in an individual who previously had a positive self-evaluation (NANDA).

Defining Characteristics

Major

Subjective

Verbalization of negative feelings about self (helplessness, uselessness)

Objective

Episodic negative self-appraisal in response to life events

Minor

Subjective

Expressed shame/guilt
Self-negating verbalizations

Objective

Evaluation of self as unable to handle situations/events
Difficulty in making decisions

Related Factors

Situational crisis (specify)

Suggestions for Use

Situational Low Self-Esteem can be differentiated from Chronic Low Self-Esteem in that the symptoms are episodic. Symptoms occur in a person with previously good self-esteem and are in response to some actual or perceived event or situation.

Suggested Alternative Diagnoses

Adjustment, Impaired
Body Image Disturbance
Coping, Ineffective Individual
Personal Identity Disturbance
Self-Esteem Disturbance
Self-Esteem, Low: Chronic

Patient Outcomes and Evaluation Criteria

Include patient-specific target date, evaluation and documentation intervals, and any other patient-specific outcomes.

Patient will:

- Acknowledge low self-esteem.
- Acknowledge personal strengths.
- Practice behaviors that generate self-confidence.
- Verbalize episodic change/loss.

NIC Priority Interventions

Self-Esteem Enhancement: Assisting a patient to increase his/her personal judgment of self-worth.

Nursing Actions

Target actions to problem etiologies. Individualize interventions to meet the unique needs of each patient.

Patient Teaching

- Teach positive behavioral skills through role play, role model, discussion, and so on.

Collaborative Activities

- Refer to appropriate community resources.
- Seek assistance from hospital resources as needed (social worker, clinical nurse specialist, pastoral care services).

Other

- Assist patient in identifying personal strengths.
- Develop a plan of care with patient/family to generate self-confidence. Plan may include:

  Assigning a primary nurse to maintain consistency for patient and to communicate plan to team members.
  Giving specific positive feedback for desired behaviors.
  Identifying positive coping behaviors.
  Providing opportunities for skill practice.

- Encourage patient to verbalize self-evaluation/feelings about self.
- Explore recent changes with patient that may have influenced low self-esteem.

Self-Mutilation: Risk for (9.2.2.1) (None)

Definition: A state in which an individual is at high risk to perform an act upon the self to injure, not kill, which produces tissue damage and possible tension relief (adapted from NANDA).

Defining Characteristics

Presence of risk factors, such as:

Command hallucinations
Drug/alcohol abuse
Dysfunctional family
Feelings of depression, rejection, self-hatred, separation anxiety, guilt, and depersonalization
Fluctuating emotions
Inability to cope with increased psychological/physiological tension in a healthy manner
Need for sensory stimuli
Parental emotional deprivation

Groups at Risk

Emotionally disturbed and/or battered children
Mentally retarded and autistic children
Patients in psychotic state—frequently males in young adulthood
Patients with a history of self-injury
Patients with Borderline Personality Disorder, especially females 16–25 years of age
Patients with history of physical, emotional, or sexual abuse
Patients with Multiple Personality Disorder

Risk Factors

See defining characteristics.

Suggestions for Use

Risk for Self-Mutilation is a more specific diagnosis than Risk for Self-Directed Violence, although the two diagnoses have some of the same defining characteristics (risk factors). Self-Directed Violence includes actions such as drug and alcohol abuse and high-risk lifestyle (eg, driving fast), which are not included in Risk for Self-Mutilation.

Suggested Alternative Diagnoses

Suicide: Risk for
Violence, Self-Directed: Risk for

Patient Outcomes and Evaluation Criteria

Include patient-specific target date, evaluation and documentation intervals, and any other patient-specific outcomes.

Patient will:

- Not injure self.
- Be free from self-injury.
- Report increasing ability to control impulses to injure self.
- Verbalize feelings rather than acting on feelings to injure self.
- Verbalize reduction of command hallucinations and/or delusions.
- Verbalize absence of command hallucinations and/or delusions.

NIC Priority Interventions

Anger Control Assistance: Facilitation of the expression of anger in an adaptive nonviolent manner.

Environmental Management, Safety: Monitoring and manipulation of the physical environment to promote safety.

Nursing Actions

For All Patients

Patient Teaching

- Provide support and education to family regarding patient status and methods of treatment.

Other

- Provide the least restrictive environment that will provide safety for patient. It may be necessary to gradually decrease restrictions based on patient's self-control.

Psychotic Patient

Ongoing Assessments

- Assess patient for history of self-injury: methods used, known triggers, and so on.
- Observe for behavioral changes from baseline assessment, eg, increased withdrawal, agitation, and so on.

- Assess patient for morbid preoccupation with suicide, self-mutilation, hopelessness, worthlessness.
- Assess patient for command hallucinations to determine content and source, eg, "Whose voice is it? What is the voice telling you to do? Is the voice telling you to hurt yourself, and how? Does the voice have control over you?"
- Assess patient for religious and/or persecutory delusions that may lead to self-injury.
- Assess patient for somatic delusions that may lead to self-injury, eg, part of body believed to be diseased, rotten, unnecessary, and so on.
- Observe patient for a calmness in behavior that abruptly follows a period of agitation.
- Monitor intensity of hallucinations/delusions and attempt reality-testing q ____.

Collaborative Activities

- Administer psychotropic and/or antianxiety medications per physician order.
- Use seclusion/restraint to protect patient per physician order.
- Use protective devices (eg, mitts, helmet, jacket restraint, long-sleeved shirt, and so on).
- Obtain physician order if intervention is a denial of rights.

Other

- If patient exhibits calmness in behavior that abruptly follows a period of agitation, provide increased safety measures to prevent self-injury.
- Assist patient to differentiate internal stimuli from outside world.
- Encourage patient to describe triggers that led up to self-injury in past.
- Remove potentially dangerous items from patient and environment, recognizing that it is impossible to have a purely "safe environment." Search patient as needed for potentially harmful items.
- Trim patient's fingernails/toenails to prevent scratching.

- Contract with patient to not injure self. Renew contract q ____.
- Encourage patient to verbalize thoughts and impulses instead of storing up tension.
- Encourage physical activity.
- If patient is unable to contract or follow directions, stay with patient at all times until either patient reports a decrease in command hallucinations, delusions, or self-mutilative impulses or seclusion/restraint is used.

Personality Disorder Patient

Ongoing Assessments

- Assess patient for history of self-injury: methods used, known triggers, and so on.
- Assess patient's level of impulsivity and frustration tolerance.

Patient Teaching

- Teach patient alternative stress/tension relieving measures, eg, relaxation techniques, physical exercise, journal writing, self-affirmations, distracting techniques such as music, TV, conversation, and so on.

Collaborative Activities

- Consider antianxiety or neuroleptic medications per physician order.
- Use seclusion/restraint with physician order.
- Provide consistent responses to patient by collaborating closely with other health care providers. Review treatment plan frequently to prevent staff splitting and conflict regarding treatment goals.

Other

- Encourage patient to seek out staff and peers, not use alcohol or drugs.
- Contract with patient to not harm self and to talk with staff about self-injury thoughts or impulses as they occur.
- Establish regular and frequent check-in times with assigned staff.

- Provide patient safety with least restrictive measures, eg, environmental manipulation (removal of harmful objects as feasible, roommate, room close to nursing station, and so on), family/visitor restriction, patient within eyesight at all times, patient within arm's length, other interventions specific to patient (specify).

Retarded/Autistic Patient

Ongoing Assessments

- Assess patient for history of self-injury behaviors: methods used, known triggers, and so on.
- Assess patient's response to environment to determine if there is a stressor that may lead to self-injury.

Other

- Alter environmental situations that may produce stress that provokes self-injury behaviors.
- Remove reinforcement that may induce self-injury behavior (eg, comforting patient after head-banging, excusing patient from perceived unpleasant tasks, and so on).
- Develop behavioral plan that will prevent or decrease incidence of self-injury.
- Use protective devices to prevent self-injury (eg, mitts, helmet, jacket restraint, protective clothing, and so on).

Sensory/Perceptual Alterations (specify) (7.2) (Y62)*

Definition: A state in which an individual experiences a change in the amount or interpretation of incoming stimuli accompanied by an absent, diminished, exaggerated, distorted response to such stimuli.

*Visual (Y62.5), Auditory (Y62.0), Kinesthetic (Y62.2), Gustatory (Y62.1), Tactile (Y62.4), Olfactory (Y62.3)

Defining Characteristics

Subjective

Altered abstraction

Complaints of fatigue

Reported change in sensory acuity

Objective

Alteration in posture

Altered communication pattern

Altered conceptualization

Anxiety

Apathy

Change in behavior pattern

Change in muscular tension

Change in problem-solving abilities

Change in usual response to stimuli

Disorientation to person, place, time, or situation

Inappropriate responses

Indication of alteration in body image

Irritability

Measured change in sensory acuity

Restlessness

Related Factors

Alcohol/substance abuse (specify)

Altered environmental stimuli

Altered sensory reception, transmission, and/or integration secondary to CVA, brain trauma, increased intracranial pressure, and so on

Electrolyte imbalance

Sensory deficit (specify)

Sensory overload

Stress

Suggestions for Use

These altered responses are a change from the individual's usual response to stimuli and are not a result of mental or personality disorders. Use this label to describe patients whose perceptions have been influenced by physiologic factors such as pain, sleep deprivation, or immobility. Altered cognition and perception can be symptoms of both Sensory/Perceptual Alterations and Altered Thought Processes. When a person's ability to interpret stimuli is affected by physical or physiologic factors, use Sensory/Perceptual Alterations; when the ability to interpret stimuli is affected by mental disorders, use Altered Thought Processes. To further help differentiate between the two diagnoses, note that the following defining characteristics and related factors may be present in Altered Thought Processes, but not in Sensory/Perceptual Alterations:

Obsessive thinking
Loss of memory
Impaired judgment

In addition, the following defining characteristics are present in Sensory/Perceptual Alteration, but not in Altered Thought Processes:

Visual and auditory distortions
Discoordinated motor activity
Changes in sensory acuity

When Sensory/Perceptual Alteration exists as a result of Immobility, consider using Risk for Disuse Syndrome.

This label may be more useful as the etiology of other problems. For example:

Risk for Injury related to Visual Sensory/Perceptual Alteration

Self-Care Deficit related to Visual Sensory/Perceptual Alteration

Impaired Communication related to Auditory Sensory/Perceptual Alteration

Risk for Injury related to Kinesthetic or Tactile Sensory/Perceptual Alteration

Altered Nutrition related to Olfactory or Gustatory Sensory/Perceptual Alteration

Suggested Alternative Diagnoses

Disuse Syndrome, Risk for
Peripheral Neurovascular Dysfunction: Risk for
Thought Processes, Altered
Unilateral Neglect

Patient Outcomes and Evaluation Criteria

Include patient-specific target date, evaluation and documentation intervals, and any other patient-specific outcomes.

Patient will:

- Be oriented to person, place, time, and situation.
- Demonstrate improving perception of environment.
- Demonstrate orientation to environment.
- Demonstrate the ability to compensate for sensory deficits by maximizing the use of unimpaired senses.
- Interact appropriately with the environment.

Other outcomes specific to the particular deficit (ie, visual, auditory, kinesthetic, gustatory, tactile, olfactory).

NIC Priority Interventions

Auditory

Communication Enhancement, Hearing Deficit: Assistance in accepting and learning alternate methods for living with diminished hearing.

Gustatory, Olfactory

Nutrition Management: Assisting with or providing a balanced dietary intake of foods and fluids.

Kinesthetic

Body Mechanics Promotion: Facilitating the use of posture and movement in daily activities to prevent fatigue and musculoskeletal strain or injury.

Tactile

Peripheral Sensation Management: Prevention or minimization of injury or discomfort in the patient with altered sensation.

Surveillance, Safety: Purposeful and ongoing collection and analysis of information about the patient and the environment for use in promoting and maintaining patient safety.

Visual

Communication Enhancement, Visual Deficit: Assistance in accepting and learning alternate methods for living with diminished vision.

Environmental Management: Manipulation of the patient's surroundings for therapeutic benefit.

Nursing Actions

Ongoing Assessments

- Assess changes in patient's neurologic status q ____, and document.
- Assess patient's ability to follow directions.
- Assess patient's level of consciousness q ____.
- Identify factors that contribute to sensory/perceptual alterations, such as sleep deprivation, chemical dependence, medications, treatments, electrolyte imbalance, and so on.
- Monitor amount of sleep in 24-hour period.

Other

- Develop a plan for self-care, maximizing abilities and acknowledging limitations. Plan is ____.
- Develop a plan that maximizes patient's use of unimpaired senses. Plan is ____.
- Encourage patient/family to verbalize anxiety.
- Ensure access to and use of sensory assistive devices, such as hearing aid, glasses.
- Explain reason for, and describe location of, surrounding equipment, furniture, and alarms.
- Increase number of stimuli to achieve appropriate sensory input (for example, increase social interaction, schedule contacts, provide radio, television, clock with large numbers).
- Orient to person, place, time, and situation with each interaction.

- Reassure patient/family that sensory/perceptual deficit is temporary, whenever appropriate.
- Reduce number of stimuli to achieve appropriate sensory input (for example, dim lights, provide a private room, limit visitors, establish rest periods for patient).

Sexual Dysfunction (3.2.1.2.1) (None)

Definition: The state in which an individual experiences a change in sexual function that is viewed as unsatisfying, unrewarding, or inadequate (NANDA).

Defining Characteristics

Subjective

Change in sexual desire
Change of interest in self or others
Concern over adequacy in meeting sexual desire of partner
Painful coitus
Seeking confirmation of desirability
Verbalization of problem

Objective

Alteration in achieving perceived sex role
Alteration in orgasm/ejaculation
Change in relationship with significant other
Conflicts involving values
Impotence
Limitations imposed by disease and/or therapy
Phobic avoidance of sexual experience
Vaginal dryness

Related Factors

Altered body function or structure
Body image disturbance
Disease

Disturbance in self-esteem
Drugs
Hormonal changes
Illness/medical treatment
Impaired relationship
Ineffectual or absent role models
Lack of knowledge
Lack of privacy
Lack of significant other
Misinformation
Pain
Physical/emotional abuse
Pregnancy
Recent childbirth
Sexual trauma/exploitation
Surgery
Trauma
Unrealistic expectations of self and partner
Values conflict
Vulnerability

Suggestions for Use

If patient data does not fit the defining characteristics, consider the more general label Altered Sexuality Patterns. Note that Sexual Dysfunction may be a symptom of other diagnoses, such as Rape-Trauma Syndrome.

Suggested Alternative Diagnoses

Body Image Disturbance
Rape-Trauma Syndrome: Silent Reaction
Self-Esteem Disturbance
Sexuality Patterns, Altered

Patient Outcomes and Evaluation Criteria

Include patient-specific target date, evaluation and documentation intervals, and any other patient-specific outcomes.

Patient will:

- Demonstrate willingness to discuss changes in sexual function.
- Request needed information about changes in sexual function.

Patient/partner will:

- Actively participate in counseling.
- Participate in problem solving.
- Verbalize understanding of medically imposed restrictions.

NIC Priority Interventions

Sexual Counseling: Use of an interactive helping process focusing on the need to make adjustments in sexual practice or to enhance coping with a sexual event/disorder.

Nursing Actions

Target actions to problem etiologies. Individualize interventions to meet the unique needs of each patient.

Patient Teaching

- Inform patient/partner of need for medically imposed limitations on sexual activity and possible consequences (drug side-effects; normal aspects of aging; postsurgical adjustments, especially after surgery on sexual organs or ostomy; post–myocardial infarction).
- Encourage verbalization of sexual concerns by utilizing caregivers who have an established rapport with patient and are comfortable discussing patient's sexual concerns. Specify caregiver.
- Instruct patient in physical illness and treatment interventions that affect sexual function.
- Provide information necessary to enhance sexual function (anticipatory guidance, education materials, stress reduction exercises, sensation-enhancing exercises, prosthetics, implants, focused counseling).
- Provide written information that patient/partner can use as a resource.

Collaborative Activities

- Confer with social services to identify appropriate referral for counseling.
- Encourage continuation of counseling after discharge.
- Inform physician of patient's need for information so that teaching may be reinforced.

Other

- Alert patient/partner to possibility of disinterest in, decreased capacity for, or discomfort during sexual activity.
- Allow time and privacy to address patient's sexual concerns.
- Encourage communication between patient and sexual partner.

Sexuality Patterns, Altered (3.3) (None)

Definition: The state in which an individual expresses concern regarding his or her sexuality patterns (adapted from NANDA).

Defining Characteristics

Subjective

Reported difficulties, limitations, or changes in sexual behaviors or activities

Related Factors

Body image disturbance
Conflicts with sexual orientation or variant preferences
Disturbance in self-esteem
Fear of pregnancy or acquiring sexually transmitted disease
Illness or medical treatments
Impaired relationship with significant other
Ineffective or absent role models

Knowledge/skill deficit about alternative responses to health-related transitions
Lack of privacy
Lack of significant other

Suggestions for Use

When possible, use a more specific label, such as Sexual Dysfunction.

Suggested Alternative Diagnoses

Body Image Disturbance
Rape-Trauma Syndrome: Silent Reaction
Self-Esteem Disturbance
Sexual Dysfunction

Patient Outcomes and Evaluation Criteria

Include patient-specific target date, evaluation and documentation intervals, and any other patient-specific outcomes.

Patient will:

- Verbalize feelings about sexual identity.
- Request needed information about sexuality.
- Acknowledge importance of discussing sexual issues with partner.
- Discuss concerns about sexuality.
- Express satisfaction with sexuality.

Patient/partner actively participates in counseling.

NIC Priority Interventions

Sexual Counseling: Use of an interactive helping process focusing on the need to make adjustments in sexual practice or to enhance coping with a sexual event/disorder.

Nursing Actions

Patient Teaching

- Inform patient/partner of need for limitations in sexual activity and possible consequences.

- Provide written information that patient/partner can use as a resource.

Collaborative Activities

- Confer with social services to identify appropriate referral for counseling.
- Encourage continuation of counseling after discharge.

Other

- Allow time and privacy to address patient's sexual concerns.
- Encourage communication between patient and sexual partner.
- Encourage verbalization of sexual concerns by utilizing caregivers who have an established rapport with patient and are comfortable discussing patient's sexual concerns. Specify caregiver.
- Explore with patient possible causes of altered sexuality pattern (sexual partner, sexual orientation, physical setting, fear of pregnancy or disease).

Skin Integrity, Impaired (specify) (1.6.2.1.2.1) (Y27.1)

Definition: A state in which the individual's skin is adversely altered (NANDA).

Defining Characteristics as manifested by

Objective

Disruption of skin surface
Destruction of skin layers
Invasion of body structures

Related Factors

Signs + symptoms

External (Environmental)

Chemical substance
Humidity
Hyperthermia
Hypothermia
Mechanical factors (shearing forces, pressure, restraint)
Physical immobilization
Radiation

Internal (Somatic)

Alterations in skin turgor (decreased elasticity)
Altered metabolic state
Altered nutritional state (obesity, emaciation)
Altered pigmentation
Altered sensation
Developmental factors
Immunologic deficit
Impaired circulation
Medication
Skeletal prominence

Suggestions for Use

Impaired Skin Integrity is rather nonspecific, even though it is at the sixth level of the taxonomy. A disruption of the skin surface could be a surgical incision, abrasion, blisters, or decubitus ulcers. When this label is used, the type of disruption should be specified in the problem, not in the etiology. Note in the following example that dermal ulcer is a specific *type* of Impaired Skin Integrity, not a cause of Impaired Skin Integrity.

Correct: Impaired Skin Integrity: *dermal ulcer* related to complete immobility

Incorrect: Impaired Skin Integrity related to *dermal ulcer*

When an ulcer is deeper than the epidermis, use Impaired Tissue Integrity instead of Impaired Skin Integrity. Deeper ulcers may require a collaborative approach (ie, surgical treatment).

Do not use Impaired Skin Integrity as a label for a surgical incision, because there are no independent nursing actions to treat this type of "impairment" and the condition is usually self-limiting. The usual nursing care for a surgical incision is to prevent and detect infection; therefore, a diagnosis of Risk for Infection of Surgical Incision might be used instead of Impaired Skin Integrity. Note that "risk" problems should be diagnosed only when the patient is at higher risk than the general population. Thus, Risk for Infection should not be used routinely for every surgery patient.

Suggested Alternative Diagnoses

Infection: Risk for
Tissue Integrity, Impaired

Patient Outcomes and Evaluation Criteria

Include patient-specific target date, evaluation and documentation intervals, and any other patient-specific outcomes.

- Patient's skin will be healed and intact.
- Patient will be free of further skin breakdown.
- Patient/family will demonstrate optimal skin/wound care routine.

NIC Priority Interventions

Incision Site Care: Cleansing, monitoring, and promotion of healing in a wound that is closed with sutures, clips, or staples.

Skin Surveillance: Collection and analysis of patient data to maintain skin and mucous membrane integrity.

Wound Care: Prevention of wound complications and promotion of wound healing.

Nursing Actions

Target actions to problem etiologies. Individualize interventions to meet the unique needs of each patient.

Ongoing Assessments

- Assess condition of skin over bony prominences for breakdown q2 hours and prn, and document.
- Assess functioning of equipment such as pressure-relieving devices, including static air mattress, low-air loss therapy, air-fluidized therapy, and water bed.
- Include the following in assessment and documentation of wound/skin breakdown:

  Location, dimensions, and depth of wound.

  Presence and character of exudate, including tenacity, color, odor.

  Presence or absence of granulation/epithelialization.

  Presence or absence of necrotic tissue. Describe color, odor, amount.

  Presence or absence of symptoms of local wound infection. Consider: presence or absence of pain on palpation, edema, pruritus, induration, warmth, foul odor, eschar, exudate.

  Presence or absence of systemic infection.

  Presence or absence of undermining and/or sinus tract formation.

Patient Teaching

- Instruct patient/family in skin care routine, including signs and symptoms of tissue repair, nutritional enhancements to healing, and reportable signs and symptoms.

Collaborative Activities

- Consult dietitian for foods high in proteins, minerals, calories, and vitamins. Maintain adequate hydration.
- Consult physician regarding implementation of enteral feedings or parenteral nutrition to increase wound healing potential.
- Refer to enterostomal therapy nurse for assistance with assessment, staging, treatment, and documentation of wound care/skin breakdown.

Other

- Assess topical dressing/treatment measures, which may include moisture vapor permeable dressings, hydrocolloid dressings, hydrophilic dressings, absorbent dressings.
- Establish local wound care measures, which include removal of eschar and necrotic debris, a moist physiologic environment attainable by a variety of dressings and treatment regimens, and consistency in local wound care to achieve the most advantageous wound healing environment.
- Establish a wound/skin care routine, which may include:

  Frequent turning and repositioning of patient.
  Keeping surrounding tissue free from excess moisture, drainage.
  Protecting patient from fecal/urinary contamination.
  Protecting patient from other wound/drain-tube excretions into wound.

- Include in treatment measures pressure-relieving devices such as static air mattress, low-air loss therapy, air-fluidized therapy, water bed.

Skin Integrity, Impaired: Risk for (1.6.2.1.2.2) (Y27.2)

Definition: A state in which the individual's skin is at risk of being adversely altered (NANDA).

Defining Characteristics

Presence of risk factors, such as:

External (Environmental)

Chemical substance
Excretions/secretions
Humidity
Hyperthermia
Hypothermia
Mechanical factors (shearing forces, pressure, restraint)

Physical immobilization
Radiation

Internal (Somatic)
Alterations in skin turgor (decreased elasticity)
Altered metabolic state
Altered nutritional state (obesity, emaciation)
Altered pigmentation
Altered sensation
Developmental factors
Immunologic deficit
Impaired circulation
Medication
Psychogenic
Skeletal prominence

Risk Factors

See defining characteristics.

Suggestions for Use

Use this diagnosis for patients who have no symptoms, but who are at risk of developing disruption of skin surface or destruction of skin layers if preventive measures are not instituted. The presence of more than one risk factor increases the likelihood of skin damage. When Risk for Impaired Skin Integrity occurs as a result of Immobility, and when other body systems are also at risk for impairment, consider using Risk for Disuse Syndrome.

Suggested Alternative Diagnosis

Disuse Syndrome, Risk for

Patient Outcomes and Evaluation Criteria

Include patient-specific target date, evaluation and documentation intervals, and any other patient-specific outcomes.

Patient's skin will remain intact.

Patient/family will:

- Demonstrate effective skin care routine.
- Understand prevention of skin breakdown.
- Demonstrate understanding of risk factors that increase chance of acquiring skin breakdown.
- Maintain and improve tissue tolerance to pressure in order to prevent injury.

NIC Priority Interventions

Pressure Management: Minimizing pressure to body parts.

Pressure Ulcer Prevention: Prevention of decubitus ulcers for a patient at high risk for developing them.

Skin Surveillance: Collection and analysis of patient data to maintain skin and mucous membrane integrity.

Nursing Actions

Target actions to problem etiologies. Individualize interventions to meet the unique needs of each patient.

For All Patients at Risk

Ongoing Assessments

- Assess patient for risk factors (eg, bed/chair confinement, inability to move, loss of bowel/bladder control, poor nutrition, and lowered mental awareness) that may lead to skin breakdown on admission and whenever physical condition changes. Document assessment.
- Perform systematic skin inspection on all patients at least qd, paying particular attention to the bony prominences. Document assessment.

Collaborative Activities

- Refer to enterostomal therapy nurse for assistance with prevention, assessment, and treatment of skin breakdown/wounds.

For Mobility/Activity Deficit

Ongoing Assessments

- Assess for any changes in mobility.
- Assess for extent of limitations in ability to transfer or move about in bed.

Other

Bed-bound individuals:

- Avoid positioning directly on the trochanter.
- Elevate the head of the bed as little and for as short a time as possible.
- Place at-risk individuals on a pressure-reducing mattress. *Do not use donut-type devices.*
- Reposition at least q2 hours.
- Use devices that totally relieve pressure on the heels.
- Use lifting devices to move, rather than drag, individuals during transfers and position changes.
- Use lubricants to reduce friction injuries.
- Use pillows or foam wedges to keep bony prominences from direct contact.
- Use proper positioning, transferring, and turning techniques.

Chair-bound individuals:

- Consider postural alignment, distribution of weight, balance and stability, and pressure relief when positioning individuals in chairs or wheelchairs.
- Have patient shift weight q15 minutes if able.
- Use pressure-reducing devices for seating surfaces. *Do not use donut-type devices.*

Presence of Moisture or Incontinence

Ongoing Assessments

- Assess need for indwelling or condom catheter.
- Assess need for protective barrier ointments/creams.
- Check for urinary or fecal incontinence q ____.
- Inspect skin at least once/day.

Other

- Avoid massage over bony prominences.
- Check for diaphoresis.
- Cleanse skin at time of soiling.
- Individualize bathing schedule. Avoid hot water. Use mild cleansing agent.

- Minimize environmental factors such as low humidity and cold air. Use moisturizers for dry skin.
- Minimize skin exposure to moisture.
- When moisture cannot be controlled, use underpads or briefs that are absorbent and present a quick-drying surface to the skin.

Presence of Nutritional Deficit

Collaborative Activities

- Consult dietitian for foods high in protein, minerals, and vitamins.
- Request physician order for serum albumin level, packed cell volume, transferrin levels. When albumin level is low, wound healing is impaired and people have increased susceptibility to breakdown.

Other

- Compare actual weight to ideal body weight.
- Investigate factors that compromise an apparently well-nourished individual's dietary intake (especially protein or calories) and offer support with eating.
- Plan and implement a nutritional support and/or supplementation program.

Panel for the Prediction and Prevention of Pressure Ulcers in Adults. Pressure Ulcers in Adults: Prediction and Prevention. *Clinical Practice Guideline,* Number 3. AHCPR Pub. No. 92-0047. Rockville, MD: Agency for Health-Care Policy and Research, Public Health Service, U.S. Department of Health and Human Services, May, 1992.

Sleep Pattern Disturbance (6.2.1) (Y50.5)

Definition: A state in which the individual experiences a disruption in the amount and/or quality of sleep, which interferes with desired life-style (adapted from NANDA).

Defining Characteristics

Subjective

*Awakening earlier or later than desired
*Complaints of difficulty in falling asleep
*Complaints of not feeling well rested

Objective

*Interrupted sleep
Advanced pregnancy
Dark circles under eyes
Decreased attention span
Disorientation
Easy arousal
Flat affect
Frequent daytime napping
Frequent yawning
Irritability
Lethargy
Listlessness
Mild, fleeting nystagmus
Mood alterations
Newborn at home
Nighttime muscle cramps
Nocturia
Ptosis of eyelid
Regular use of medications that can change sleep patterns
Regular use of sedative/hypnotic medications
Restlessness
Slight hand tremor
Thick speech with mispronunciation and incorrect words

*Critical

Related Factors

Anxiety
Effect of depressants or stimulants
Emotional state
Environmental changes
Inactivity

Medications (specify)
Pain/discomfort
Psychologic stress (specify)
Sensory alterations
Sleep deprivation secondary to ____ (specify)
Unfamiliar surroundings

Suggestions for Use

Sleep Pattern Disturbance is used when disruption of sleep causes discomfort or interferes with the patient's desired lifestyle.

Sleep Pattern Disturbance is a general diagnosis. The etiological factors can sometimes make it specific enough to direct nursing intervention, as in: Sleep Pattern Disturbance related to frequent awakening of infant during the night. When possible, the specific type of Sleep Pattern Disturbance should be identified (on the problem-side of the diagnosis) in order to better direct nursing care. For example:

Sleep Pattern Disturbance (*Early Awakening*) related to depression

Sleep Pattern Disturbance (*Delayed Onset of Sleep*) related to overstimulation prior to bedtime

Suggested Alternative Diagnoses

Activity Intolerance
Fatigue

Patient Outcomes and Evaluation Criteria

Include patient-specific target date, evaluation and documentation intervals, and any other patient-specific outcomes.

Patient will:

- Identify measures that will increase rest/sleep.
- Decrease daytime napping to (specify).
- Report adequate rest.
- Sleep ____ hours per night.

NIC Priority Interventions

Sleep Enhancement: Facilitation of regular sleep/wake cycles.

Nursing Actions

Target actions to problem etiologies. Individualize interventions to meet the unique needs of each patient.

Ongoing Assessments

- Assess and document patient's sleeping pattern.
- Assess patient's need for sleeping aids.

Patient Teaching

- Inform patient of necessary interruptions during hospitalization.

Collaborative Activities

- Confer with physician regarding need to revise medication regimen when it interferes with sleep pattern.

Other

- Avoid loud noises and use of overhead lights during nighttime sleep, providing quiet, peaceful environment and minimizing interruptions.
- Develop plan to decrease daytime napping. Plan is ____ (specify).
- Discourage daytime napping by involving patient in activity.
- Evaluate need for sleep medication, taking into account necessary activities during nighttime.
- Find a compatible roommate for the patient, if possible.
- Help patient identify possible underlying causes of sleeplessness, such as fear, unresolved problems, and conflicts.
- Plan activities to allow time for sleep/rest, avoid unnecessary procedures during sleep period, and limit visiting during rest periods.
- Provide comfort measures, such as pain medication, back rub, warm milk, and soft music at hour of sleep and nap time. Specify.
- Reassure patient that irritability and mood alterations are common consequences of sleep deprivation.

Social Interaction, Impaired (3.1.1) (None)

Definition: The state in which an individual participates in an insufficient or excessive quantity or quality of social exchange (NANDA).

Defining Characteristics

Major

Subjective

Verbalization of discomfort in social situations

Verbalization of inability to achieve a satisfying sense of belonging, caring, interest, or shared history

Objective

Demonstrated unsuccessful interaction with others

Dysfunctional interaction with others

Minor

Subjective

Family report of change of style or pattern of interaction

Related Factors

Absence of significant others/peers
Altered thought processes
Chemical dependence
Communication barriers
Developmental disability
Environmental barriers
Knowledge/skill deficit
Limited physical mobility
Psychologic impairment (specify)
Self-concept disturbance
Sociocultural conflict
Therapeutic isolation

Suggestions for Use

Differentiate between Impaired Social Interaction and Social Isolation. A diagnosis of Impaired Social Interaction focuses more on the patient's social skills and abilities, whereas Social Isolation focuses on the patient's feelings of aloneness and may not be a result of her/his ineffective social skills. Compare the following defining characteristics and related factors:

	Impaired Social Interaction	*Social Isolation*
Shared Defining Characteristics	Verbalized or observed discomfort in social situations	Verbalized or observed discomfort in social situations
Differentiating	Ineffective social behaviors	Feelings of aloneness imposed by others
Defining Characteristics	Feelings of rejection	Dysfunctional interactions
Related Factors	Lack of knowledge of social skills Communication barriers	Mental impairment Physical disabilities

Suggested Alternative Diagnoses

Communication, Impaired: Verbal
Social Isolation
Thought Processes, Altered

Patient Outcomes and Evaluation Criteria

Include patient-specific target date, evaluation and documentation intervals, and any other patient-specific outcomes.

Patient will:

- Acknowledge the effect of own behavior on social interactions.

- Demonstrate behaviors that may increase/improve social interactions.
- Express a desire for social contact with others.
- Verbalize a sense of belonging.

NIC Priority Interventions

Socialization Enhancement: Facilitation of another person's ability to interact with others.

Nursing Actions

Target actions to problem etiologies. Individualize interventions to meet the unique needs of each patient.

Ongoing Assessments

- Assess established pattern of interaction between patient and others.

Patient Teaching

- Provide information on community resources that will assist the patient to continue with increasing social interaction after discharge.

Collaborative Activities

- Confer with other disciplines and patient to establish, implement, and evaluate a plan to increase/improve the patient's interactions with others. Include the following in plan:

  Assigning primary nurse.
  Assigning scheduled interactions.
  Establishing evaluation checkpoints.
  Establishing structured quiet time.
  Identifying specific behavior change.
  Identifying tasks that will increase/improve social interactions.
  Involving supportive peers in giving feedback to patient on social interactions.

Other

- Mediate between patient and others when patient exhibits negative behavior.

Social Isolation (3.1.2) (None)

Definition: A state in which an individual experiences aloneness, which is perceived as a negative or threatened state imposed by others (adapted from NANDA).

Defining Characteristics

Subjective

*Expressed feelings of aloneness imposed by others
*Expressed feelings of rejection
Expressed anger
Expressed feelings of difference from others
Projection of hostility in voice

Objective

Absence of significant purpose in life
*Absence of supportive significant other, family, friends, group
Display of behavior unacceptable to dominant cultural group
Evidence of physical/mental handicap
Expressed values acceptable to the subculture but unacceptable to the dominant cultural group
Inappropriate or immature activities/interests for developmental stage
Insecurity in public
No eye contact
Preoccupation with own thoughts
Repetitive meaningless actions
Sad, dull affect
Withdrawal

*Critical

Related Factors

Alteration in physical appearance
Chemical dependence
Delay in accomplishing developmental tasks
Disease/illness
Immature interests
Inadequate personal resources
Life-style changes (specify)
Medical condition (specify)
Psychologic impairment (specify)
Treatment-imposed isolation
Unacceptable social behavior or values

Suggestions for Use

Differentiate between Social Isolation and Impaired Social Interaction. A diagnosis of Impaired Social Interaction focuses more on the patient's social skills and abilities, whereas Social Isolation focuses on the patient's feelings of aloneness and may not be a result of her/his ineffective social skills. Compare the following defining characteristics and related factors:

	Impaired Social Interaction	*Social Isolation*
Shared Defining Characteristic	Verbalized or observed discomfort in social situations	Verbalized or observed discomfort in social situations
Differentiating	Ineffective social behaviors	Feelings of aloneness imposed by others
Defining Characteristics	Feelings of rejection	Dysfunctional interactions
Related Factors	Lack of knowledge of social skills Communication barriers	Mental impairment Physical disabilities

Suggested Alternative Diagnoses

Communication, Impaired
Post-Trauma Response
Rape-Trauma Syndrome
Relocation Stress Syndrome
Social Interaction, Impaired
Thought Processes, Altered

Patient Outcomes and Evaluation Criteria

Include patient-specific target date, evaluation and documentation intervals, and any other patient-specific outcomes.

Patient will:

- Demonstrate beginning acceptance of own personal characteristics that are perceived to contribute to social isolation.
- Demonstrate behaviors that may decrease social isolation.
- Identify behaviors that produce social isolation.
- Identify community resources that will assist in decreasing social isolation after discharge.

NIC Priority Interventions

Socialization Enhancement: Facilitation of another person's ability to interact with others.

Nursing Actions

Target actions to problem etiologies. Individualize interventions to meet the unique needs of each patient.

Patient Teaching

- Provide information on community resources that may decrease patient's social isolation after discharge (community agencies, social agencies, self-improvement classes, counseling). Specify.

Collaborative Activities

- Confer with other disciplines to establish, implement, and evaluate a plan to decrease the patient's social isolation with others. Specify plan.

Other

- Assist patient to distinguish reality from perceptions.
- Identify with patient those factors that may be contributing to feelings of social isolation.
- Reduce stigma of isolation by respecting patient's dignity.
- Reduce visitor anxiety by explaining reason for isolation precautions and/or equipment.
- Reinforce efforts by patient/family/friends to establish interactions.
- Schedule time with patient for social interaction. Scheduled times are ____.

Spiritual Distress (4.1.1) (Y80.0)

Definition: A state in which an individual experiences a disruption in his/her belief and value system that is a usual source of security and strength for the person.

Defining Characteristics

Subjective

Asking, "Why did this happen to me?"

Expressing concern about nonadherence to dietary laws

*Expressing concern with meaning of life/death and/or belief system

Feeling hopeless/abandoned

Questioning existence or fairness of deity

Questioning moral/ethical implications of therapeutic regimen

Requesting objects associated with worship

*Critical

Objective

Anger toward God

Seeking spiritual counseling

Disruption in sleep pattern

Inability to participate in usual spiritual rituals
Refusing to accept visits from priest, minister, rabbi, and so on

Related Factors

Challenge to belief and value system (eg, due to moral/ethical implications of therapy or intense suffering)
Discrepancy between spiritual beliefs and prescribed treatment
Separation from religious/cultural ties
Test of spiritual beliefs

Suggestions for Use

None

Suggested Alternative Diagnoses

Coping, Ineffective Individual
Decisional Conflict

Patient Outcomes and Evaluation Criteria

Include patient-specific target date, evaluation and documentation intervals, and any other patient-specific outcomes.

Patient will:

- Acknowledge that illness is a challenge to belief system.
- Acknowledge that treatment conflicts with belief system.
- Demonstrate coping techniques to deal with spiritual distress.
- Express acceptance of limited religious/cultural ties.
- Express reconciliation with usual belief system.

NIC Priority Interventions

Spiritual Support: Assisting the patient to feel balance and connection with a greater power.

Nursing Actions

Target actions to problem etiologies. Individualize interventions to meet the unique needs of each patient.

Collaborative Activities

- Communicate dietary needs (such as kosher food, vegetarian diet, pork-free diet) to dietitian.

- Contact denominational representative in community and/or hospital on request of patient/family.
- Request spiritual consultation to help patient/family determine posthospitalization needs and community resources for support.

Other

- Clarify patient's religious needs/conflicts:

  Encourage patient to express thoughts and feelings.
  Encourage patient to talk about conflicts and what may be causing them.
  Explain limitations that hospitalization imposes on religious observances.

- Identify supportive/helpful measures:

  Assist patient to identify objects, rites/rituals, and services that provide spiritual comfort.
  Communicate acceptance of and respect for patient's religious beliefs by involving the patient in the planning of care.

- Make immediate changes necessary to accommodate patient's needs:

  Encourage patient's family or friends to bring special food.
  Provide privacy and time for patient to observe religious practices.
  Provide religious reading material on patient's request.

Spontaneous Ventilation, Inability to Sustain (1.5.1.3.1) (None)

Definition: A state in which the response pattern of decreased energy reserves results in an individual's inability to maintain breathing adequate to support life (NANDA).

Defining Characteristics

Major

Subjective

Dyspnea

Objective

Increased metabolic rate

Minor

Objective

Apprehension
Decreased cooperation
Decreased PaO_2
Decreased PO_2
Decreased tidal volume
Increased heart rate
Increased PCO_2
Increased restlessness
Increased use of accessory muscles

Related Factors

Metabolic factors (alkalemia, hypokalemia, hypochloremia, hypophosphatemia, anemia)
Respiratory muscle fatigue

Suggestions for Use

Impaired Gas Exchange is one of the defining characteristics for this label. When blood gases are altered, but the patient is able to breathe without mechanical assistance, a diagnosis of Impaired Gas Exchange should be made instead of Inability to Sustain Spontaneous Ventilation.

Suggested Alternative Diagnoses

Dysfunctional Ventilatory Weaning Response (DVWR)
Gas Exchange, Impaired

Patient Outcomes and Evaluation Criteria

Include patient-specific target date, evaluation and documentation intervals, and any other patient-specific outcomes.

Patient will:

- Demonstrate necessary metabolic and physical energy levels to achieve weaning goals.
- Have adequate energy level to sustain spontaneous breathing.
- Maintain adequate energy level during weaning process from ventilator.
- Receive adequate nutrition prior to, during, and following weaning process.

NIC Priority Interventions

Artificial Airway Management: Maintenance of endotracheal and tracheostomy tubes and preventing complications associated with their use.

Mechanical Ventilation: Use of an artificial device to assist a patient to breathe.

Respiratory Monitoring: Collection and analysis of patient data to ensure airway patency and adequate gas exchange.

Ventilation Assistance: Promotion of an optimal spontaneous breathing pattern that maximizes oxygen and carbon dioxide exchange in the lungs.

Nursing Actions

Target actions to problem etiologies. Individualize interventions to meet the unique needs of each patient.

Ongoing Assessments

- Assess patient's readiness to wean by considering the following respiratory indicators:

  Arterial blood gases stable with $PaO_2 > 60$ on 40–60% oxygen.
  Cough effectively enough to handle secretions.
  Length of time on ventilator.
  Maximum inspiratory force > –30 cm H_2O (normal –80 to –1000) so independent respiration can be initiated.

Minute volume (VE) > 5–10 L/minute.
Unassisted tidal volume > 5 ml/kg ideal body weight.
Vital capacity > 13 ml/kg ideal body weight.

- Assess patient's readiness to wean by considering the following nonrespiratory indicators:

Absence of constipation, diarrhea, or ileus.
Absence of fever and/or infection.
Adequate nutritional status as evidenced by acceptable serum albumin, transferrin, midarm muscle circumference > 15th percentile.
Adequate rest and sleep.
Electrolytes within normal limits for patient.
Hemoglobin and hematocrit within normal limits for patient.
Improving body strength and endurance.
Normal blood pressure for patient.
Psychological/emotional readiness.
Stable heart rate and rhythm.
Tolerable pain or discomfort level.

- Monitor patient's response to current medications and correlate with weaning goals.

Patient Teaching

- Instruct patient/family in weaning process and goals, which should include:

How patient may feel as process evolves.
Participation of family.
Participation required by patient.
What patient can expect from nurse.
Why weaning is necessary.

Collaborative Activities

- Discuss weaning process and goals with physician and respiratory therapist, including patient's present and preexisting medication condition(s).
- Reevaluate appropriateness of weaning process with physician if weaning goals are not attainable.

Other

- Document in nursing care plan those strategies that promote success with weaning process to ensure consistency (eg, communication method with patient, family participation, coaching methods, and so on).
- Encourage increase in self-care and evaluate patient's response to higher levels of use of energy.
- Establish a trusting relationship that instills patient's confidence in nurse to assist patient with weaning process.
- Establish methods of communication between patient and others (eg, writing, blinking eyes, squeezing hand).

The Weaning Process

Initiate the weaning process by:

- Understanding the rationale for weaning orders (use of CPAP [Continuous Positive Airway Pressure], SIMV [Synchronized Intermittent Mandatory Ventilation], PSV [Pressure Support Ventilation], MMV [Mandatory Minute Ventilation], or T-piece).
- Explaining procedure to patient and family.

Assessments for the Weaning Process

- Check equipment to make sure it is attached to gas source.
- Check for presence of bilateral breath sounds.
- Check that settings are as ordered.
- Check tubing for kinks and excessive moisture.
- Measure and record baseline respiratory rate, heart rate, blood pressure, EKG, rhythm, lung sounds, vital capacity, tidal volume, inspiratory force.

Other Actions Specific to the Weaning Process

- Document weaning process and patient's tolerance in nurses' notes or flow sheet.
- Evaluate vital signs and patient for indicators of nontolerance or fatigue q5–15 minutes. Reconnect patient to ventilator at preweaning setting if indicators of nontolerance occur.
- Preoxygenate, hyperinflate, suction, reoxygenate patient prior to weaning.

- Provide a quiet environment during weaning time.
- Provide diversions such as television or radio.
- Sit patient in an upright position to decrease abdominal pressure on the diaphragm, allowing for better lung expansion.
- Start the weaning time when patient is rested and awake and alert.
- Stay with patient during weaning time to provide coaching and reassurance.

Suffocation: Risk for (1.6.1.1) (Y23.3)

Definition: Accentuated risk of accidental suffocation (inadequate air available for inhalation) (NANDA).

Defining Characteristics

Presence of risk factors such as the following:

Internal (Individual)

Cognitive or emotional difficulties
Disease or injury process
Lack of safety education
Lack of safety precautions
Reduced motor abilities
Reduced olfactory sensation

External (Environmental)

Children left unattended in bathtubs or pools
Children playing with plastic bags or inserting small objects into their mouths or noses
Discarded or unused refrigerators or freezers without removed doors
Eating large mouthfuls of food
Household gas leaks
Low-strung clothesline
Pacifier hung around infant's head
Pillow placed in an infant's crib

Propped bottle placed in an infant's crib
Smoking in bed
Use of fuel-burning heaters not vented to outside
Vehicle warming in closed garage

Risk Factors

See defining characteristics.

Suggestions for Use

Use the most specific label that matches the patient's defining characteristics. This label is more specific than Risk for Injury or Risk for Trauma, for example.

Suggested Alternative Diagnoses

Injury: Risk for
Trauma: Risk for

Patient Outcomes and Evaluation Criteria

Include patient-specific target date, evaluation and documentation intervals, and any other patient-specific outcomes.

Patient/family will:

- Identify appropriate safety factors that protect individual/child from suffocation.
- Identify risks that increase possibility of suffocation.
- Identify strategies for prevention of suffocation.

NIC Priority Interventions

Airway Management: Facilitation of patency of air passages.
Environmental Management, Safety: Monitoring and manipulation of the physical environment to promote safety.
Respiratory Monitoring: Collection and analysis of patient data to ensure airway patency and adequate gas exchange.

Nursing Actions

Target actions to problem etiologies. Individualize interventions to meet the unique needs of each patient.

Ongoing Assessments

- Assess high-risk areas that may lead to injury to patient/family.

Patient Teaching

- Provide educational materials related to strategies and countermeasures and to emergency measures.
- Provide information on environmental hazards and characteristics (eg, stairs, windows, cupboard locks, swimming pools, streets, gates).
- Provide information on the local poison control center and exposure to medications and household products.

Collaborative Activities

- Refer to educational classes in the community (CPR, first aid, swimming classes).

Other

- Explore strategies to prevent injury.

Swallowing, Impaired (6.5.1.1) (Y53.1)

Definition: The state in which an individual has decreased ability to voluntarily pass fluids and/or solids from the mouth to the stomach (NANDA).

Defining Characteristics

Major

Objective

Observed evidence of difficulty in swallowing (eg, stasis of food in oral cavity, coughing/choking)

Minor

Objective

Evidence of aspiration

Related Factors

Altered sensory reception, transmission, and/or integration
Fatigue
Irritated oropharyngeal cavity
Limited awareness
Mechanical obstruction (eg, edema, tracheostomy tube, tumor)
Neuromuscular impairment (eg, decreased or absent gag reflex, decreased strength or excursion of muscles involved in mastication, perceptual impairment, facial paralysis)
Psychologic impairment (specify)

Suggestions for Use

None

Suggested Alternative Diagnoses

Aspiration: Risk for
Infant Feeding Pattern, Ineffective

Patient Outcomes and Evaluation Criteria

Include patient-specific target date, evaluation and documentation intervals, and any other patient-specific outcomes.

Patient will

- Demonstrate increasing improvement in swallowing.
- Eat independently without choking.
- Identify emotional/psychologic factors that interfere with swallowing.
- Tolerate food ingestion without aspiration.

Patient/family identifies appropriate diet and feeding routine.

NIC Priority Interventions

Aspiration Precautions: Prevention or minimization of risk factors in the patient at risk for aspiration.

Swallowing Therapy: Facilitating swallowing and preventing complications of impaired swallowing.

Nursing Actions

Target actions to problem etiologies. Individualize interventions to meet the unique needs of each patient.

Ongoing Assessments

- Assess ability to swallow.
- Evaluate family's comfort level.
- Monitor food ingestion q ____.

Patient Teaching

- Instruct family about feeding techniques and food preparation.
- Review with patient/family signs and symptoms of aspiration and preventive measures.
- Teach patient adaptive measures that may help reduce embarrassment.

Collaborative Activities

- Administer pain medication prior to mealtimes to ensure maximal comfort.
- Consult dietitian for development of meal plan to provide food easily swallowed.
- Request occupational therapy consultation.
- Request social service consultation to help the family determine posthospitalization needs and identify sources of community support.

Other

- Acknowledge patient's feelings of embarrassment regarding impaired swallowing.
- Crush medications to facilitate swallowing.
- Have suction catheter available at bedside, and suction during meals as needed.
- Involve family during ingestion of food/medications to provide support and reassurance.
- Place food on unaffected side of mouth.
- Place patient in semi- or high-Fowler's position when eating.
- Provide opportunities to discuss fears related to swallowing.

- Provide positive reinforcement for attempts to swallow independently.
- Reassure patient during episodes of choking.
- When feeding patient, use syringe, if necessary, to facilitate swallowing.

Therapeutic Regimen Management, Ineffective Individual (5.2.1) (None)

Definition: A pattern of regulating and integrating into daily living a program for treatment of illness and the sequelae of illness that is unsatisfactory for meeting specific health goals (NANDA).

Defining Characteristics

Major

Subjective

Choices of daily living ineffective for meeting the goals of a treatment or prevention program

Minor

Subjective

Statements that patient/family did not take action to include treatment regimens in daily routines

Statements that patient/family did not take action to reduce risk factors for progression of illness and sequelae

Verbalized desire to manage the treatment of illness and prevention of sequelae

Verbalized difficulty with regulation/integration of one or more prescribed regimens for treatment of illness and its effects or prevention of complications

Objective

Acceleration (expected or unexpected) of illness symptoms

Related Factors

Complexity of health care system
Complexity of therapeutic regimen
Decisional conflict
Economic difficulties
Excessive demands made on individual or family
Family conflict
Family patterns of health care
Inadequate number and types of cues to action
Knowledge deficits
Mistrust of regimen and/or health care personnel
Perceived barriers
Perceived benefits
Perceived seriousness
Perceived susceptibility
Powerlessness
Social support deficits

Suggestions for Use

Use this diagnosis for patients or families who wish to follow a therapeutic regimen and are motivated to do so, but who are having difficulty doing so. For example, the diagnosis is appropriate for a patient who is trying to lose weight and has the necessary information, but finds it difficult to adhere to a low calorie diet because her business requires her to eat out frequently. It is not appropriate for an obese patient who is not interested in dieting or losing weight.

Suggested Alternative Diagnoses

Adjustment, Impaired
Health Maintenance, Altered
Noncompliance (specify)

Patient Outcomes and Evaluation Criteria

Include patient-specific target date, evaluation and documentation intervals, and any other patient-specific outcomes.

Patient will:

- Develop plan to achieve therapeutic regimen.
- Follow plan to achieve therapeutic regimen.
- Identify obstacles that interfere with adherence to the therapeutic regimen.

NIC Priority Interventions

Behavior Modification: Promotion of a behavior change.

Self-Modification Assistance: Reinforcement of self-directed change initiated by the patient to achieve personally important goals.

Nursing Actions

Target actions to problem etiologies. Individualize interventions to meet the unique needs of each patient.

Ongoing Assessments

- Assess patient's level of understanding of illness, complications, recommended treatments to determine knowledge deficit.
- Interview patient/family to determine "problem areas" in integrating treatment regimen into life-style.

Patient Teaching

- Identify essential treatments.
- Offer information on community resources specific to health goals of patient (eg, support groups). Assist patient to identify situational obstacles that interfere with adherence to therapeutic regimen.
- Provide information on illness, complications, recommended treatments.

Collaborative Activities

- Collaborate with other health care providers to determine how to modify therapeutic regimen without jeopardizing patient's health.

Other

- Assist patient to develop realistic plan of care to achieve adherence to therapeutic regimen. Plan to include:

  Identification of modifications/adaptations in ADLs.
  Identification of support systems to achieve therapeutic goals.
  Identification of what patient/family is willing to do (eg, dietary changes, exercise modification, sleep pattern changes, medication schedule, treatment schedules, sexual activity modifications, role change).

- Provide coaching and support to motivate patient's continued adherence to therapy.

Thermoregulation, Ineffective (1.2.2.4) (Y25.4)

Definition: The state in which an individual's temperature fluctuates between hypothermia and hyperthermia (NANDA).

Defining Characteristics

Objective

Fluctuations in body temperature above or below normal range.

(See also major and minor defining characteristics present in Hypothermia and Hyperthermia.)

Related Factors

Aging
Fluctuating environmental temperature
Immaturity
Trauma or illness

Suggestions for Use

This label is most appropriate for patients who are especially vulnerable to environmental conditions (ie, newborns and the elderly).

Suggested Alternative Diagnoses

For specific patient outcomes and evaluation criteria, refer to these diagnoses:

Body Temperature, Altered: Risk for
Hyperthermia
Hypothermia

NIC Priority Interventions

Temperature Regulation: Attaining and/or maintaining body temperature within a normal range.

Nursing Actions

Nursing interventions focus on teaching for prevention and on maintaining a normal body temperature by manipulating external factors such as clothing and room temperature.

Thought Processes, Altered (8.3) (Y41)

Definition: A state in which an individual experiences an impairment in cognitive operations, such as conscious thought, reality orientation, problem solving, and judgment.

Defining Characteristics

Subjective

Fearful thoughts
Hallucinations

Inaccurate interpretation of environment
Nonreality-based thinking

Objective

Distractibility
Egocentricity
Hyper- or hypovigilance
Irritability
Memory deficit/problems

Related Factors

Mental disorder (specify)
Organic mental disorder (specify)
Personality disorder (specify)
Substance abuse

Suggestions for Use

These impairments are a result of mental/personality or chronic organic disorders that may be exacerbated by situational crises. Altered Thought Processes may be the etiology of other problems, such as Self-Care Deficit, Impaired Home Maintenance Management, Risk for Injury, or Impaired Social Interaction.

Suggested Alternative Diagnoses

Communication, Impaired: Verbal
Sensory/Perceptual Alterations: Visual, Auditory, Kinesthetic, Gustatory, Tactile, Olfactory (specify)

Patient Outcomes and Evaluation Criteria

Include patient-specific target date, evaluation and documentation intervals, and any other patient-specific outcomes.

Patient will:

- Be oriented to person, place, and time.
- Be oriented to situation.
- Demonstrate improved ability to solve problems.
- Demonstrate improved mental status.

- Respond appropriately to questions/situation.
- Sustain no injury or harm.

Patient/family will identify community resources for care after discharge.

NIC Priority Interventions

Confusion Management: Provision of a modified environment for the patient who is experiencing a chronic confusional state.

Nursing Actions

Target actions to problem etiologies. Individualize interventions to meet the unique needs of each patient.

Ongoing Assessments

- Assess and document patient's orientation to person, place, time, and situation q ____.

Patient Teaching

- Demonstrate reorientation techniques to family.

Collaborative Activities

- Communicate patient's skill level in ADLs to other members of the health care team.
- Identify community resources.
- Involve social services for additional support.

Other

- Assist family to identify coping skills.
- Develop plan for ADLs:

  Involve patient in development.
  Post schedule of activities in room; plan is ____ (specify).

- Establish a plan for patient's discharge; involve patient/family in development.
- Orient patient as needed:

  Call patient by preferred name.
  Refer to calendar and clock often.

Remind patient where he/she is.
Selectively use TV and radio to assist with orientation.
Tell patient your name.
Use familiar items from home provided by family.

- Provide a safe environment:
  Apply soft restraints as necessary.
  Assist patient with ambulation and activities as needed.
  Keep frequently used items in same location.
  Leave bed in low position and use siderails.
  Provide adequate lighting (night light).
- Provide positive feedback and reinforcement of appropriate behavior.
- Provide simple explanations while providing care to patient.
- Provide support to patient/family during patient's periods of disorientation.

Tissue Integrity, Impaired (1.6.2.1) (Y27)

Definition: A state in which an individual experiences damage to mucous membranes or to corneal, integumentary, or subcutaneous tissue (NANDA).

Defining Characteristics

Objective

Damaged or destroyed tissue (cornea, mucous membrane, integumentary, or subcutaneous)

Related Factors

Altered circulation
Chemical irritants (body excretions and secretions, medications)
Fluid deficit/excess
Impaired physical mobility

Knowledge deficit
Mechanical factors (pressure, shear, friction)
Nutritional deficit/excess
Radiation (including therapeutic radiation)
Thermal factors (temperature extremes)

Suggestions for Use

If tissue integrity is at risk because of immobility and if other systems are also at risk, consider using Risk for Disuse Syndrome.

Suggested Alternative Diagnoses

Disuse Syndrome: Risk for
Oral Mucous Membrane, Altered
Skin Integrity, Impaired

NIC Priority Interventions

Wound Care: Prevention of wound complications and promotion of wound healing.

Nursing Actions

For patient outcomes, evaluation criteria, and specific nursing actions, refer to these diagnoses:

- Infection: Risk for
- Oral Mucous Membrane, Altered
- Pain [Acute]
- Sensory/Perceptual Alterations: Visual
- Skin Integrity, Impaired

Tissue Perfusion, Altered: Peripheral (1.4.1.1) (Y28.3)

Definition: The state in which an individual experiences a decrease in nutrition and oxygenation at the cellular level due to a deficit in capillary blood supply (NANDA).

Defining Characteristics

	Chances that characteristics will be present in given diagnosis	*Estimated sensitivities and specificities. Chances that characteristic will not be explained by any other diagnosis.*
Objective: Data		
Skin temperature, cold extremities	High	Low
Skin color, dependent blue or purple	Moderate	Low
*Pale on elevation, color does not return on lowering of leg	High	High
*Diminished arterial pulsations	High	High
Skin quality: shining	High	Low
Lack of lanugo, round scars covered with atrophied skin.	High	Moderate
Gangrene	Low	High
Slow-growing, dry brittle nails	High	Moderate
Claudication	Moderate	High
Blood pressure changes in extremities; bruits	Moderate	Moderate
Slow healing of lesions	High	Low

*Critical

Related Factors

Exchange problems
Hypo- or hypervolemia
Interruption of arterial flow
Interruption of venous flow

Suggestions for Use

Because some of the nursing interventions are different, it is important to determine whether Altered Peripheral Tissue Perfusion is of arterial or venous origin.

Suggested Alternative Diagnoses

Injury, Risk for
Skin Integrity, Impaired: Risk for
Tissue Integrity, Impaired

Patient Outcomes and Evaluation Criteria

Include patient-specific target date, evaluation and documentation intervals, and any other patient-specific outcomes.

Patient will:

- Be able to describe plan for care at home.
- Have decreased edema.
- Report acceptable level of comfort.
- Report decreased numbness and tingling in extremity.
- Report increased sensation in extremity.

NIC Priority Interventions

Circulatory Care: Promotion of arterial and venous circulation.

Neurologic Monitoring: Collection and analysis of patient data to prevent or minimize neurologic complications.

Peripheral Sensation Management: Prevention or minimization of injury or discomfort in the patient with altered sensation.

Nursing Actions

Ongoing Assessments

- Assess affected extremity for color, temperature, sensation, movement, and pain; assess rate, rhythm, and volume of peripheral pulses to evaluate circulation to limb.
- Assess and document presence of edema on scale from 1+ to 4+.
- Assess effects of medications on tissue perfusion.
- Assess need for antiembolus (TED) hose.

Patient Teaching

- Instruct patient/family regarding:

  Avoiding extremes of temperature to extremities.
  Importance of exercise program, correct diet, and adherence to medication regimen.
  Methods to provide meticulous hygiene to extremities.
  Reportable signs and symptoms that may require notification of physician.

- Instruct patient to inform nurse of presence or absence of numbness or tingling in extremity.

Collaborative Activities

- Consult dietitian for diet instruction.
- Correlate daily assessment with baseline, reporting any increase or decrease in circulation to extremities.
- Offer pain medications q ____, and document response to pain medication. Notify physician if pain is unrelieved.

Other

- Avoid chemical, mechanical, or thermal trauma to involved extremity.
- Discourage leg crossing or sitting for long periods to avoid compromising circulation to extremities.
- Discourage smoking and use of stimulants.
- Elevate extremity above heart q ___ to improve venous blood return.
- Encourage active/passive range-of-motion exercises to affected extremities q ___.

- Place extremity in dependent position q ___ to improve arterial blood flow.
- Use foot cradle to avoid pressure of covers on extremities.

Tissue Perfusion, Altered: (specify) (1.4.1.1)*

Definition: The state in which an individual experiences a decrease in nutrition and oxygenation at the cellular level due to a deficit in capillary blood supply (NANDA).

Defining Characteristics

Further work and development are required for these subcomponents of Altered Tissue Perfusion: cardiopulmonary, cerebral, renal, and gastrointestinal (NANDA, 1992).

Related Factors

Exchange problems
Hypo- or hypervolemia
Interruption of arterial flow
Interruption of venous flow

Suggestions for Use

The patient outcomes, evaluation criteria, and nursing interventions for these diagnoses have not been developed, because the outcomes and interventions are medical/surgical treatments. Nursing's role is to monitor and detect changes in the patient's condition, and nursing care may be better directed by the use of other nursing diagnoses. The following list offers the nurse alternative nursing diagnoses that specifically address responses to impaired perfusion of renal, cerebral, cardiopulmonary, and gastrointestinal tissue.

*Renal (Y28.4), Cerebral (Y28.1), Cardiopulmonary (Y28.0), Gastrointestinal (Y28.2)

Renal

Fluid Volume Excess

Cerebral

Communication, Impaired: Verbal

Injury: Risk for

Sensory/Perceptual Alterations: All

Cardiopulmonary

Activity Intolerance

Activity Intolerance: Risk for

Breathing Pattern, Ineffective

Cardiac Output, Decreased

Dysfunctional Ventilatory Weaning Response (DVWR)

Fatigue

Gas Exchange, Impaired

Spontaneous Ventilation, Inability to Sustain

Gastrointestinal

Infection: Risk for

Pain [Acute]

Trauma: Risk for (1.6.1.3) (Y23.4)

Definition: Accentuated risk of accidental tissue injury (eg, wound, burn, fracture) (NANDA).

Defining Characteristics

Presence of risk factors such as:

Internal (individual): Weakness, poor vision, balancing difficulties, reduced temperature or tactile sensation, reduced large or small muscle coordination, reduced hand-eye coordination, lack of safety education, lack of safety precautions, insufficient finances to purchase safety equipment or effect repairs, cognitive or emotional difficulties, history of previous trauma.

External (environmental): Slippery floors (eg, wet or highly waxed), snow or ice collected on stairs or walkways, unanchored rugs, bathtub without handgrip or antislip equipment, use of unsteady ladders or chairs, entering unlighted rooms, unsturdy or absent stair rails, unanchored electrical wires, litter or liquid spills on floors or stairways, high beds, children playing without a gate at the top of stairs, obstructed passageways, unsafe window protection in homes with young children, inappropriate call-for-aid mechanisms for bed-resting patients, pot handles facing toward front of stove, bathing in very hot water (eg, unsupervised bathing of young children), potential igniting gas leaks, delayed lighting of gas burner or oven, experimenting with chemicals or gasoline, unscreened fires or heaters, wearing plastic apron or flowing clothes around open flame, children playing with matches or candles or cigarettes, inadequately stored combustibles or corrosives (eg, matches, oily rags, lye), highly flammable children's toys or clothing, overloaded fuse boxes, contact with rapidly moving machinery, industrial belts or pulleys, sliding on coarse bed linen or struggling within bed restraints, faulty electrical plugs, frayed wires or defective appliances, contact with acids or alkalis, playing with fireworks or gunpowder, contact with intense cold, overexposure to sun or sun lamps, radiotherapy, use of cracked dishware or glasses, knives stored uncovered, guns or ammunition stored unlocked, large icicles hanging from roof, exposure to dangerous machinery, children playing with sharp-edged toys, vulnerable patient in a high-crime neighborhood, driving a mechanically unsafe vehicle, driving after partaking of alcoholic beverage or drugs, driving at excessive speeds, driving without necessary visual aids, children riding in the front seat in car, smoking in bed or near oxygen, overloaded electrical outlets, grease waste collected on stoves, use of thin or worn pot holders or mitts, unrestrained babies riding in car, nonuse or misuse of necessary headgear for motorized cyclists or young children carried on adult bicycles, unsafe road or road-crossing conditions, play or work near vehicle pathways (eg, driveways, railroad tracks), nonuse or misuse of seat re-straints.

Risk Factors

See defining characteristics.

Suggestions for Use

None

Suggested Alternative Diagnoses

Aspiration, Risk for
Home Maintenance Management, Impaired
Injury: Risk for
Poisoning: Risk for

Patient Outcomes and Evaluation Criteria

Include patient-specific target date, evaluation and documentation intervals, and any other patient-specific outcomes.

Patient/family will:

- Identify appropriate safety factors that protect individual/child from injury.
- Identify risks that increase susceptibility to injury.

Patient will:

- Avoid physical injury.
- Identify strategies that prevent injury.

NIC Priority Interventions

Environmental Management: Manipulation of the patient's surroundings for therapeutic benefit.

Skin Surveillance: Collection and analysis of patient data to maintain skin and mucous membrane integrity.

Nursing Actions

Target actions to problem etiologies. Individualize interventions to meet the unique needs of each patient.

Ongoing Assessments

- Assess risk areas that may lead to injury to patient/family.

Patient Teaching

- Instruct patient/family in safety measures specific to risk area.
- Provide educational materials related to strategies and countermeasures.
- Provide information on environmental hazards and characteristics (eg, stairs, windows, cupboard locks, swimming pools, streets, gates).
- Provide information on poison control center and exposure to medications and household products.

Collaborative Activities

- Refer to educational classes in the community (CPR, first aid, swimming classes).

Other

- Explore strategies to prevent injury.

Unilateral Neglect (7.2.1.1) (None)

Definition: The state in which an individual is perceptually unaware of and inattentive to one side of the body (NANDA).

Defining Characteristics

Major

Objective

Consistent inattention to stimuli on affected side

Minor

Objective

Inadequate self-care

Failure to look toward affected side

Leaving food on plate on affected side

Unsafe physical activity

Related Factors

Anesthesia of one side of the body (hemianesthesia)
Blindness in half of the field of vision in one or both eyes (hemianopia)
Neurologic illness or trauma
One-sided blindness
Paralysis of one side of body (hemiplegia)
Real or pretended ignorance of presence of paralysis (anosognosia)
Weakness of one side of body (hemiparesis)

Suggestions for Use

None

Suggested Alternative Diagnoses

Self-Care Deficit
Sensory/Perceptual Alterations

Patient Outcomes and Evaluation Criteria

Include patient-specific target date, evaluation and documentation intervals, and any other patient-specific outcomes.

Patient will:

- Acknowledge extent of deficit.
- Modify behavior/environment to accommodate deficit.
- Demonstrate ability to manage ADLs.
- Demonstrate improving perception of environment.
- Not experience falls or other accidents.

NIC Priority Interventions

Unilateral Neglect Management: (No definition given)

Nursing Actions

Target actions to problem etiologies. Individualize interventions to meet the unique needs of each patient.

Ongoing Assessments

- Assess the nature and extent of deficit.
- Monitor for changes in deficit.

Patient Teaching

- Explain and reinforce nature and extent of deficit to patient/family.
- Provide information about community resources.

Collaborative Activities

- Consult with OT/PT for assistance in developing a plan of care that challenges the affected side. Consider:

  Modification of the environment.
  Most effective methods of providing instruction.
  Performance of ADLs.
  Safety.
  Visual, olfactory, and tactile stimulation.

Other

- If patient does not respond to aggressive treatment, initiate plan of care directed at safety, simplification of tasks, and environmental adaptations. Consider:

  Approaching patient from the unaffected side.
  Placing food in patient's visual field.
  Placing frequently used items within view and reach.
  Positioning patient so that unaffected side faces activity.

- Include family in plan of care.

Urinary Elimination, Altered (1.3.2) (Y29)

Definition: The state in which the individual experiences a disturbance in urine elimination (NANDA).

Defining Characteristics

Subjective

Dysuria

Hesitancy

Urgency

Objective

Frequency

Incontinence

Nocturia

Retention

Related Factors

Multiple causality including anatomic obstruction, sensory or motor impairment, urinary tract infection

Suggestions for Use

Use a more specific label when possible. For specific patient outcomes, evaluation criteria and nursing interventions, refer to the suggested alternative diagnoses.

Suggested Alternative Diagnoses

Urinary Incontinence, Functional

Urinary Incontinence, Reflex

Urinary Incontinence, Stress

Urinary Incontinence, Total

Urinary Incontinence, Urge

Urinary Retention

Urinary Incontinence, Functional (1.3.2.1.4) (Y29.0)

Definition: The state in which an individual experiences an involuntary, unpredictable passage of urine (NANDA).

Defining Characteristics

Major

Urge to void or bladder contractions sufficiently strong to result in loss of urine before reaching an appropriate receptacle

Related Factors

Cognitive impairment
Disorientation
Environmental barriers
Impaired manual dexterity
Impaired physical mobility
Sensory deficit
Unfamiliar environment

Suggestions for Use

None

Suggested Alternative Diagnoses

Urinary Elimination, Altered
Urinary Incontinence, Reflex
Urinary Incontinence, Stress
Urinary Incontinence, Total
Urinary Incontinence, Urge
Urinary Retention

Patient Outcomes and Evaluation Criteria

Include patient-specific target date, evaluation and documentation intervals, and any other patient-specific outcomes.

Patient will:

- Recognize urge to void.
- Improve in ability to manipulate clothing in time for toileting.
- Experience less frequent episodes of incontinence.

NIC Priority Interventions

Environmental Management: Manipulation of the patient's surroundings for therapeutic benefit.

Urinary Elimination Management: Maintenance of an optimum urinary elimination pattern.

Urinary Incontinence Care: Institution of a program to promote continence and to maintain perineal skin integrity.

Nursing Actions

Target actions to problem etiologies. Individualize interventions to meet the unique needs of each patient.

Patient Teaching

- Consider:

  Improving environmental lighting to enhance vision.
  Installing raised toilet seat, hand rails.
  Providing bedside commode, bedpan, hand-held urinal.
  Removing loose rugs.
  Using assistive devices, eg, wheelchairs, canes, walkers, nonskid walking shoes.

- Discuss with patient/family ways to modify environment to reduce number of wetness episodes.
- Instruct patient/family in prompted voiding routine based on patient's pattern of toileting. Frequent reminders to toilet will decrease wetness episodes.
- Instruct patient/family in skin care–hygiene routine to prevent skin breakdown.
- Offer strategies for bladder management during activities away from home.

Collaborative Activities

- Consult with physical/occupational therapy for assistance with manual dexterity.

Other

- Obtain clothing that is easily removed.
- Substitute elastic waistbands and Velcro for zippers, buttons, snap devices, hooks whenever feasible.

Urinary Incontinence, Reflex (1.3.2.1.2) (Y29.1)

Definition: The state in which an individual experiences an involuntary loss of urine occurring at somewhat predictable intervals when a specific bladder volume is reached (NANDA).

Defining Characteristics

Major

Subjective

No awareness of bladder filling

No urge to void or feelings of bladder fullness

Uninhibited bladder contraction/spasm at regular intervals

Related Factors

Neurologic impairment (eg, spinal cord lesion that interferes with conduction of cerebral messages above the level of the reflex arc)

Suggestions for Use

None

Suggested Alternative Diagnoses

Urinary Elimination, Altered

Urinary Incontinence, Functional

Urinary Incontinence, Stress

Urinary Incontinence, Total

Urinary Incontinence, Urge

Urinary Retention

Patient Outcomes and Evaluation Criteria

Include patient-specific target date, evaluation and documentation intervals, and any other patient-specific outcomes.

Patient will:

- Demonstrate appropriate voiding schedule.
- Demonstrate intermittent self-catheterization procedure.
- Be free of urinary tract infection.
- Be free of skin breakdown.
- Describe plan for care at home.

NIC Priority Interventions

Urinary Elimination Management: Maintenance of an optimum urinary elimination pattern.

Urinary Retention Care: Assistance in relieving bladder distention.

Nursing Actions

Target actions to problem etiologies. Individualize interventions to meet the unique needs of each patient.

Ongoing Assessments

- Identify voiding pattern (either voiding after specified intake or voiding after a specified interval).

Patient Teaching

- Instruct patient regarding:

  Reportable signs/symptoms of urinary tract infection (fever, chills, flank pain, hematuria, change in consistency and odor of urine).

  Reportable signs/symptoms of autonomic dysreflexia such as severe hypertension, severe headache, diaphoresis above level of injury, tachycardia of sudden onset.

  Self-administration drug therapy program, which may include calcium channel blocking drugs, tricyclic antidepressant in combination with antispasmodic drug, and/or alpha sympathomimetic antagonist drugs.

Collaborative Activities

- Refer to enterostomal therapy nurse for instruction in clean intermittent self-catheterization, approximately q4–6 hours while awake.

Other

- Assist patient in maintaining adequate hygiene and skin care routine.
- Consider:

  Application of moisture barrier ointment or skin sealant.
  Keeping skin dry.
  Use of collection device.

- Establish a bladder management program:

  Attempt a programmed voiding schedule.
  Consider condom catheter collection device with leg bag.
  Maintain fluid intake of approximately 2000 cc/day.

Urinary Incontinence, Stress (1.3.2.1.1) (Y29.2)

Definition: The state in which an individual experiences a loss of urine of less than 50 ml occurring with increased abdominal pressure (NANDA).

Defining Characteristics

Major

Subjective

Reported dribbling with increased abdominal pressure

Objective

Observed dribbling with increased abdominal pressure

Minor

Subjective

Urinary urgency

Objective

Urinary frequency (more often than every 2 hours)

Related Factors

Degenerative changes in pelvic muscles and structural supports associated with increased age

High intra-abdominal pressure (eg, obesity, gravid uterus)
Incompetent bladder outlet
Overdistention between voidings
Weak pelvic muscles and structural supports

Suggestions for Use

None

Suggested Alternative Diagnoses

Urinary Elimination, Altered
Urinary Incontinence, Functional
Urinary Incontinence, Reflex
Urinary Incontinence, Total
Urinary Incontinence, Urge
Urinary Retention

Patient Outcomes and Evaluation Criteria

Include patient-specific target date, evaluation and documentation intervals, and any other patient-specific outcomes.

Patient will:

- Demonstrate ability to implement a timed voiding schedule.
- Describe plan for improved urinary elimination pattern.

NIC Priority Interventions

Urinary Elimination Management: Maintenance of an optimum urinary elimination pattern.

Urinary Incontinence Care: Institution of a program to promote continence and to maintain perineal skin integrity.

Nursing Actions

Target actions to problem etiologies. Individualize interventions to meet the unique needs of each patient.

Patient Teaching

- Teach patient not to limit fluid intake in effort to decrease incontinence.
- Instruct patient in:

Hygiene and skin care measures.

Techniques that strengthen the sphincter and structural supports of the bladder, eg, pelvic muscle exercises.

Self-administration of oral or topical estrogens to ameliorate symptoms.

Collaborative Activities

- Consult with physician regarding surgical or medical management of incontinent episodes.
- Consult with physician regarding use of biofeedback in conjunction with pelvic muscle exercises and electrostimulation therapy. Consider insertion of pessary if surgical correction not possible.

Other

- Assist patient to identify and choose appropriate urinary containment devices/pads.
- Encourage patient to void on a timed schedule.

Urinary Incontinence, Total (1.3.2.1.5) (Y29.4)

Definition: The state in which an individual experiences a continuous and unpredictable loss of urine (NANDA).

Defining Characteristics

Major

Objective

Constant flow of urine occurring at unpredictable times without distention or uninhibited bladder contractions/spasms

Nocturia

Unsuccessful refractory treatments

Minor

Objective

Lack of awareness of incontinence

Lack of perineal or bladder-filling awareness

Related Factors

Anatomic (fistula)

Independent contraction of detrusor reflex due to surgery, trauma, or disease affecting spinal cord nerves

Neurologic dysfunction causing triggering of micturition at unpredictable times

Neuropathy preventing transmission of reflex indicating bladder fullness

Suggestions for Use

None

Suggested Alternative Diagnoses

Urinary Elimination, Altered
Urinary Incontinence, Functional
Urinary Incontinence, Reflex
Urinary Incontinence, Stress
Urinary Incontinence, Urge
Urinary Retention

Patient Outcomes and Evaluation Criteria

Include patient-specific target date, evaluation and documentation intervals, and any other patient-specific outcomes.

Patient will:

- Maintain adequate skin integrity.
- Remain free of urinary tract infection.

Patient/family will describe a plan of care for indwelling foley catheter at home.

NIC Priority Interventions

Urinary Incontinence Care: Institution of a program to promote continence and to maintain perineal skin integrity.

Nursing Actions

Target actions to problem etiologies. Individualize interventions to meet the unique needs of each patient.

Ongoing Assessments

- Assess patient for presence of fistula (ie, urethral, vaginal, rectovaginal).
- Assess patient for skin breakdown and maintenance of adequate hygiene and skin care routine.

Patient Teaching

- Instruct patient/family in use of indwelling catheter management at home.
- Instruct patient/family in reportable signs/symptoms of urinary tract infection (fever, chills, flank pain, hematuria, change in consistency and odor of urine).

Collaborative Activities

- Consult physician about use of indwelling catheter.

Other

- Consider:

  Adequate drying of skin.
  Application of moisture barrier.
  Frequent perineal care.
  Ointment or skin sealant.

Urinary Incontinence, Urge (1.3.2.1.3) (Y29.3)

Definition: The state in which an individual experiences involuntary passage of urine occurring soon after a strong sense of urgency to void (NANDA).

Defining Characteristics

Major

Subjective

Bladder contraction/spasm

Objective

Frequency (voiding more often than every 2 hours)
Urinary urgency

Minor

Objective

Inability to reach toilet in time

Nocturia (urination more than 2 times per night)

Voiding in small amounts (less than 100 cc) or in large amounts (more than 500 cc)

Related Factors

Alcohol intake

Caffeine intake

Decreased bladder capacity (eg, history of PID, abdominal surgery, indwelling urinary catheter)

Increased fluid intake

Increased urine concentration

Irritation of bladder stretch receptors, causing spasm (eg, bladder infection)

Overdistention of bladder

Suggestions for Use

None

Suggested Alternative Diagnoses

Urinary Elimination, Altered

Urinary Incontinence, Functional

Urinary Incontinence, Reflex

Urinary Incontinence, Stress

Urinary Incontinence, Total

Urinary Retention

Patient Outcomes and Evaluation Criteria

Include patient-specific target date, evaluation and documentation intervals, and any other patient-specific outcomes.

Patient will :

- Describe bladder management program to restore satisfactory urinary elimination pattern.
- Have less frequent incontinent episodes.

NIC Priority Interventions

Urinary Incontinence Care: Institution of a program to promote continence and to maintain perineal skin integrity.

Nursing Actions

Patient Teaching

- Teach patient that limiting fluid intake is not a good way to decrease incontinence.
- Instruct patient regarding:

  Hygiene and skin care measures.

  Techniques that will increase bladder capacity, such as pelvic floor raising when feeling urge to void and bladder-training schedule that lengthens time between voids.

  Use of drug therapy.

Collaborative Activities

- Consult with physician regarding:

  Antispasmodic/anticholinergic medications.

  Medical management, eg, electrostimulation therapy, investigation of underlying irritative or inflammatory bladder disorders, and surgical therapy.

Other

- Consider:

  Assisting patient to void prior to sleep and encourage nighttime voids to reduce urgency.

  Assisting patient/family to identify and choose appropriate urinary collection/containment devices.

  Discouraging use of bladder irritants, such as caffeine, alcohol, citrus juices, carbonated drinks, cigarette smoke, and certain spicy foods.

  Encouraging a voiding schedule based on voiding diary.

  Encouraging fluid intake: ____ cc for day; ____ cc for PMs; ____ cc for nights.

  Increasing intervals between voiding gradually.

  Providing bedpan, bedside commode, urinal nearby to encourage frequent voiding episodes.

- Encouraging patient to complete a voiding diary for several days to create awareness of voiding patterns.
- Implementing a bladder management program.

Urinary Retention (1.3.2.2) (Y29.5)

Definition: The state in which an individual experiences incomplete emptying of the bladder (NANDA).

Defining Characteristics

Major

Objective

Bladder distention
Small, frequent voiding or absence of urine output

Minor

Subjective

Sensation of bladder fullness

Objective

Dribbling
Overflow incontinence
Residual urine

Related Factors

Blockage
High urethral pressure caused by weak detrusor
Inhibition of reflex arc
Strong sphincter

Suggestions for Use

None

Suggested Alternative Diagnoses

Urinary Elimination, Altered
Urinary Incontinence, Functional

Urinary Incontinence, Reflex
Urinary Incontinence, Stress
Urinary Incontinence, Total
Urinary Incontinence, Urge

Patient Outcomes and Evaluation Criteria

Include patient-specific target date, evaluation and documentation intervals, and any other patient-specific outcomes.

Patient will:

- Demonstrate bladder evacuation by clean intermittent self-catheterization procedure.
- Demonstrate reduced retention by voiding at least ____ cc each time he/she urinates.
- Describe plan of care at home.
- Remain free of urinary tract infection.
- Report a decrease in bladder spasms.

NIC Priority Interventions

Urinary Catheterization: Insertion of a catheter into the bladder for temporary or permanent drainage of urine.

Urinary Retention Care: Assistance in relieving bladder distention.

Nursing Actions

Ongoing Assessments

- Identify and document patient's bladder evacuation pattern.
- Palpate bladder to determine presence of bladder distention q ____.

Patient Teaching

- Instruct patient in reportable signs/symptoms of urinary tract infection (fever, chills, flank pain, hematuria, change in consistency and odor of urine).

Collaborative Activities

- Refer to enterostomal therapy nurse for instruction in clean intermittent self-catheterization q4–6 hours while awake.

Other

- Establish a bladder-evacuation training program.
- Consider:

Implementing techniques that may encourage voiding, such as running water in sink, running warm water over hands, having patient inhale oil of peppermint, providing warm blanket to pelvis, Crede's maneuver, timed voiding schedule.

Inserting indwelling catheter for use at home. Instruct in use of leg bag for urinary collection while ambulating.

Spacing fluids throughout the day to ensure adequate intake without bladder overdistention. Encourage oral intake of fluids: ____ cc for day; ____ cc for PMs; ____ cc for nights.

Violence, Risk for: Self-Directed or Directed at Others (9.2.2) (Y35)

Definition: A state in which an individual experiences behaviors that can be physically harmful either to self or others (NANDA).

Defining Characteristics

Presence of risk factors such as:

Body Language

Clenched fists
Rigid posture
Tautness indicating effort to control
Tense facial expression

Hostile Threatening Verbalizations

Continued complaints, requests, demands

Increased Motor Activity

Agitation
Excitement
Irritation
Pacing

Overt and Aggressive Acts

Active aggressive suicidal acts
Delusions, hallucinations
Goal-directed destruction of objects in environment
Paranoid ideation
Possession of destructive means (gun, knife, weapon)
Rage
Self-destructive behavior
Substance abuse/withdrawal
Suspicion of others

Other Possible Characteristics

Subjective

Anger
Continued complaints, requests, and demands
Fear of self or others
Increasing anxiety levels
Repetition of verbalizations

Objective

Depression (specifically active, aggressive, suicidal acts)
Inability to verbalize feelings
Provocative behavior (argumentative, dissatisfied, overreactive, hypersensitive)
Vulnerable self-esteem

Risk Factors

See defining characteristics. Also:

Arrest/conviction pattern
Catatonic excitement

History of abuse by spouse
History of physical/mental abuse by others
History of suicide attempts
History of violence
Manic excitement
Organic brain syndrome
Pain states
Panic states
Rage reaction
Substance abuse (specify)
Suicidal ideation
Temporal lobe epilepsy
Toxic reactions to medications

Suggestions for Use

None

Suggested Alternative Diagnosis

Self-Mutilation: Risk for

Patient Outcomes and Evaluation Criteria

Include patient-specific target date, evaluation and documentation intervals, and any other patient-specific outcomes.

Patient will:

- Demonstrate increasing ability to control impulses to harm self or others.
- Identify alternative ways to cope with problems.
- Identify effective way to express anger in a nondestructive manner.
- Identify support systems in the community.
- Not harm self/others.
- Report a decrease in suicidal thoughts.
- Report increasing ability to control anger.
- Verbalize anger.

NIC Priority Interventions

Anger Control Assistance: Facilitation of the expression of anger in an adaptive nonviolent manner.

Environmental Management: Violence Prevention: Monitoring and manipulation of the physical environment to decrease the potential for violent behavior directed toward self, others, or environment.

Nursing Actions

Target actions to problem etiologies. Individualize interventions to meet the unique needs of each patient.

Ongoing Assessments

- Assess and document patient's potential for suicide q ____.
- Identify behaviors that signal impending violence against self and others. Specify.

Collaborative Activities

- Clarify use of 72-hour hold for evaluation and treatment in psychiatric unit in the event of abuse against self or others.
- Confer with physician on use of appropriate restraining measures when necessary to prevent injury to patient and others.
- Confer with physician regarding a psychiatric consultation.
- Follow hospital/agency policy regarding legal responsibility for reporting abuse to authorities.
- Initiate a multidisciplinary patient care conference to develop a plan of care.

Other

- Discuss with patient/family the role of anger in self-harm.
- Encourage patient to verbalize anger.
- Encourage the use of positive coping mechanisms, such as relaxation techniques, exercise; specify.
- Explore with patient alternative ways of expressing anger.
- Help patient to control anger by anticipating events that may precipitate aggressive episodes.

- Identify situations that provoke violence. Specify.
- Institute suicide precautions as needed (such as 24-hour attendant, room close to nurses' station, removal of potentially harmful objects from room).
- Provide positive feedback when patient adheres to behavior limits.
- Set limits on patient's behavior; specify limits.
- Reassure patient that you will protect him/her against own suicidal impulses until able to regain control by:

  Constantly observing patient.
  Frequently checking patient.
  Removing harmful objects.
  Taking patient's suicidal ideation seriously.

Clinical Conditions Guide to Nursing Diagnoses

Medical Conditions

Surgical Conditions

Psychiatric Conditions

Antepartum and Postpartum Conditions

Newborn Conditions

Pediatric Conditions

This section contains lists of nursing diagnoses associated with selected conditions (eg, medical, surgical). However, because nursing diagnoses represent *human responses,* and because human beings respond in infinite ways, *any* nursing diagnosis could occur with *any* disease process or condition. Therefore, when using these lists, keep in mind that for each condition (for example, congestive heart failure): (1) a patient may have nursing diagnoses that are not included in the list, and (2) the list may include many nursing diagnoses that the patient does not have.

For the nursing diagnoses in this section, the etiologies ("related to") are stated in broad, general terms. Etiologies, like problems, are highly individual. Therefore, when writing a nursing diagnosis for a particular patient, the nurse will need to use the list as a starting point and expand the etiology to describe fully that patient's pathophysiology, disease process, situation, or other related factors.

Medical Conditions

Abdominal pain
Acquired immune deficiency syndrome (AIDS)
Angina/coronary insufficiency
Arthritis
Autoimmune disorders
Blood disorders
Burns
Cancer
Cerebrovascular accident (stroke)
Chest injury
Congestive heart failure
Endocrine disorders
Gastrointestinal bleeding
Immobilized patient
Liver disease
Myocardial infarction (chest pain, arrhythmias)
Neurologic disorders
Obesity
Pancreatitis
Pericarditis/endocarditis
Pneumonia
Pulmonary edema
Pulmonary embolism
Renal failure, Acute
Renal failure, Chronic
Respiratory disorders, Chronic
Terminal patient
Urologic disorders
Vascular disease

Abdominal Pain

Breathing Pattern, Ineffective Related factors: Acute pain, Chronic pain

Constipation Related factors: Decreased activity, Decreased fluid intake, Dietary changes, Decreased motility, Medications (specify)

Diarrhea Related factors: Dietary changes, Increased intestinal motility, Impaction, Medications (specify), Excessive alcohol intake

Fluid Volume Deficit Related factors: Abnormal fluid loss (specify), Inadequate fluid intake, Abnormal blood loss (specify), Excessive continuous consumption of alcohol

Nutrition, Altered: Less Than Body Requirements Related factors: Loss of appetite, Nausea and vomiting, Food intolerance

Pain [Acute] Related factors: Injury, Noxious stimulus

Pain, Chronic Related factors: Specific to patient

Sleep Pattern Disturbance Related factors: Pain/discomfort, Anxiety

Urinary Retention Related factor: Urethral obstruction

Acquired Immune Deficiency Syndrome (AIDS)

Adjustment, Impaired Related factors: Inadequate support system, Necessity for major life-style/behavior changes

Airway Clearance, Ineffective Related factors: Decreased energy/fatigue, Tracheobronchial secretions

Body Image Disturbance Related factor: Chronic illness

Caregiver Role Strain (Actual/Risk for) Related factors/risk factors: Illness severity of the care receiver, Unpredictable illness course or instability in the care receiver's health, Duration of caregiving required, Inadequate physical environment for providing care, Lack of respite and recreation for caregiver, Complexity/number of caregiving tasks

Coping, Ineffective Family: Compromised Related factors: Inadequate or incorrect information or understanding by family member/close friend, Chronic illness

Coping, Ineffective Family: Disabling Related factor: Chronically unresolved feelings

Coping, Ineffective Individual Related factor: Personal vulnerability in a situational crisis (terminal illness)

Decisional Conflict (specify) Related factors: Lack of experience with decision making, Lack of support system, Interference with support system

Diversional Activity Deficit Related factors: Frequent/lengthy medical treatments, Long-term hospitalization, Prolonged bed rest

Family Processes, Altered Related factors: Illness/disability of family member, Lack of adequate support system

Fatigue Related factors: Disease process, Overwhelming psychologic or emotional demands

Fear Related factors: Powerlessness, Real threat to own well-being

Fluid Volume Deficit Related factor: Inadequate fluid intake

Fluid Volume Deficit: Risk for Risk factor: Excessive loss through normal route

Gas Exchange, Impaired Related factor: Decreased functional lung tissue secondary to *Pneumocystis* pneumonia

Grieving, Anticipatory Related factor: Impending death of self

Grieving, Dysfunctional Related factors: Terminal illness, Loss of body function

Home Maintenance Management, Impaired Related factors: Inadequate support systems, Lack of knowledge, Lack of familiarity with community resources

Hopelessness Related factor: Failing or deteriorating physical condition

Infection: Risk for Risk factor: Inadequate acquired immunity

[Infection transmission: Risk for] Risk factor: Contagious nature of body fluids

Knowledge Deficit Related factors: Information misinterpretation, Limited exposure to information (specify)

Mobility, Impaired Physical Related factor: Decreased strength and endurance

Nutrition, Altered: Less Than Body Requirements Related factors: Difficulty in swallowing, Loss of appetite, Oral lesions

Oral Mucous Membrane, Altered: Risk for Risk factor: Compromised immune system

Pain [Acute] Related factors: Progression of disease process, Terminal stage of illness

Powerlessness Related factors: Terminal illness, Treatment regimen

Role Performance, Altered Related factors: Chronic illness, Situational crisis, Treatment side-effects

Self-Care Deficit: Bathing/Hygiene, Dressing/Grooming, Feeding, Toileting (specify) Related factors: Decreased strength and endurance, Intolerance to activity

Self-Esteem Disturbance Related factors: Chronic illness, Situational crisis

Skin Integrity, Impaired Related factors: Altered nutritional state, Skeletal prominence

Skin Integrity, Impaired: Risk for Risk factors: Alterations in nutritional state, Skeletal prominence, Diarrhea

Social Interaction, Impaired Related factors: Self-concept disturbance, Absence of significant other/peers

Social Isolation Related factors: Fear by others of contracting disease, Medical condition

Spiritual Distress Related factors: Challenged belief and value system, Test of spiritual beliefs

Thought Processes, Altered Related factor: Organic mental disorder

Violence, Risk for: Self-Directed Risk factor: Suicidal ideation

Angina/Coronary Insufficiency

Activity Intolerance Related factors: Anxiety, Arrhythmias, Acute pain, Weakness/fatigue

Adjustment, Impaired Related factors: Assault to self-esteem, Necessity for major life-style/behavior change

Anxiety Related factors: Threat to self-concept, Threat of death, Threat to or change in role functioning

Body Image Disturbance Related factors: Chronic illness, Treatment side-effects

Breathing Pattern, Ineffective Related factors: Acute pain, Anxiety

Cardiac Output, Decreased Related factors: Dysfunctional electrical conduction, Drug toxicity, Ventricular ischemia, Ventricular damage, Ventricular restriction

Coping, Ineffective Individual Related factor: Personal vulnerability to situational crisis (new diagnosis of illness, declining health)

Denial, Ineffective Related factor: Fear of consequences

Family Processes, Altered Related factors: Change in family roles, Hospitalization/changes in environment, Illness/disability of family member

Fear Related factors: Environmental stressors/hospitalization, Powerlessness, Real or imagined threat to well-being

Hopelessness Related factor: Failing or deteriorating physical condition

Knowledge Deficit Related factors: Information misinterpretation, Limited exposure to information, Unreadiness to learn

Noncompliance Related factors: Denial of illness, Negative consequences of treatment regimen, Negative perception of treatment regimen, Perceived benefits of continued illness, Dysfunctional patient/provider relationship

Pain [Acute] Related factor: Injury

Personal Identity Disturbance Related factor: Chronic illness

Powerlessness Related factors: Illness-related regimen, Chronic illness

Role Performance, Altered Related factors: Chronic illness, Treatment side-effects

Self-Care Deficit: Bathing/Hygiene, Dressing/Grooming, Feeding, Toileting (specify) Related factors: Depression, Severe anxiety, Pain/discomfort, Intolerance to activity

Self-Esteem Disturbance Related factor: Chronic illness

Sexual Dysfunction Related factors: Pain, Illness/medical treatment

Sleep Pattern Disturbance Related factors: Pain/discomfort, Anxiety, Inactivity

Arthritis

Includes but is not limited to rheumatoid arthritis, osteoarthritis, juvenile rheumatoid arthritis, gouty arthritis.

Activity Intolerance Related factors: Chronic pain, Weakness, Fatigue

Body Image Disturbance Related factors: Chronic illness, Progression of joint abnormalities

Coping, Ineffective Individual Related factor: Personal vulnerability in a situational crisis (new diagnosis of illness, declining health)

Family Processes, Altered Related factors: Change in family roles, Disability of family member, Lack of support system

Fatigue Related factors: Pain, Overwhelming psychologic or emotional demand

Home Maintenance Management, Impaired Related factor: Physical impairment

Knowledge Deficit (specify) Related factor: Limited exposure to information (side-effects of medication, prevention of further injury)

Mobility, Impaired Physical Related factors: Musculoskeletal impairment, Pain/discomfort

Pain [Acute] Related factor: Progression of joint abnormalities

Role Performance, Altered Related factor: Chronic illness

Self-Care Deficit: Bathing/Hygiene, Dressing/Grooming, Feeding, Toileting (specify) Related factors: Musculoskeletal impairment, Pain/discomfort

Autoimmune Disorders

Includes but is not limited to systemic lupus erythematosus (SLE), scleroderma, vasculitis, rheumatic fever, glomerulonephritis, multiple sclerosis.

Activity Intolerance Related factors: Anxiety, Acute pain, Chronic pain, Weakness/fatigue

Adjustment, Impaired Related factors: Necessity for major lifestyle/behavior change

Aspiration: Risk for Risk factors: Impaired swallowing, Presence of tracheostomy or endotracheal tube

Body Image Disturbance Related factors: Chronic illness, Chronic pain

Cardiac Output, Decreased Related factors: Ventricular restriction, Increased ventricular workload

Caregiver Role Strain (Actual/Risk for) Related factors/risk factors: Illness severity of care receiver, Duration of caregiving required, Lack of respite and recreation for caregiver, Complexity/number of caregiving tasks

Constipation Related factors: Decreased activity, Medications (specify)

Coping, Ineffective Family: Compromised Related factors: Chronic illness or disability

Coping, Ineffective Individual Related factor: Personal vulnerability in a situational crisis (declining health)

Denial, Ineffective Related factor: Fear of consequences

Diversional Activity Deficit Related factors: Long-term hospitalization, Frequent/lengthy treatments, Forced inactivity

Family Processes, Altered Related factors: Complex therapies, Change in family roles, Hospitalization/change in environment, Illness/disability of family member

Fear Related factors: Environmental stressors/hospitalization, Powerlessness, Real or imagined threat to own well-being

Fluid Volume Excess Related factor: Decreased urine output secondary to sodium retention

Gas Exchange, Impaired Related factor: Decreased functional lung tissue

Grieving, Anticipatory Related factors: Potential loss of body function, Potential loss of social role

Grieving, Dysfunctional Related factors: Actual loss, Terminal illness, Chronic illness

Home Maintenance Management, Impaired Related factor: Physical impairment

Hopelessness Related factors: Failing or deteriorating physical condition, Long-term stress

Infection: Risk for Risk factors: Immunosuppression, Chronic disease, Pharmaceutical agents

Knowledge Deficit Related factors: Information misinterpretation (disease process and treatment), Limited exposure to information (disease process and treatment)

Mobility, Impaired Physical Related factors: Pain/discomfort, Medically prescribed limitations, Musculoskeletal impairment, Neuromuscular impairment

Noncompliance Related factors: Denial of illness, Negative perception of treatment regimen, Perceived benefits of continued illness, Negative consequences of treatment regimen

Nutrition, Altered: Less Than Body Requirements Related factors: Difficulty in chewing, Difficulty in swallowing, Loss of appetite, Nausea and vomiting

Pain [Acute] Related factor: Paresthesia

Pain, Chronic Related factor: Altered body function

Personal Identity Disturbance Related factor: Chronic illness

Powerlessness Related factors: Chronic illness, Terminal illness, Treatment regimen

Protection, Altered Related factor: Corticosteroid therapy

Role Performance, Altered Related factors: Chronic illness, Chronic pain

Self-Care Deficit: Bathing/Hygiene, Dressing/Grooming, Feeding, Toileting (specify) Related factors: Decreased strength and endurance, Pain/discomfort, Intolerance to activity, Neuromuscular impairment, Musculoskeletal impairment

Self-Esteem Disturbance Related factors: Chronic illness, Chronic pain, Altered role performance

Sensory/Perceptual Alterations: Visual, Kinesthetic, Tactile Related factor: Disease process

Skin Integrity, Impaired (Actual/Risk for) Related factors/risk factors: Medication, Altered circulation, Physical immobilization, Immunologic deficit

Sleep Pattern Disturbance Related factors: Pain/discomfort, Anxiety, Inactivity

Social Interaction, Impaired Related factors: Self-concept disturbance, Limited physical mobility

Urinary Incontinence, Functional Related factor: Impaired mobility

Blood Disorders

Includes but is not limited to anemias and coagulation disorders.

Activity Intolerance Related factors: Imbalance between oxygen supply and demand, Acute pain, Weakness/fatigue, Decreased strength and endurance

Family Processes, Altered Related factors: Hospitalization/change in environment, Illness/disability of family member

Fear Related factors: Environmental stressors/hospitalization

Injury: Risk for Risk factors: Abnormal blood profile, Sickle cell, Decreased hemoglobin

Nutrition, Altered: Less Than Body Requirements Related factor: Loss of appetite

Pain [Acute] Related factor: Altered body function

Protection, Altered Related factors: Abnormal clotting, Bleeding

Self-Esteem, Low: Chronic Related factor: Chronic illness

Burns

Activity Intolerance Related factors: Anxiety, Acute pain

Aspiration: Risk for Risk factors: Presence of tracheostomy or endotracheal tube, Tube feeding, Impaired swallowing, Hindered elevation of upper body

Body Image Disturbance Related factor: Physical impairment

Body Temperature, Altered: Risk for Risk factor: Dehydration secondary to impairment in skin integrity

Breathing Pattern, Ineffective Related factor: Pain

Caregiver Role Strain (Actual/Risk for) Related factors/risk factors: Illness severity of care receiver, Duration of caregiving required, Lack of respite and recreation for caregiver, Complexity/number of caregiving tasks

Constipation Related factors: Decreased activity, Medications (specify)

Coping, Ineffective Individual Related factor: Personal vulnerability to situational crisis (presence of burns)

Disuse Syndrome: Risk for Risk factor: Severe pain

Diversional Activity Deficit Related factors: Long-term hospitalization, Frequent/lengthy treatments

Family Processes, Altered Related factors: Complex therapies, Hospitalization/change in environment, Illness/disability of family member

Fatigue Related factors: Pain, Disease process, Overwhelming psychologic or emotional demands

Fear Related factors: Environmental stressors/hospitalization, Real or imagined threat to own well-being

Fluid Volume Deficit Related factor: Abnormal fluid loss (specify)

Infection: Risk for Risk factors: Tissue destruction and increased environmental exposure

Mobility, Impaired Physical Related factors: Pain/discomfort, Musculoskeletal impairment

Nutrition, Altered: Less Than Body Requirements Related factors: Difficulty in swallowing, High metabolic rate

Pain [Acute] Related factor: Injury

Powerlessness Related factors: Treatment regimen, Health care environment

Self-Care Deficit: Bathing/Hygiene, Dressing/Grooming, Feeding, Toileting (specify) Related factors: Pain/discomfort, Intolerance to activity, Decreased strength and endurance, Musculoskeletal impairment

Sensory/Perceptual Alterations: Visual, Auditory, Kinesthetic, Gustatory, Tactile, Olfactory (specify) Related factor: Sensory deficit

Skin Integrity, Impaired Related factors: Burns, Physical immobilization

Sleep Pattern Disturbance Related factors: Pain/discomfort, Anxiety

Cancer

Activity Intolerance Related factors: Chronic pain, Weakness, Fatigue

Activity Intolerance: Risk for Risk factors: Pain, Fatigue, Frail or debilitated state

Adjustment, Impaired Related factors: Necessity for major life-style changes, Incomplete grieving

Airway Clearance, Ineffective Related factors: Tracheobronchial obstruction, Decreased energy/fatigue, Pain

Anxiety Related factors: Threat of death, Threat to or change in role functioning, Change in health status

Body Image Disturbance Related factors: Chronic illness, Treatment side-effects

Bowel Incontinence Related factors: Decreased awareness of need to defecate, Disease process, Loss of sphincter control

Breathing Pattern, Ineffective Related factors: Medication, Chronic pain, Decreased energy/fatigue

Caregiver Role Strain (Actual/Risk for) Related factors/risk factors: Illness severity of care receiver, Duration of caregiving required, Lack of respite and recreation for caregiver, Complexity/number of caregiving tasks

Constipation Related factors: Decreased activity, Dietary changes, Medication (specify), Painful defecation

Coping, Ineffective Family: Disabling Related factor: Chronically unresolved feelings

Coping, Ineffective Individual Related factors: Personal vulnerability in a maturational crisis (terminal illness in childhood), Personal vulnerability in a situational crisis (terminal illness)

Decisional Conflict Related factors: Perceived threat to value system, Lack of relevant information, Multiple or divergent sources of information, Lack of support system

Diarrhea Related factors: Dietary changes, Impaction, Medication (specify), Stress

Disuse Syndrome: Risk for Risk factors: Severe pain, Altered level of consciousness

Diversional Activity Deficit Related factors: Frequent/lengthy medical treatments, Forced inactivity, Long-term hospitalization

Family Processes, Altered Related factors: Change in family roles, Complex therapies, Hospitalization/change in environment, Illness/disability of family member, Separation of family members

Fatigue Related factors: Pain, Disease process, Overwhelming psychologic or emotional demands

Fear Related factors: Real or imagined threat to own well-being, Environmental stressors/hospitalization

Fluid Volume Deficit Related factors: Inadequate fluid intake, Abnormal fluid loss (specify)

Fluid Volume Deficit: Risk for Risk factor: Excessive losses through normal routes

Gas Exchange, Impaired Related factor: Decreased functional lung tissue secondary to tumor mass or fluid accumulation

Grieving, Anticipatory Related factor: Impending death of self

Grieving, Dysfunctional Related factor: Terminal illness

Hopelessness Related factors: Failing or deteriorating physical condition, Long-term stress, Lost spiritual belief

Infection: Risk for Risk factors: Immunosuppression, Pharmaceutical agents

Knowledge Deficit (specify) Related factors: Limited exposure to prescribed treatment information (specify), Cognitive limitations of child (specify)

Mobility, Impaired Physical Related factors: Decreased strength and endurance, Musculoskeletal impairment, Neuromuscular impairment, Pain/discomfort

Nutrition, Altered: Less Than Body Requirements Related factors: Difficulty in swallowing, Nausea/vomiting, Loss of appetite

Oral Mucous Membrane, Altered Related factors: Chemotherapy, Radiation to head and neck

Pain [Acute] Related factor: Ongoing tissue destruction

Powerlessness Related factor: Terminal illness

Role Performance, Altered Related factors: Chronic pain, Treatment side-effects

Self-Care Deficit: Bathing/Hygiene, Dressing/Grooming, Feeding, Toileting (specify) Related factors: Developmental disability, Maturational age, Pain/discomfort, Intolerance to activity, Decreased strength and endurance

Sexual Dysfunction Related factors: Pain, Disease, Illness/medical treatment

Skin Integrity, Impaired Related factors: Radiation, Skeletal prominence, Immunologic deficit

Skin Integrity, Impaired: Risk for Risk factors: Radiation, Skeletal prominence, Immunologic deficit

Sleep Pattern Disturbance Related factors: Anxiety, Emotional state, Medically induced regimen, Pain/discomfort

Social Interaction, Impaired Related factors: Developmental disability, Self-concept disturbance, Therapeutic isolation

Spiritual Distress Related factors: Test of spiritual beliefs, Challenged belief and value system

Swallowing, Impaired Related factors: Irritated oropharyngeal cavity, Mechanical obstruction

Cerebrovascular Accident (Stroke)

Activity Intolerance Related factors: Anxiety, Weakness/fatigue

Airway Clearance, Ineffective Related factors: Decreased energy and fatigue, Tracheobronchial secretions

Anxiety Related factors: Change in health status, Change in role functioning, Change in interaction patterns

Aspiration: Risk for Risk factors: Reduced level of consciousness, Impaired swallowing, Depressed cough and gag reflexes

Body Image Disturbance Related factors: Chronic illness, Diminished physical function, Loss of control over body

Bowel Incontinence Related factors: Decreased awareness of need to defecate, Loss of sphincter control

Caregiver Role Strain (Actual/Risk for) Related factors/risk factors: Illness severity of care receiver, Duration of caregiving required, Lack of respite and recreation for caregiver, Complexity/number of caregiving tasks

Communication, Impaired: Verbal Related factors: Aphasia, Inability to speak, Inability to speak clearly

Constipation Related factors: Decreased activity, Medications (specify)

Coping, Ineffective Family: Compromised Related factors: Temporary family disorganization and role changes, Chronic illness/disability

Coping, Ineffective Individual Related factor: Personal vulnerability in a situational crisis (declining health)

Diarrhea Related factor: Impaction

Disuse Syndrome: Risk for Risk factors: Altered level of consciousness, Paralysis

Family Processes, Altered Related factors: Hospitalization/change in environment, Illness/disability of family member, Change in family roles

Fatigue Related factors: Overwhelming psychologic or emotional demands

Fluid Volume Deficit Related factor: Inadequate fluid intake

Fluid Volume Deficit: Risk for Risk factor: Deviations affecting access to or intake or absorption of fluids

Grieving, Dysfunctional Related factors: Actual loss, Chronic illness

Health Maintenance, Altered Related factor: Motor/perceptual impairment

Home Maintenance Management, Impaired Related factors: Home environment obstacles, Inadequate support system, Lack of familiarity with community resources

Hopelessness Related factor: Failing or deteriorating physical condition

Injury: Risk for Risk factors: Altered mobility, Sensory dysfunction

Knowledge Deficit (specify) Related factors: Cognitive deficit, Information misinterpretation

Mobility, Impaired Physical Related factors: Musculoskeletal impairment, Neuromuscular impairment

Nutrition, Altered: Less Than Body Requirements Related factors: Difficulty in chewing, Difficulty in swallowing, Nausea/vomiting

Powerlessness Related factor: Treatment regimen

Relocation Stress Syndrome Related factors: Change in environment/location, Anxiety, Depression, Verbalization of being concerned/upset about transfer

Role Performance, Altered Related factor: Chronic illness

Self-Care Deficit: Bathing/Hygiene, Dressing/Grooming, Feeding, Toileting (specify) Related factors: Neuromuscular impairment, Musculoskeletal impairment, Decreased strength and endurance, Intolerance to activity

Self-Esteem Disturbance Related factor: Chronic illness

Sensory/Perceptual Alterations: Visual, Auditory, Kinesthetic, Gustatory, Tactile, Olfactory (specify) Related factors: Altered sensory reception, transmission, and/or integration

Skin Integrity, Impaired: Risk for Risk factors: Altered sensation, Immobility, Incontinence of stool or urine

Spiritual Distress Related factors: Challenged belief and value system, Test of spiritual values

Swallowing, Impaired Related factors: Neuromuscular impairment, Impaired sensory integration

Therapeutic Regimen Management, Ineffective Individual Related factors: Complexity of therapeutic regimen, Knowledge deficit, Excessive demands made on individual or family, Social support deficits, Decisional conflict

Urinary Incontinence, Functional Related factors: Cognitive impairment, Mobility deficit

Urinary Incontinence, Total Related factor: Neurologic dysfunction

Chest Injury

Includes but is not limited to hemothorax, pneumothorax.

Activity Intolerance Related factors: Acute pain, Anxiety, Weakness/fatigue

Aspiration: Risk for Risk factor: Presence of tracheostomy or endotracheal tube

Breathing Pattern, Ineffective Related factors: Acute pain, Anxiety

Dysfunctional Ventilatory Weaning Response (DVWR) Related factors: Anxiety, History of ventilator dependence > 1 week, Inappropriate pacing of diminished ventilatory support, Uncontrolled episodic energy demands or problems

Fear Related factor: Real or imagined threat to own well-being

Fluid Volume Deficit Related factor: Abnormal fluid loss (specify)

Gas Exchange, Impaired Related factor: Decreased functional lung tissue

Mobility, Impaired Physical Related factor: Pain/discomfort

Pain [Acute] Related factor: Chest injury

Self-Care Deficit: Bathing/Hygiene, Dressing/Grooming, Feeding, Toileting (specify) Related factor: Pain/discomfort

Sleep Pattern Disturbance Related factors: Pain/discomfort, Medically induced regimen

Congestive Heart Failure

Activity Intolerance Related factors: Weakness/fatigue, Imbalance between oxygen supply and demand

Adjustment, Impaired Related factor: Necessity for major lifestyle/behavior change

Anxiety Related factor: Shortness of breath, dyspnea

Cardiac Output, Decreased Related factors: Dysfunctional electrical conduction, Increased ventricular workload, Ventricular ischemia, Ventricular damage

Family Processes, Altered Related factors: Hospitalization/change in environment, Illness/disability of family member

Fatigue Related factor: Disease process

Fear Related factor: Real or imagined threat to own well-being

Fluid Volume Excess Related factor: Decreased urine output secondary to heart failure

Gas Exchange, Impaired Related factor: Decreased pulmonary blood supply secondary to congestive heart failure

Health Maintenance, Altered Related factors: Lack of social supports, Lack of material resources

Home Maintenance Management, Impaired: Risk for Risk factor: Fatigue

Hopelessness Related factor: Failing or deteriorating physical condition

Knowledge Deficit (specify) Related factors: Information misinterpretation, Limited exposure to information

Nutrition, Altered: Less Than Body Requirements Related factors: Nausea, Anorexia, Fatigue

Powerlessness Related factors: Chronic illness, Treatment regimen

Self-Care Deficit: Bathing/Hygiene, Dressing/Grooming, Feeding, Toileting (specify) Related factors: Decreased strength and endurance, Intolerance to activity

Sleep Pattern Disturbance Related factors: Anxiety, Medically induced regimen

Endocrine Disorders

Includes but is not limited to Cushing's disease, diabetes mellitus, hyperthyroidism, hypothyroidism, hypoglycemia, pancreatic tumors.

Adjustment, Impaired Related factors: Necessity for major lifestyle/behavior changes, Inadequate support systems

Body Image Disturbance Related factors: Chronic illness, Treatment side-effects

Coping, Ineffective Individual Related factor: Personal vulnerability in situational crisis

Family Processes, Altered Related factors: Change in family roles, Hospitalization/change in environment

Fear Related factor: Real or imagined threat to own well-being

Fluid Volume Deficit Related factors: Abnormal fluid loss, Inadequate fluid intake, Failure of regulatory mechanisms

Health Maintenance, Altered Related factors: Lack of material resources, Lack of social supports

Knowledge Deficit (specify) Related factors: Limited exposure to information, Limited practice of skill, Information misinterpretation

Nutrition, Altered: Less Than Body Requirements Related factor: Nausea/vomiting

Nutrition, Altered: More Than Body Requirements Related factor: Increased appetite

Role Performance, Altered Related factors: Chronic illness, Treatment side-effects

Self-Esteem Disturbance Related factor: Chronic illness

Sensory/Perceptual Alterations: Visual, Tactile Related factor: Sensory deficit

Sexual Dysfunction Related factor: Disease

Skin Integrity, Impaired: Risk for Risk factors: Altered circulation, Medications (specify)

Therapeutic Regimen Management, Ineffective Individual Related factors: Complexity of therapeutic regimen, Knowledge deficit, Perceived seriousness, Decisional conflict

Tissue Perfusion, Altered: Peripheral Related factor: Impaired arterial circulation

Gastrointestinal Bleeding

Includes but is not limited to hematemesis, melena.

Activity Intolerance Related factor: Weakness/fatigue

Adjustment, Impaired Related factor: Necessity for major lifestyle/behavior changes secondary to alcoholism

Coping, Ineffective Individual Related factor: Personal vulnerability to situational crisis (acute illness)

Diarrhea Related factor: Increased intestinal motility

Fatigue Related factors: Disease process, Low hemoglobin level

Fear Related factor: Real or imagined threat to own well-being

Fluid Volume Deficit Related factor: Abnormal fluid loss (specify, eg, emesis, diarrhea)

Nutrition, Altered: Less Than Body Requirements Related factors: Loss of appetite, Nausea/vomiting

Pain [Acute] Related factor: Injury

Skin Integrity, Impaired: Risk for Risk factor: Stool incontinence

Sleep Pattern Disturbance Related factors: Pain/discomfort, Sleep deprivation

Immobilized Patient

Activity Intolerance Related factors: Weakness/fatigue, Acute pain, Chronic pain

Aspiration: Risk for Risk factor: Hindered elevation of upper body

Constipation Related factor: Decreased activity

Coping, Ineffective Individual Related factor: Personal vulnerability to a situational crisis (specify)

Disuse Syndrome: Risk for Risk factors: Paralysis, Mechanical immobilization, Prescribed immobility

Diversional Activity Deficit Related factor: Prolonged bed rest

Dysreflexia Related factor: Spinal cord injury T7 or above

Fear Related factor: Real or imagined threat to own well-being

Infection: Risk for Risk factors: Broken skin, Environmental exposure to ____ (specify), Trauma

Mobility, Impaired Physical Related factors: Decreased strength and endurance, Pain/discomfort

Noncompliance Related factor: Dysfunctional patient/provider relationship

Peripheral Neurovascular Dysfunction: Risk for Risk factor: Immobilization

Self-Care Deficit: Bathing/Hygiene, Dressing/Grooming, Feeding, Toileting (specify) Related factors: Pain/discomfort, Intolerance to activity, Decreased strength and endurance

Skin Integrity, Impaired: Risk for Risk factors: Physical immobilization, Altered circulation

Sleep Pattern Disturbance Related factors: Sleep deprivation, Pain/discomfort

Urinary Incontinence, Functional Related factor: Neurologic impairment

Urinary Incontinence, Stress Related factor: Overdistention between voidings

Urinary Incontinence, Total Related factor: Neurologic dysfunction

Liver Disease

Includes but is not limited to cirrhosis, hepatitis.

Activity Intolerance Related factor: Weakness and fatigue

Body Image Disturbance Related factors: Change in appearance, Chronic illness

Coping, Ineffective Individual Related factor: Personal vulnerability to situational crisis (new diagnosis of illness, declining health)

Diarrhea Related factors: Dietary changes, Medication (specify), Stress

Family Processes, Altered Related factors: Change in family roles, Illness/disability of family member

Fatigue Related factor: Disease process

Fear Related factor: Real or imagined threat to own well-being

Fluid Volume Deficit Related factors: Abnormal fluid loss (specify), Inadequate fluid intake

Fluid Volume Excess Related factors: Malnutrition, Portal hypertension

Knowledge Deficit (specify) Related factors: Information misinterpretation, Unreadiness to learn

Mobility, Impaired Physical Related factors: Pain/discomfort, Decreased strength and endurance

Nutrition, Altered: Less Than Body Requirements Related factors: Loss of appetite, Nausea/vomiting

Pain [Acute] Related factor: Injury

Role Performance, Altered Related factor: Chronic illness

Self-Care Deficit: Bathing/Hygiene, Dressing/Grooming, Feeding, Toileting (specify) Related factors: Pain/discomfort, Intolerance to activity

Self-Esteem Disturbance Related factors: Chronic illness, Situational crisis

Skin Integrity, Impaired: Risk for Risk factor: Physical immobility

Social Interaction, Impaired Related factor: Chemical dependence

Thought Processes, Altered Related factors: Chronic organic disorder, Substance abuse

Myocardial Infarction (Chest Pain, Arrhythmias)

Activity Intolerance Related factors: Acute pain, Weakness/fatigue, Arrhythmias

Anxiety Related factors: Threat to or change in health status, Threat to or change in role functioning

Cardiac Output, Decreased Related factors: Dysfunctional electrical conduction, Increased ventricular workload, Ventricular ischemia, Ventricular damage

Coping, Ineffective Individual Related factor: Personal vulnerability to situational crisis (new diagnosis of illness, declining health)

Denial, Ineffective Related factor: Fear of consequences

Family Processes, Altered Related factors: Change in family roles, Hospitalization/change in environment

Fatigue Related factor: Disease process

Fear Related factor: Real or imagined threat to own well-being

Fluid Volume Excess Related factor: Decreased urine output secondary to heart failure

Gas Exchange, Impaired Related factor: Decreased pulmonary blood supply secondary to pulmonary hypertension/congestive heart failure

Health Maintenance, Altered Related factor: Lack of social supports

Pain [Acute] Related factor: Myocardial ischemia

Powerlessness Related factor: Treatment regimen

Role Performance, Altered Related factors: Situational crisis, Treatment side-effects

Self-Care Deficit: Bathing/Hygiene, Dressing/Grooming, Feeding, Toileting (specify) Related factors: Pain/discomfort, Intolerance to activity

Self-Esteem Disturbance Related factor: Treatment side-effects

Sexual Dysfunction Related factors: Disease, Health-related transitions, Illness/medical treatment

Sleep Pattern Disturbance Related factors: Sleep deprivation, Pain/discomfort

Neurologic Disorders

Includes but is not limited to multiple sclerosis, amyotrophic lateral sclerosis, brain tumors, Guillain-Barré syndrome, myasthenia gravis, seizure disorders, Alzheimer's disease, coma, head injury, cerebral thrombosis, and transient ischemic attack.

Associated psychiatric diagnoses: central nervous system infections (tertiary neurosyphilis, viral encephalitis, Jakob-Creutzfeldt disease, and so on), brain trauma, Huntington's chorea, Parkinson's disease, and meningitis.

Activity Intolerance Related factors: Acute pain, Chronic pain, Weakness/fatigue

Adjustment, Impaired Related factors: Inadequate support systems, Necessity for major life-style/behavior changes

Airway Clearance, Ineffective Related factor: Decreased energy/fatigue

Anxiety Related factors: Change in health status, Threat to or change in role functioning, Change in interaction pattern

Aspiration: Risk for Risk factors: Impaired swallowing, Presence of tracheostomy or endotracheal tube, Reduced level of consciousness, Depressed cough and gag reflexes, Tube feedings, Hindered elevation of upper body

Body Image Disturbance Related factors: Chronic illness, Surgery, Treatment side-effects

Bowel Incontinence Related factors: Decreased awareness of need to defecate, Loss of sphincter control

Breathing Pattern, Ineffective Related factors: Neuromuscular paralysis/weakness, Decreased energy/fatigue

Communication, Impaired: Verbal Related factors: Psychologic impairment, Aphasia, Inability to speak, Inability to speak clearly, Tracheostomy

Constipation Related factor: Decreased activity

Coping, Ineffective Family: Compromised Related factors: Temporary family disorganization and role changes, Chronic illness/disability

Coping, Ineffective Individual Related factor: Personal vulnerability to situational crisis (new diagnosis of illness, declining health, terminal illness)

Disuse Syndrome: Risk for Risk factors: Paralysis, Altered level of consciousness

Diversional Activity Deficit Related factors: Forced inactivity, Long-term hospitalization

Dysfunctional Ventilatory Weaning Response (DVWR) Related factors: History of ventilator dependence > 1 week, Ineffective airway clearance, Anxiety

Family Processes, Altered Related factors: Change in family roles, Change in family structure, Illness/disability of family member, Hospitalization/change in environment

Fatigue Related factor: Disease process

Fear Related factor: Real threat to well-being

Fluid Volume Deficit Related factor: Inadequate fluid intake

Fluid Volume Deficit: Risk for Risk factor: Deviation affecting access to intake or absorption of fluid

Home Maintenance Management, Impaired Related factors: Home environment obstacles, Inadequate support system, Insufficient family organization or planning, Psychologic impairment, Lack of familiarity with community resources

Hopelessness Related factor: Failing or deteriorating physical condition

Injury: Risk for Risk factors: Sensory dysfunction; Orientation, cognitive, affective, and psychomotor factors

Knowledge Deficit (specify) Related factor: Cognitive limitations

Mobility, Impaired Physical Related factors: Neuromuscular impairment, Decreased strength and endurance, Pain/discomfort, Medically prescribed treatment

Noncompliance Related factors: Denial of illness, Negative perception of treatment regimen

Nutrition, Altered: Less Than Body Requirements Related factors: Difficulty in chewing, Difficulty in swallowing, Psychologic impairment, Loss of appetite

Pain, Chronic Related factor: Neurologic injury

Powerlessness Related factor: Chronic illness

Role Performance, Altered Related factors: Chronic illness, Treatment side-effects

Self-Care Deficit: Bathing/Hygiene, Dressing/Grooming, Feeding, Toileting (specify) Related factors: Pain/discomfort, Decreased strength and endurance, Neuromuscular impairment, Psychologic impairment

Self-Esteem Disturbance Related factor: Chronic illness

Sensory/Perceptual Alterations: Visual, Auditory, Kinesthetic, Gustatory, Tactile, Olfactory (specify) Related factors: Altered sensory reception, transmission, and/or integration; Sensory deficit; Sensory overload

Skin Integrity, Impaired Related factors: Physical immobilization, Altered circulation

Skin Integrity, Impaired: Risk for Risk factors: Physical immobilization, Altered circulation

Sleep Pattern Disturbance Related factor: Psychologic impairment

Social Interaction, Impaired Related factors: Communication barriers, Self-concept disturbance, Therapeutic isolation

Swallowing, Impaired Related factors: Neuromuscular impairment; Psychologic impairment; Altered sensory transmission, reception, and/or integration

Thought Processes, Altered Related factor: Chronic organic disorder

Urinary Incontinence, Functional Related factors: Cognitive impairment, Mobility deficit, Disorientation

Urinary Incontinence, Total Related factor: Neurologic dysfunction

Violence, Risk for: Self-Directed or Directed at Others Risk factor: Organic mental disorder

Obesity

Activity Intolerance Related factor: Sedentary life-style

Body Image Disturbance Related factors: Eating disorder, Psychologic impairment

Coping, Ineffective Individual Related factor: Personal vulnerability in situational crisis

Fatigue Related factor: Energy requirements to perform activities of daily living

Health Maintenance, Altered Related factor: Lack of ability to make deliberate and thoughtful judgments

Health-Seeking Behaviors (specify) Related factors: Specific to patient

Mobility, Impaired Physical Related factor: Decreased strength and endurance

Nutrition, Altered: More Than Body Requirements Related factors: Eating disorder, Lack of physical exercise, Decreased metabolic requirements, Lack of basic nutritional knowledge

Self-Esteem Disturbance Related factor: Psychologic impairment

Sexuality Patterns, Altered Related factor: Body image disturbance

Skin Integrity, Impaired: Risk for Risk factor: Alterations in nutritional state

Sleep Pattern Disturbance Related factors: Discomfort, Activity

Social Interaction, Impaired Related factor: Self-concept disturbance

Therapeutic Regimen Management, Ineffective Individual Related factors: Decisional conflict, Perceived barriers, Perceived susceptibility, Social support deficits, Family patterns of health care

Pancreatitis

Activity Intolerance Related factors: Acute pain, Weakness/fatigue

Diarrhea Related factor: Medication (specify)

Family Processes, Altered Related factors: Hospitalization/change in environment, Change in family roles

Fatigue Related factors: Disease process, Pain

Fear Related factor: Real or imagined threat to own well-being

Fluid Volume Deficit Related factors: Abnormal fluid loss (specify), Inadequate fluid intake

Health Maintenance, Altered Related factor: Lack of ability to make deliberate and thoughtful judgments

Noncompliance Related factors: Negative perception of treatment regimen, Dysfunctional relationship between patient and provider

Nutrition, Altered: Less Than Body Requirements Related factors: Loss of appetite, Nausea/vomiting, Chemical dependence

Pain [Acute] Related factor: Injury

Self-Care Deficit: Bathing/Hygiene, Dressing/Grooming, Feeding, Toileting (specify) Related factors: Pain/discomfort, Intolerance to activity

Self-Esteem Disturbance Related factor: Chronic illness

Sleep Pattern Disturbance Related factor: Sleep deprivation

Therapeutic Regimen Management, Ineffective Individual Related factors: Perceived susceptibility, Family conflict, Mistrust of regimen and/or health care personnel, Decisional conflict

Thought Processes, Altered Related factor: Substance abuse

Pericarditis/Endocarditis

Anxiety Related factor: Threat to health status

Breathing Pattern, Ineffective Related factor: Acute pain

Cardiac Output, Decreased Related factors: Dysfunctional electrical conduction, Increased ventricular workload

Fear Related factor: Real or imagined threat to own well-being

Pain [Acute] Related factor: Inflammation

Self-Care Deficit: Bathing/Hygiene, Dressing/Grooming, Feeding, Toileting (specify) Related factors: Pain/discomfort, Decreased strength and endurance

Pneumonia

Activity Intolerance Related factor: Weakness/fatigue

Airway Clearance, Ineffective Related factor: Pain

Anxiety Related factors: Threat to or change to health status, Dyspnea

Fluid Volume Deficit: Risk for Risk factor: Factors affecting fluid needs

Gas Exchange, Impaired Related factor: Decreased functional lung tissue secondary to pneumonia

Nutrition, Altered: Less Than Body Requirements Related factor: Loss of appetite

Pain [Acute] Related factor: Injury

Self-Care Deficit: Bathing/Hygiene, Dressing/Grooming, Feeding, Toileting (specify) Related factors: Pain/discomfort, Intolerance to activity

Sleep Pattern Disturbance Related factors: Sleep deprivation, Dyspnea, Pain

Pulmonary Edema

Activity Intolerance Related factors: Imbalance between oxygen supply and demand, Weakness/fatigue

Cardiac Output, Decreased Related factor: Increased ventricular workload

Fatigue Related factor: Disease process

Fear Related factor: Environmental stressors/hospitalization

Fluid Volume Excess Related factor: Decreased urine output secondary to pulmonary edema

Nutrition, Altered: Less Than Body Requirements Related factor: Loss of appetite

Self-Care Deficit: Bathing/Hygiene, Dressing/Grooming, Feeding, Toileting (specify) Related factors: Pain/discomfort, Intolerance to activity

Sleep Pattern Disturbance Related factors: Sleep deprivation, Dyspnea

Pulmonary Embolism

Activity Intolerance Related factors: Acute pain, Imbalance between oxygen supply and demand

Diversional Activity Deficit Related factors: Prolonged bed rest, Forced inactivity

Fear Related factor: Real or imagined threat to own well-being

Gas Exchange, Impaired Related factor: Decreased pulmonary blood supply secondary to pulmonary embolus

Self-Care Deficit: Bathing/Hygiene, Dressing/Grooming, Feeding, Toileting (specify) Related factors: Pain/discomfort, Intolerance to activity

Renal Failure, Acute

Body Image Disturbance Related factors: Treatment side-effects, Situational crisis

Breathing Pattern, Ineffective Related factors: Decreased energy/fatigue, Fluid overload

Cardiac Output, Decreased Related factor: Increased ventricular workload

Coping, Ineffective Individual Related factor: Personal vulnerability in situational crisis (new diagnosis of illness)

Denial, Ineffective Related factor: Fear of consequences

Family Processes, Altered Related factors: Hospitalization/change in environment, Change in family roles, Illness/disability of family member

Fear Related factors: Environmental stressors/hospitalization, Powerlessness, Real threat to own well-being, Real threat to child

Fluid Volume Excess Related factors: Increased fluid intake, Decreased urine output

Infection: Risk for Risk factor: Invasive therapy

Nutrition, Altered: Less Than Body Requirements Related factors: Loss of appetite, Nausea/vomiting, Dietary restrictions

Personal Identity Disturbance Related factor: Situational crisis

Powerlessness Related factor: Treatment regimen

Role Performance, Altered Related factor: Treatment side-effects

Self-Esteem Disturbance Related factor: Treatment side-effects

Therapeutic Regimen Management, Ineffective Individual Related factors: Complexity of therapeutic regimen, Knowledge deficits, Perceived seriousness, Perceived benefits

Renal Failure, Chronic

Activity Intolerance Related factor: Weakness/fatigue secondary to anemia

Adjustment, Impaired Related factors: Assault to self-esteem, Pattern of dependence

Body Image Disturbance Related factors: Altered growth and development, Treatment side-effects, Chronic illness, Surgery (hemodialysis blood access, peritoneal catheter, amputations)

Breathing Pattern, Ineffective Related factors: Anemia, Volume overload

Cardiac Output, Decreased Related factors: Drug toxicity, Increased ventricular workload

Caregiver Role Strain (Actual/Risk for) Related factors/risk factors: Complexity/amount of caregiving tasks; Illness severity of the health care receiver; Care receiver exhibits deviant, bizarre behavior; Situational stressors within the family; Chronicity of caregiving; Caregiver's health, knowledge, skills, experience, competing role commitments, coping styles, isolation, opportunity for respite and recreation

Communication, Impaired: Verbal Related factor: Acute confusion

Constipation Related factor: Medication (specify)

Coping, Ineffective Family: Disabling Related factors: Chronically unresolved feelings, Conflicting coping styles

Coping, Ineffective Individual Related factor: Personal vulnerability in situational crisis (new diagnosis of chronic illness, declining health, terminal illness)

Denial, Ineffective Related factor: Fear of consequences

Diversional Activity Deficit Related factor: Frequent/lengthy medical treatments

Family Processes, Altered Related factor: Illness/disability of family member

Fatigue Related factor: Overwhelming psychologic or emotional demands

Fear Related factors: Environmental stressors/hospitalization, Powerlessness, Real or imagined threat to well-being

Fluid Volume Deficit Related factors: Abnormal fluid loss (specify), Abnormal blood loss secondary to hemodialysis procedure, Inadequate fluid intake

Fluid Volume Excess Related factors: Increased fluid intake secondary to excess sodium intake, Sodium retention, Hyperglycemia, Noncompliance with fluid restriction

Grieving, Dysfunctional Related factors: Chronic illness, Loss, Terminal illness

Health Maintenance, Altered Related factors: Lack of social supports, Lack of material resources

Hopelessness Related factors: Failing or deteriorating physical condition, Lack of social supports, Long-term stress

Infection: Risk for Risk factors: Immunosuppression, Malnutrition, Invasive therapy

Injury: Risk for Risk factors: Altered mobility, Sensory dysfunction, Hypotension, Weakness

Knowledge Deficit (specify) Related factors: Limited understanding of prescribed treatment, Limited practice of skill (specify)

Mobility, Impaired Physical Related factors: Decreased strength and endurance secondary to anemia, Musculoskeletal impairment, Neuromuscular impairment

Noncompliance Related factors: Denial of illness, Dysfunctional relationship between patient and provider, Negative consequence of treatment regimen, Negative perception of treatment regimen, Perceived benefits of continued illness

Nutrition, Altered: Less Than Body Requirements Related factors: Loss of appetite, Nausea/vomiting

Pain [Acute] Related factors: Paresthesia, Muscle cramps, Pruritus

Powerlessness Related factors: Treatment regimen, Chronic illness

Role Performance, Altered Related factors: Chronic illness, Treatment side-effects

Self-Care Deficit: Bathing/Hygiene, Dressing/Grooming, Feeding, Toileting (specify) Related factors: Depression, Pain/discomfort, Intolerance to activity, Decreased strength and endurance, Neuromuscular impairment, Musculoskeletal impairment

Self-Esteem Disturbance Related factors: Altered growth and development, Chronic illness, Surgery (hemodialysis blood access, peritoneal catheter, amputations), Treatment side-effects

Sensory/Perceptual Alterations: Visual, Kinesthetic, Gustatory, Tactile (specify) Related factor: Sensory deficit secondary to diabetic retinopathy, peripheral neuropathy

Sexual Dysfunction Related factors: Disturbance in self-esteem, Impotence, Loss of libido

Skin Integrity, Impaired: Risk for Risk factors: Alterations in nutritional state, Altered circulation

Sleep Pattern Disturbance Related factor: Sleep deprivation secondary to insomnia

Social Isolation Related factors: Medical condition, Alteration in physical appearance, Life-style changes

Therapeutic Regimen Management, Ineffective Individual Related factors: Complexity of therapeutic regimen, Knowledge deficits, Perceived seriousness, Perceived benefits

Tissue Perfusion, Altered: Peripheral Related factors: Impaired venous circulation secondary to surgical creation of hemodialysis blood access, Impaired arterial circulation secondary to hypertension, Diabetes

Respiratory Disorders, Chronic

Includes but is not limited to asthma, chronic obstructive pulmonary disease, and chronic restrictive pulmonary disease.

Activity Intolerance Related factors: Weakness/fatigue, Imbalance between oxygen supply and demand, Anxiety

Adjustment, Impaired Related factors: Necessity for major lifestyle/behavior change secondary to chronic illness, Pattern of dependence

Airway Clearance, Ineffective Related factors: Decreased energy/fatigue, Tracheobronchial obstruction, Tracheobronchial secretions

Aspiration: Risk for Risk factor: Presence of tracheostomy or endotracheal tube

Body Image Disturbance Related factor: Chronic illness

Breathing Pattern, Ineffective Related factors: Decreased energy/fatigue, Anxiety

Caregiver Role Strain (Actual/Risk for) Related factors/risk factors: Illness severity of the care receiver, Unpredictable illness course or instability in the care receiver's health, Duration of caregiving required, Inadequate physical environment for providing care, Lack of respite and recreation for caregiver, Complexity/amount of caregiving tasks

Coping, Ineffective Individual Related factor: Personal vulnerability in situational crisis (declining health)

Dysfunctional Ventilatory Weaning Response (DVWR) Related factors: Ineffective airway clearance, Inadequate nutrition, Patient perceived inefficacy about the ability to wean, Decreased motivation, Decreased self-esteem, Anxiety, Inappropriate pacing of diminished ventilator support, Adverse environment, History of ventilatory dependence > 1 week, History of multiple unsuccessful weaning attempts

Family Processes, Altered Related factors: Change in family roles, Change in family structure, Hospitalization/change in environment, Illness/disability of family member

Fear Related factors: Environmental stressors/hospitalization, Real or imagined threat to own well-being

Fluid Volume Deficit: Risk for Risk factors: Inadequate fluid intake secondary to difficulty in breathing, Medications

Gas Exchange, Impaired Related factor: Decreased functional lung tissue secondary to chronic lung disease

Health Maintenance, Altered Related factors: Health beliefs, Lack of social supports

Infection: Risk for Risk factors: Malnutrition, Environmental exposure to ____ (specify)

Knowledge Deficit (specify) Related factors: Information misinterpretation, Limited exposure to information (specify)

Nutrition, Altered: Less Than Body Requirements Related factors: Loss of appetite, Nausea/vomiting

Powerlessness Related factors: Treatment regimen, Chronic illness

Role Performance, Altered Related factor: Chronic illness

Self-Care Deficit: Bathing/Hygiene, Dressing/Grooming, Feeding, Toileting (specify) Related factors: Decreased strength and endurance, Intolerance to activity

Self-Esteem Disturbance Related factor: Chronic illness

Sleep Pattern Disturbance Related factors: Anxiety, Medically induced regimen

Social Interaction, Impaired Related factor: Self-concept disturbance

Therapeutic Regimen Management, Ineffective Individual Related factors: Complexity of therapeutic regimen, Decisional conflict, Family patterns of health care, Knowledge deficits, Perceived seriousness, Powerlessness, Social support deficits

Terminal Patient

Activity Intolerance Related factors: Chronic pain, Weakness/fatigue

Adjustment, Impaired Related factors: Inadequate support systems, Incomplete grieving

Airway Clearance, Ineffective Related factors: Decreased energy/fatigue, Pain, Tracheobronchial obstruction

Body Image Disturbance Related factor: Treatment side-effects

Bowel Incontinence Related factors: Loss of sphincter control, Decreased awareness of need to defecate

Breathing Pattern, Ineffective Related factor: Chronic pain

Caregiver Role Strain (Actual/Risk for) Related factors/risk factors: Illness severity of the care receiver, Unpredictable illness course or instability in the care receiver's health, Duration of caregiving required, Inadequate physical environment for providing care, Lack of respite and recreation for caregiver, Complexity/amount of caregiving tasks

Communication, Impaired: Verbal Related factors: Inability to speak, Inability to speak clearly

Constipation Related factors: Decreased activity, Decreased motility secondary to medications

Coping, Ineffective Family: Compromised Related factor: Family member's temporary preoccupation with own emotional conflicts and personal suffering

Coping, Ineffective Individual Related factor: Personal vulnerability to situational crisis (terminal illness)

Denial, Ineffective Related factor: Fear of consequences

Diarrhea Related factor: Impaction

Family Processes, Altered Related factors: Change in family roles, Hospitalization/change in environment, Illness/disability of family member

Fatigue Related factors: Disease process, Overwhelming psychologic or emotional demands

Fear Related factors: Powerlessness, Environmental stressors/hospitalization

Fluid Volume Deficit Related factor: Inadequate fluid intake

Fluid Volume Deficit: Risk for Risk factors: Excessive losses through normal routes, Loss of fluid through abnormal routes, Deviations affecting access to or intake or absorption of fluids

Gas Exchange, Impaired Related factors: Decreased functional lung tissue, Decreased pulmonary blood supply

Grieving, Anticipatory Related factor: Impending death of self

Home Maintenance Management, Impaired Related factors: Home environment obstacles, Inadequate support system, Insufficient family organization or planning, Insufficient finances, Lack of familiarity with community resources

Hopelessness Related factors: Failing or deteriorating physical condition, Lack of social support

Infection: Risk for Risk factors: Immunosuppression, Environmental exposure to ___ (specify)

Mobility, Impaired Physical Related factors: Pain/discomfort, Decreased strength and endurance

Nutrition, Altered: Less Than Body Requirements Related factors: Difficulty in swallowing, Loss of appetite, Nausea/vomiting

Oral Mucous Membrane, Altered Related factors: Chemotherapy, Inadequate oral hygiene, Radiation to head and neck

Pain, Chronic Related factors: Specific to patient

Powerlessness Related factor: Terminal illness

Role Performance, Altered Related factors: Chronic pain, Treatment side-effects

Self-Care Deficit: Bathing/Hygiene, Dressing/Grooming, Feeding, Toileting (specify) Related factors: Pain/discomfort, Intolerance to activity, Decreased strength and endurance

Self-Esteem Disturbance Related factor: Treatment side-effects

Sensory/Perceptual Alterations: Visual, Auditory, Kinesthetic, Gustatory, Tactile, Olfactory (specify) Related factors: Altered sensory reception, transmission, and/or integration

Skin Integrity, Impaired Related factors: Physical immobilization, Incontinence of stool/urine, Radiation therapy

Skin Integrity, Impaired: Risk for Risk factors: Physical immobilization, Incontinence of stool/urine, Radiation therapy

Sleep Pattern Disturbance Related factors: Sleep deprivation, Pain/discomfort

Social Isolation Related factors: Medical condition, Alteration in physical appearance

Spiritual Distress Related factors: Challenged belief and value system, Separation from religious/cultural ties, Test of spiritual beliefs

Urinary Incontinence, Functional Related factors: Disorientation, Mobility deficit

Urinary Incontinence, Total Related factor: Neurologic dysfunction

Urologic Disorders

Includes but is not limited to cystitis, glomerulonephritis, pyelonephritis, urolithiasis.

Anxiety Related factor: Threat to or change in health status

Fear Related factor: Real or imagined threat to own well-being

Knowledge Deficit (specify) Related factor: Limited exposure to information

Pain [Acute] Related factor: Inflammation

Urinary Incontinence, Urge Related factor: Bladder irritation

Urinary Retention Related factors: Blockage, Strong sphincter, Inhibition of reflex arc, High urethral pressure caused by weak detrusor

Vascular Disease

Includes but is not limited to deep vein thrombosis, hypertension, stasis ulcers, varicosities, peripheral vascular disease, thrombophlebitis.

Activity Intolerance Related factors: Weakness/fatigue, Acute pain

Anxiety Related factors: Threat to or change in role functioning, Threat to or change in health status

Body Image Disturbance Related factor: Chronic illness

Disuse Syndrome: Risk for Risk factor: Prescribed immobilization

Fear Related factor: Real or imagined threat to own well-being

Fluid Volume Deficit: Risk for Risk factor: Medication

Injury: Risk for Risk factors: Sensory dysfunction, Altered mobility

Mobility, Impaired Physical Related factor: Pain/discomfort

Pain [Acute] Related factor: Disease process

Role Performance, Altered Related factor: Chronic pain

Self-Care Deficit: Bathing/Hygiene, Dressing/Grooming, Feeding, Toileting (specify) Related factors: Pain/discomfort, Intolerance to activity

Self-Esteem Disturbance Related factor: Chronic illness

Skin Integrity, Impaired Related factors: Draining wound, Altered circulation, Physical immobilization

Skin Integrity, Impaired: Risk for Risk factors: Draining wound, Altered circulation, Physical immobilization

Tissue Perfusion, Altered: Peripheral Related factor: Impaired venous circulation

Surgical Conditions

Abdominal surgery
Breast surgery
Chest surgery
Craniotomy
Ear surgery
Eye surgery
Musculoskeletal surgery
Neck surgery
Rectal surgery
Skin graft
Spinal surgery
Urologic surgery
Vascular surgery

Abdominal Surgery

Includes but is not limited to appendectomy, cholecystectomy, colectomy, colon resection, colostomy, gastrectomy, gastric resection, gastroenterostomy, abdominal hysterectomy with or without salpingo-oophrectomy, ileostomy, laparotomy, lysis of adhesions, Marshall-Marchetti-Krantz operation, ovarian cystectomy, salpingotomy, small bowel resection, splenectomy, vagotomy, and hiatal hernia repair.

Activity Intolerance Related factors: Acute pain, Weakness/fatigue

Activity Intolerance: Risk for Risk factors: Limited mobility, Pain, Fatigue

Aspiration: Risk for Risk factors: Depressed cough and gag reflexes, Presence of endotracheal tube, Incomplete lower esophageal sphincter, Gastrointestinal tubes, Tube feedings, Increased intragastric pressure, Increased gastric residual, Decreased gastrointestinal motility, Delayed gastric emptying, Hindered elevation of upper body

Body Image Disturbance Related factors: Surgery, Situational crisis, Treatment side-effects, Cultural or spiritual factors

Bowel Incontinence Related factor: Loss of sphincter control

Breathing Pattern, Ineffective Related factor: Pain

Caregiver Role Strain (Actual/Risk for) Related factors/risk factors: Illness severity of care receiver, Discharge of family member with significant home care needs, Past history of poor relationship between caregiver and care receiver

Constipation, Colonic Related factors: Decreased activity, Decreased fluid intake, Lack of adequate fiber, Immobility, Lack of privacy, Change in daily routine

Diarrhea Related factors: Dietary changes, Increased intestinal motility, Medication, Stress

Fear Related factors: Environmental stressors/hospitalization, Powerlessness, Real or imagined threat to own well-being

Fluid Volume Deficit Related factors: Abnormal blood loss, Abnormal fluid loss, Failure of regulatory mechanisms

Fluid Volume Deficit: Risk for Risk factors: Excessive losses through normal routes, Loss of fluid through abnormal routes, Deviations affecting access to or intake or absorption of fluids

Gas Exchange, Impaired Related factors: Decreased functional lung tissue secondary to atelectasis, Ventilation-perfusion imbalance

Grieving, Anticipatory Related factor: Potential loss of body part or function

Grieving, Dysfunctional Related factors: Actual loss, Terminal illness

Infection: Risk for Risk factors: Stasis of body fluids, Altered peristalsis, Suppressed inflammatory response, Invasive procedures

Knowledge Deficit (specify) Related factors: Limited practice of skill, Unreadiness to learn

Nutrition, Altered: Less Than Body Requirements Related factors: Loss of appetite, Nausea/vomiting

Protection, Altered Related factors: Deficient immunity secondary to ____, Impaired healing secondary to ____, Altered clotting secondary to ____

Role Performance, Altered Related factors: Surgery, Situational crisis (specify), Treatment side-effects

Sexual Dysfunction Related factors: Pain, Health-related transitions, Body image disturbance, Surgery, Altered body function or structure

Skin Integrity, Impaired: Risk for Risk factors: Mechanical factors, Physical immobilization, Excretions/secretions, Alterations in nutritional state, Altered sensation, Skeletal prominence

Therapeutic Regimen Management, Ineffective Individual Related factors: Complexity of therapeutic regimen, Economic difficulties, Knowledge deficits

Tissue Perfusion, Altered: Gastrointestinal Related factors: Interruption of arterial flow, Exchange problems, Hypervolemia, Hypovolemia

Breast Surgery

Includes but is not limited to augmentation, mastectomy, reconstruction, lumpectomy, biopsy.

Activity Intolerance Related factors: Acute pain, Anxiety

Anxiety Related factors: Threat to self-concept, Threat to or change in health status, Threat to or change in interaction pattern, Situational/maturational crisis

Body Image Disturbance Related factors: Surgery, Treatment side-effects, Cultural or spiritual factors

Caregiver Role Strain (Actual/Risk for) Related factor/risk factor: Caregiver is spouse

Family Processes, Altered Related factors: Complex therapies, Hospitalization/change in environment

Fear Related factors: Disease process/prognosis, Powerlessness, Real or imagined threat to own well-being

Grieving, Anticipatory Related factor: Potential loss of body part or function

Pain [Acute] Related factors: Surgical procedure, Paresthesia

Peripheral Neurovascular Dysfunction: Risk for Risk factor: Vascular obstruction

Powerlessness Related factor: Treatment regimen

Self-Care Deficit: Dressing/Grooming Related factors: Pain/discomfort, Neuromuscular impairment

Sexual Dysfunction Related factors: Surgery, Pain, Health-related transitions, Altered body function or structure, Illness/medical treatment, Body image disturbance, Self-esteem disturbance

Chest Surgery

Includes but is not limited to biopsy, cardiopulmonary bypass, coronary artery bypass, lobectomy, and thoracotomy.

Activity Intolerance Related factors: Imbalance between oxygen supply and demand, Acute pain, Weakness/fatigue

Activity Intolerance: Risk for Risk factors: Limited mobility, Pain, Fatigue

Adjustment, Impaired Related factor: Necessity for major lifestyle/behavior changes

Airway Clearance, Ineffective Related factors: Decreased energy/fatigue, Tracheobronchial secretions

Aspiration: Risk for Risk factor: Presence of endotracheal tube

Breathing Pattern, Ineffective Related factors: Decreased energy/fatigue, Acute pain

Cardiac Output, Decreased Related factors: Dysfunctional electrical conduction, Ventricular ischemia, Ventricular damage

Caregiver Role Strain (Actual/Risk for) Related factors/risk factors: Discharge of family member with significant home care needs, Caregiver's competing role commitments

Communication, Impaired: Verbal Related factor: Intubation

Coping, Ineffective Individual Related factor: Personal vulnerability in situational crisis (specify)

Dysfunctional Ventilatory Weaning Response (DVWR) Related factors: Uncontrolled pain/discomfort, Moderate/severe anxiety, Fear, History of ventilatory dependence > 1 week

Fatigue Related factors: Pain, Disease process

Fear Related factors: Environmental stressors/hospitalization, Real or imagined threat to own well-being

Fluid Volume Deficit Related factors: Abnormal fluid loss, Abnormal blood loss

Fluid Volume Deficit: Risk for Risk factors: Excessive losses through normal routes, Loss of fluid through abnormal routes, Deviations affecting access to or intake or absorption of fluids

Gas Exchange, Impaired Related factors: Decreased functional lung tissue secondary to pneumonia, Thoracotomy, Respiratory distress syndrome, Ventilation-perfusion imbalance

Noncompliance Related factors: Denial of illness, Negative perception of treatment regimen

Pain [Acute] Related factor: Surgical procedure

Powerlessness Related factor: Treatment regimen

Protection, Altered Related factor: Altered clotting secondary to ___

Role Performance, Altered Related factors: Surgery, Treatment side-effects

Self-Care Deficit: Bathing/Hygiene, Dressing/Grooming Related factors: Pain/discomfort, Intolerance to activity, Decreased strength and endurance

Skin Integrity, Impaired Related factors: Altered circulation, Altered sensation, Mechanical factors

Sleep Pattern Disturbance Related factors: Pain/discomfort, Unfamiliar surroundings, Medically induced regimen

Craniotomy

Includes but is not limited to acoustic neuroma removal, cerebral aneurysm clipping, cerebral bleed, cerebral trauma.

Activity Intolerance Related factor: Weakness/fatigue

Airway Clearance, Ineffective Related factor: Tracheobronchial secretions

Body Image Disturbance Related factors: Surgery, Treatment side-effects

Body Temperature, Altered: Risk for Risk factors: Altered metabolic rate, Trauma, Sedation

Bowel Incontinence Related factor: Decreased awareness of need to defecate

Breathing Pattern, Ineffective Related factors: Depression of respiratory center secondary to ___, Neuromuscular paralysis/weakness

Caregiver Role Strain (Actual/Risk for) Related factors/risk factors: Illness severity of care receiver, Discharge of family member with significant home care needs, Unpredictable illness course, Psychologic or cognitive problems in care receiver

Communication, Impaired: Verbal Related factors: Aphasia, Acute confusion, Intubation

Coping, Ineffective Individual Related factor: Personal vulnerability in situational crisis (specify)

Disuse Syndrome: Risk for Risk factors: Paralysis, Mechanical immobilization, Prescribed immobilization, Altered level of consciousness

Fear Related factors: Environmental stressors/hospitalization, Powerlessness, Real or imagined threat to own well-being

Fluid Volume Deficit Related factor: Failure of regulatory mechanisms (diabetes insipidus)

Fluid Volume Deficit: Risk for Risk factors: Excessive losses through normal routes, Loss of fluid through abnormal routes, Deviations affecting access to or intake or absorption of fluids

Fluid Volume Excess Related factor: Decreased urine output secondary to renal dysfunction

Injury: Risk for Risk factor: Sensory dysfunction

Mobility, Impaired Physical Related factors: Neuromuscular impairment, Perceptual/cognitive impairment, Depression/severe anxiety

Pain [Acute] Related factors: Surgical procedure, Paresthesia

Peripheral Neurovascular Dysfunction: Risk for Related factors: Trauma, Vascular obstruction

Protection, Altered Related factors: Neurosensory alterations secondary to ____, Altered clotting secondary to ____ (specify)

Role Performance, Altered Related factors: Surgery, Psychologic impairment, Treatment side-effects, Assumption of new role

Self-Care Deficit: Bathing/Hygiene, Dressing/Grooming, Feeding, Toileting (specify) Related factors: Intolerance to activity, Neuromuscular impairment

Sensory/Perceptual Alterations: Visual, Auditory, Kinesthetic, Gustatory, Tactile, Olfactory (specify) Related factors: Altered sensory reception, transmission, and/or integration; Sensory deficit; Sensory overload

Swallowing, Impaired Related factors: Altered sensory reception, transmission, and/or integration; Neuromuscular impairment

Tissue Perfusion, Altered: Cerebral Related factor: Interruption of arterial flow

Urinary Incontinence, Functional Related factors: Cognitive impairment, Disorientation, Mobility deficits

Urinary Incontinence, Total Related factors: Neuropathy preventing transmissions of reflex indicating bladder fullness, Neurologic dysfunction causing triggering of micturition at unpredictable times, Independent contraction of detrusor reflex due to surgery

Ear Surgery

Includes but is not limited to myringotomy, reconstruction, stapedectomy.

Body Image Disturbance Related factor: Surgery

Fear Related factor: Real or imagined threat to own well-being

Mobility, Impaired Physical Related factor: Neuromuscular impairment

Self-Care Deficit: Bathing/Hygiene, Dressing/Grooming, Feeding, Toileting (specify) Related factor: Intolerance to activity secondary to dizziness

Sensory/Perceptual Alterations: Auditory, Tactile Related factors: Sensory deficit, Sensory overload

Eye Surgery

Includes but is not limited to blepharoplasty, cataract removal, cryosurgery for retinal detachment, iridectomy, iridotomy, lens implant.

Body Image Disturbance Related factor: Surgery

Fear Related factor: Real or imagined threat to own well-being

Injury: Risk for Risk factors: Sensory deficit, Unsafe ambulation secondary to limited vision

Mobility, Impaired Physical Related factor: Medically prescribed treatment

Sensory/Perceptual Alteration: Visual Related factor: Sensory deficit

Tissue Integrity, Impaired Related factor: Irritants

Musculoskeletal Surgery

Includes but is not limited to amputation, arthrotomy, bunionectomy, casts, hip pinning, hip prosthesis, open reduction/internal fixation of fracture, shoulder repair, total ankle replacement, total hip replacement, total knee replacement, traction.

Activity Intolerance Related factors: Acute pain, Weakness/fatigue

Adjustment, Impaired Related factor: Necessity for major lifestyle/behavior change

Anxiety Related factors: Threat to self-concept, Threat to or change in health status, Threat to or change in role functioning

Body Image Disturbance Related factors: Surgery, Treatment side-effects

Caregiver Role Strain (Actual/Risk for) Related factors/risk factors: Illness severity of care receiver, Presence of situational stressors, Duration of caregiving required

Constipation Related factors: Decreased activity, Dietary changes, Medication

Disuse Syndrome: Risk for Risk factor: Prescribed immobilization

Diversional Activity Deficit Related factor: Prolonged bed rest

Fatigue Related factor: Increased energy requirement to perform activities of daily living

Fluid Volume Deficit: Risk for Risk factors: Excessive losses through normal routes, Loss of fluid through abnormal routes, Deviations affecting access to or intake or absorption of fluids

Injury: Risk for Risk factor: Altered mobility

Mobility, Impaired Physical Related factors: Pain/discomfort, Decreased strength and endurance

Nutrition, Altered: More Than Body Requirements Related factors: Lack of physical exercise, Decreased metabolic requirements

Pain [Acute] Related factors: Muscle cramps, Paresthesia

Peripheral Neurovascular Dysfunction: Risk for Risk factors: Fractures, Mechanical compression, Orthopedic surgery, Trauma, Immobilization

Role Performance, Altered Related factors: Surgery, Situational crisis, Chronic pain

Self-Care Deficit: Bathing/Hygiene, Dressing/Grooming, Feeding, Toileting (specify) Related factors: Pain/discomfort, Intolerance to activity, Decreased strength and endurance

Skin Integrity, Impaired: Risk for Risk factors: Mechanical factors, Physical immobilization, Altered circulation, Altered sensation

Sleep Pattern Disturbance Related factors: Pain/discomfort, Unfamiliar surroundings, Medically induced regimen

Tissue Perfusion, Altered: Peripheral Related factors: Interruption of arterial flow, Interruption of venous flow

Neck Surgery

Includes but is not limited to carotid endarterectomy, laryngectomy, parathyroidectomy, radical neck dissection, thyroidectomy, tonsillectomy, and tracheostomy.

Activity Intolerance Related factors: Imbalance between oxygen supply and demand, Anxiety, Acute pain, Weakness/fatigue

Activity Intolerance: Risk for Risk factors: Limited mobility, Fatigue

Adjustment, Impaired Related factors: Assault to self-esteem, Necessity for major life-style/behavior change

Airway Clearance, Ineffective Related factors: Decreased energy/fatigue, Edema, Pain, Tracheobronchial obstruction, Tracheobronchial secretions

Aspiration: Risk for Risk factors: Depressed cough or gag reflex, Presence of tracheostomy or endotracheal tube, Impaired swallowing, Hindered elevation of upper body

Body Image Disturbance Related factors: Surgery, Depression, Treatment side-effects

Breathing Pattern, Ineffective Related factors: Anxiety, Decreased energy/fatigue

Caregiver Role Strain (Actual/ Risk for) Related factors/risk factors: Illness severity of care receiver, Duration of caregiving required, Inadequate physical environment for providing care, Complexity/amount of caregiving tasks

Communication, Impaired: Verbal Related factors: Acute confusion, Inability to speak, Inability to speak clearly, Tracheostomy

Coping, Ineffective Individual Related factor: Personal vulnerability in situational crisis (specify)

Dysfunctional Ventilatory Weaning Response (DVWR) Related factors: Ineffective airway clearance, Decreased motivation, Moderate/severe anxiety, Fear, Uncontrolled episodic energy demands or problems

Family Processes, Altered Related factors: Change in family roles, Illness/disability of family member

Fear Related factors: Real or imagined threat to own well-being, Powerlessness

Fluid Volume Deficit: Risk for Risk factors: Loss of fluid through abnormal routes, Hypermetabolic state

Fluid Volume Excess Related factor: Insufficient protein secondary to decreased intake

Grieving, Dysfunctional Related factor: Actual loss

Infection: Risk for Risk factors: Tissue destruction and increased environmental exposure, Trauma

Injury: Risk for Risk factors: Sensory dysfunction, Integrative dysfunction, Altered mobility

Knowledge Deficit (specify) Related factors: Lack of motivation, Limited practice of skill (specify), Unreadiness to learn

Nutrition, Altered: Less Than Body Requirements Related factors: Difficulty in swallowing, High metabolic states, Loss of appetite, Nausea/vomiting

Oral Mucous Membrane, Altered Related factors: Inadequate oral hygiene, Tubes, Surgery in oral cavity, Infection, Radiation therapy to head and neck

Pain [Acute] Related factor: Surgical procedure

Role Performance, Altered Related factors: Surgery, Treatment side-effects

Skin Integrity, Impaired Related factors: Mechanical factors, Radiation, Altered nutritional state

Spontaneous Ventilation, Inability to Sustain Related factor: Respiratory muscle fatigue

Swallowing, Impaired Related factors: Irritated oropharyngeal cavity, Mechanical obstruction

Tissue Integrity, Impaired Related factors: Nutritional deficit, Irritants, Mechanical factors, Radiation

Rectal Surgery

Includes but is not limited to fissurectomy, hemorrhoidectomy, pilonidal cystectomy, polypectomy.

Activity Intolerance Related factor: Acute pain

Constipation Related factors: Dietary changes, Medication, Painful defecation

Pain [Acute] Related factor: Surgical procedure

Sexual Dysfunction Related factors: Surgery, Pain, Disease, Health-related transitions, Altered body function, Trauma

Tissue Integrity, Impaired Related factors: Altered circulation, Irritants, Mechanical factors

Urinary Retention Related factors: Inhibition of reflex arc, Blockage

Skin Graft

Includes but is not limited to excision of lesion with flap, excision of lesion with full thickness graft, excision of lesion with split thickness graft, excision of lesion with synthetic graft.

Activity Intolerance Related factors: Anxiety, Weakness/fatigue, Decreased activity

Body Image Disturbance Related factors: Surgery, Treatment side-effects

Constipation Related factor: Decreased activity

Diversional Activity Deficit Related factor: Prolonged bed rest

Fear Related factors: Real or imagined threat to own well-being

Mobility, Impaired Physical Related factors: Pain/discomfort

Pain [Acute] Related factors: Surgical procedure, Pruritus, Paresthesia

Peripheral Neurovascular Dysfunction: Risk for Risk factors: Immobilization, Burns

Spinal Surgery

Includes but is not limited to Harrington rod implant, laminectomy, Luque rod implant, spinal fusion.

Activity Intolerance Related factors: Anxiety, Acute pain, Weakness/fatigue, Sedentary life-style

Caregiver Role Strain (Actual/Risk for) Related factors/risk factors: Premature birth/congenital defect, Developmental delay or retardation of the care receiver/caregiver, Duration of caregiving required

Constipation, Colonic Related factors: Decreased activity, Medication, Painful defecation, Change in daily routine

Disuse Syndrome: Risk for Risk factor: Prescribed immobilization

Dysreflexia Related factors: Urinary retention, Constipation

Fear Related factor: Real or imagined threat to own well-being

Fluid Volume Deficit: Risk for Risk factors: Excessive losses through normal routes, Loss of fluid through abnormal routes, Deviations affecting access to or intake or absorption of fluids

Injury: Risk for Risk factors: Sensory dysfunction, Altered mobility

Mobility, Impaired Physical Related factors: Pain/discomfort, Neuromuscular impairment

Nutrition, Altered: More Than Body Requirements Related factors: Increased appetite, Sedentary life-style, Decreased activity

Pain [Acute] Related factors: Bed rest, Muscle cramps, Paresthesia, Surgical procedure

Pain, Chronic Related factors: Neurologic injury, Altered body function

Peripheral Neurovascular Dysfunction: Risk for Risk factors: Fractures, Mechanical compression, Trauma, Immobilization

Role Performance, Altered Related factors: Surgery, Chronic pain, Chronic illness

Urologic Surgery

Includes but is not limited to cystocele repair, rectocele repair, removal of bladder tumor, cystoscopy, nephrectomy, penile implant, percutaneous nephrostomy, retroperitoneal lymphadenotomy, transurethral resection of the prostate, ureterolithotomy, urostomy, and vasectomy.

Activity Intolerance Related factors: Anxiety, Acute pain, Weakness/fatigue

Anxiety Related factors: Threat to self-concept, Threat to or change in health status, Threat to or change in role functioning, Threat to or change in interaction pattern

Body Image Disturbance Related factors: Surgery, Depression, Treatment side-effects

Caregiver Role Strain (Actual/Risk for) Related factors/risk factors: Discharge of family member with significant home care needs, Caregiver is female, Caregiver is spouse, Duration of caregiving required

Constipation Related factor: Painful defecation

Fear Related factor: Real or imagined threat to own well-being

Fluid Volume Deficit Related factors: Abnormal fluid loss, Inadequate fluid intake

Fluid Volume Deficit: Risk for Risk factor: Loss of fluid through abnormal route

Grieving, Anticipatory Related factor: Potential loss of body parts or function

Grieving, Dysfunctional Related factor: Perceived loss

Infection: Risk for Risk factors: Stasis of body fluids, Change in pH secretions, Decreased hemoglobin, Suppressed inflammatory response, Tissue destruction and increased environmental exposure, Invasive procedures

Mobility, Impaired Physical Related factors: Pain, Discomfort

Pain [Acute] Related factors: Muscle cramps, Surgical procedure

Role Performance, Altered Related factors: Surgery, Psychologic impairment

Sexual Dysfunction Related factors: Surgery, Pain, Health-related transitions, Altered body function or structure, Body image disturbance

Urinary Incontinence, Stress Related factors: Incompetent bladder outlet, Overdistention between voidings, Weak pelvic muscles and structural supports

Urinary Incontinence, Urge Related factors: Decreased bladder capacity, Surgery, Irritation of bladder stretch receptors causing spasm, Overdistention of bladder

Urinary Retention Related factors: Inhibition of reflex arc, Blockage

Vascular Surgery

Includes but is not limited to aortic aneurysm resection, aorto-iliac bypass graft, embolectomy, femoro-iliac bypass graft, portacaval shunt, sympathectomy, and vein ligation.

Activity Intolerance Related factors: Anxiety, Acute pain, Weakness/fatigue, Imbalance between oxygen supply and demand

Adjustment, Impaired Related factor: Necessity for major lifestyle/behavior change

Cardiac Output, Decreased Related factors: Dysfunctional electrical conduction, Ventricular ischemia, Ventricular damage

Caregiver Role Strain (Actual/Risk for) Related factors/risk factors: Illness severity of care receiver, Unpredictable illness course or instability in the care receiver's health, Complexity/amount of caregiving tasks

Fear Related factor: Real or imagined threat to own well-being

Fluid Volume Deficit: Risk for Risk factors: Loss of fluid through abnormal routes, Medications

Fluid Volume Excess Related factor: Decreased urine output secondary to heart failure

Gas Exchange, Impaired Related factor: Decreased functional lung tissue, Decreased pulmonary blood supply

Grieving, Anticipatory Related factor: Potential loss of body part or function

Grieving, Dysfunctional Related factor: Perceived loss

Injury: Risk for Risk factors: Tissue hypoxia, Abnormal blood profile, Altered mobility

Pain [Acute] Related factor: Surgical procedure

Peripheral Neurovascular Dysfunction: Risk for Risk factors: Immobilization, Vascular obstruction

Role Performance, Altered Related factors: Surgery, Chronic illness, Treatment side-effects, Assumption of new role

Self-Esteem Disturbance Related factors: Surgery, Depression

Tissue Perfusion, Altered: Renal, Cerebral, Cardiopulmonary, Gastrointestinal, Peripheral (specify type) Related factors: Interruption of venous flow, Exchange problems

Psychiatric Conditions

Assaultive patient
Borderline personality disorder patient
Chronically ill psychiatric patient
Eating disorder patient
Manic patient
Paranoid patient
Phobic patient
Psychotic patient
Severely depressed patient
Substance abuse patient
Suicidal patient
Withdrawn patient

Assaultive Patient

Associated psychiatric diagnoses include but are not limited to bipolar disorder, manic; schizophrenia, disorganized type; substance abuse disorders; organic mental disorders; drug-induced psychoses; personality disorders; panic disorders; post-traumatic stress disorder.

Coping, Defensive Related factors: Psychologic impairment (specify), Situational crisis (specify)

Denial, Ineffective Related factors: Specific to patient

Fear Related factors: Real or imagined threat to own well-being, Powerlessness

Personal Identity Disturbance Related factors: Situational crisis (specify), Psychologic impairment (specify)

Post-Trauma Response Related factors: Abuse, Incest, Rape, Participation in combat

Role Performance, Altered Related factors: Situational crises (specify), Psychologic impairment (specify)

Self-Esteem, Low: Chronic Related factors: Psychologic impairment (specify), Repeatedly unmet expectations

Self-Esteem, Low: Situational Related factor: Situational crisis (specify)

Sensory/Perceptual Alterations: Visual, Auditory, Kinesthetic, Gustatory, Tactile, Olfactory (specify) Related factors: Alcohol/substance abuse (specify); Altered sensory reception, transmission, and/or integration; Sensory deficit (specify); Sensory overload

Social Interaction, Impaired Related factors: Developmental disability, Communication barriers, Psychologic impairment (specify)

Thought Processes, Altered Related factors: Mental disorder (specify), Organic mental disorder (specify), Personality disorder (specify), Substance abuse

Violence, Risk for: Self-Directed or Directed at Others Risk factors: Manic excitement, Panic states, Rage reaction, History of violence, Drug/alcohol intoxication/withdrawal, Temporal lobe epilepsy, Paranoid ideation, Organic brain syndrome, Arrest/conviction pattern, Toxic reaction to medications, Command hallucinations

Borderline Personality Disorder Patient

Anxiety Related factors: Threat to role functioning, Change in role functioning, Situational crises (specify), Maturational crisis (specify), Unmet needs, Threat to or change in environment, Threat to or change in interaction patterns

Coping, Ineffective Family: Disabling Related factors: Conflicting coping styles, Highly ambivalent family relationships, Chronically unresolved feelings (specify)

Coping, Ineffective Individual Related factors: Personal vulnerability in situational crisis (specify), Personal vulnerability in maturational crisis (specify)

Decisional Conflict Related factors: Specific to patient

Parenting, Altered Related factor: Psychologic impairment (borderline personality disorder)

Personal Identity Disturbance Related factors: Situational crises, Psychologic impairment (borderline personality disorder)

Post-Trauma Response Related factors: Abuse, Incest, Rape

Powerlessness Related factor: Pattern of helplessness

Role Performance, Altered Related factors: Situational crises, Psychologic impairment (borderline personality disorder)

Self-Esteem, Low: Chronic Related factors: Psychologic impairment (borderline personality disorder), Repeatedly unmet expectations

Self-Mutilation: Risk for Risk factors: Inability to cope with increased psychologic/physiologic tension in a healthy manner; Feelings of depression, rejection, self-hatred, separation anxiety, guilt, and depersonalization; Fluctuating emotions; Drug/alcohol abuse; History of self-injury; History of physical, emotional, or sexual abuse

Sexuality Patterns, Altered Related factors: Conflict with sexual orientation, Sexual abuse, Impaired relationship with significant person

Social Interaction, Impaired Related factor: Psychologic impairment (borderline personality disorder)

Thought Processes, Altered Related factors: Psychologic impairment (borderline personality disorder), Substance abuse

Violence, Risk for: Self-Directed or Directed at Others Risk factors: Rage reaction, Suicidal ideation, History of self-mutilation, Substance abuse (specify)

Chronically Ill Psychiatric Patient

Associated psychiatric diagnoses include but are not limited to schizophrenia: disorganized type, paranoid type, undifferentiated type; affective disorders: bipolar disorder, major depression (recurrent); eating disorders: anorexia and bulimia; borderline personality disorder; organic mental disorders; substance abuse disorders.

Caregiver Role Strain (Actual/Risk for) Related factors/risk factors: Unpredictable illness course or instability in the care receiver's health; Marginal caregiver's coping patterns; Past history of poor relationship between caregiver and care receiver; Marginal family adaptation or dysfunction prior to the caregiving situation; Psychological problems in care receiver; Care receiver exhibits deviant, bizarre behavior; Presence of abuse or violence; Duration of caregiving required; Inexperience with caregiving

Constipation, Colonic Related factors: Medications, Decreased activity, Chronic use of laxatives/enemas

Constipation, Perceived Related factor: Impaired thought processes

Coping, Ineffective Family: Disabling Related factors: Arbitrary disregard for patient's needs, Chronically unresolved feelings (specify guilt, anxiety, hostility, despair, and so on), Conflicting coping styles, Highly ambivalent family relationships

Denial, Ineffective Related factors: Specific to patient

Diversional Activity Deficit Related factors: Deficit in social skills, Disturbance in motivation, Impaired perception of reality

Fluid Volume Excess Related factor: Increased fluid intake secondary to compulsive water drinking, Medications

Health Maintenance, Altered Related factors: Lack of ability to make deliberate and thoughtful judgments, Lack of material resources, Lack of social supports

Home Maintenance Management, Impaired Related factors: Psychologic impairment (specify), Insufficient family organization or planning, Insufficient finances, Inadequate support system, Lack of knowledge

Injury: Risk for Risk factors: *Psychologic:* Affective factors, Orientation; *Chemical:* Drugs (alcohol, caffeine, nicotine); *Physical:* Exploitation by others

Knowledge Deficit (specify) Related factors: Information misinterpretation, Lack of motivation, Unreadiness to learn, Limited practice of skill (specify)

Noncompliance Related factors: Denial of illness, Negative consequence of treatment regimen, Negative perception of treatment regimen, Perceived benefits of continued illness

Nutrition, Altered: Less Than Body Requirements Related factors: Chemical dependence (specify), Psychologic impairment (specify), Economic factors

Nutrition, Altered: More Than Body Requirements Related factors: Decreased metabolic requirements secondary to medication, Lack of physical exercise, Eating disorder (bulimia)

Parenting, Altered Related factors: Psychologic impairment (specify), Lack of cognitive functioning, Substance abuse (specify), Unmet maturational needs of parent, Physical/emotional abuse of parent

Powerlessness Related factors: Chronic illness, Pattern of helplessness

Self-Care Deficit: Bathing/Hygiene, Dressing/Grooming, Feeding, Toileting (specify) Related factors: Psychologic impairment (specify), Depression, Severe anxiety

Self-Esteem, Low: Chronic Related factors: Repeatedly unmet expectations, Psychologic impairment (specify)

Sensory/Perceptual Alterations: Visual, Auditory, Kinesthetic, Gustatory, Tactile, Olfactory (specify) Related factors: Alcohol/substance abuse (specify), Electrolyte imbalance secondary to anorexia

Sexuality Patterns, Altered Related factors: Lack of significant other, Conflicts with sexual orientation, Disturbance in self-esteem, Body image disturbance, Impaired relationship with significant other

Sleep Pattern Disturbance Related factors: Anxiety, Inactivity, Psychologic impairment (specify)

Social Interaction, Impaired Related factors: Self-concept disturbance, Psychologic impairment (specify), Chemical dependency (specify), Absence of significant other/peer

Social Isolation Related factor: Psychologic impairment (specify)

Therapeutic Regimen Management, Ineffective Individual Related factors: Complexity of health care system, Complexity of therapeutic regimen, Decisional conflict, Economic difficulties, Family conflict, Mistrust of regimen and/or health care personnel, Perceived seriousness, Perceived benefits, Powerlessness, Social support deficits

Thought Processes, Altered Related factors: Mental disorder (specify), Organic mental disorder (specify), Personality disorder (specify), Substance abuse

Violence, Risk for: Self-Directed or Directed at Others Risk factors: History of violence, Panic states, Substance abuse (specify), History of suicide attempts, Arrest/conviction pattern

Eating Disorder Patient

Associated psychiatric diagnoses are limited to anorexia nervosa and bulimia.

Activity Intolerance Related factor: Weakness/fatigue

Anxiety Related factors: Threat to self-concept, Threat to or change in role functioning, Threat to or change in environment, Situational/maturational crises, Unmet needs

Body Image Disturbance Related factor: Eating disorder

Body Temperature, Altered: Risk for Risk factors: Extremes of weight, Inactivity, Vigorous activity, Altered metabolic rate

Constipation Related factor: Dietary changes

Constipation, Colonic Related factors: Less than adequate amounts of fiber and bulk-forming foods in diet, Chronic use of medication and enemas

Constipation, Perceived Related factor: Impaired thought processes

Coping, Ineffective Family: Disabling Related factors: Arbitrary disregard for patient's needs, Chronically unresolved feelings (specify guilt, anxiety, hostility, despair, and so on), Conflicting coping styles, Highly ambivalent family relationships

Coping, Ineffective Individual Related factor: Personal vulnerability in a maturational or situational crisis (specify)

Denial, Ineffective Related factors: Specific to patient

Diarrhea Related factor: Dietary changes

Fatigue Related factor: Altered body chemistry

Fear Related factors: Powerlessness, Real or imagined threat to well-being

Fluid Volume Deficit: Risk for Risk factor: Extremes of weight

Fluid Volume Excess Related factor: Insufficient protein secondary to decreased intake

Infection: Risk for Risk factors: Altered peristalsis, Malnutrition

Knowledge Deficit (specify) Related factor: Limited exposure to information (ie, balanced diet, meal planning)

Noncompliance Related factors: Denial of illness, Negative perception of treatment regimen, Perceived benefits of continued illness

Nutrition, Altered: Less Than Body Requirements Related factor: Psychologic impairment (bulimia, anorexia)

Nutrition, Altered: More Than Body Requirements Related factor: Psychologic impairment (bulimia)

Oral Mucous Membrane, Altered Related factor: Malnutrition

Post-Trauma Response Related factors: Abuse, Incest

Powerlessness Related factor: Chronic illness

Role Performance, Altered Related factor: Psychologic impairment (eating disorder)

Self-Esteem, Low: Chronic Related factors: Psychologic impairment (specify), Repeatedly unmet expectations

Sexuality Patterns, Altered Related factors: Ineffective or absent role models, Body image disturbance, Impaired relationship with significant other, Disturbance in self-esteem

Social Interaction, Impaired Related factor: Psychologic impairment (anorexia, bulimia)

Therapeutic Regimen Management, Ineffective Individual Related factors: Decisional conflict, Family conflict, Mistrust of regimen and/or health care personnel, Perceived seriousness, Perceived benefits, Powerlessness

Thought Processes, Altered Related factor: Mental disorder (anorexia, bulimia)

Manic Patient

Associated psychiatric diagnoses include but are not limited to bipolar disorders (manic, mixed), manic episode, schizophrenia (undifferentiated type, catatonic type), schizoaffective disorder, substance abuse disorders.

Anxiety Related factors: Change in role functioning, Change in environment, Change in interaction patterns, Unmet needs

Coping, Defensive Related factor: Psychologic impairment (specify)

Coping, Ineffective Individual Related factor: Personal vulnerability in a situational crisis (specify)

Denial, Ineffective Related factors: Specific to patient

Diarrhea Related factor: Medications (lithium)

Family Processes, Altered Related factor: Illness/disability of family member

Fluid Volume Deficit Related factor: Inadequate fluid intake

Fluid Volume Excess Related factor: Increased fluid intake secondary to lithium therapy

Health Maintenance, Altered Related factors: Significant alteration in communication skills, Lack of ability to make deliberate and thoughtful judgments

Home Maintenance Management, Impaired Related factor: Psychologic impairment (specify)

Injury: Risk for Risk factors: *Psychologic:* Affective factors, Orientation; *Chemical:* Drugs (alcohol, caffeine, nicotine); *Physical:* Cognitive, affective, and psychomotor factors

Noncompliance Related factors: Denial of illness, Negative perception of treatment regimen

Nutrition, Altered: Less Than Body Requirements Related factor: Psychologic impairment (specify)

Parenting, Altered Related factor: Psychologic impairment (specify)

Personal Identity Disturbance Related factor: Psychologic impairment (specify)

Role Performance, Altered Related factor: Psychologic impairment (specify)

Self-Care Deficit: Bathing/Hygiene, Dressing/Grooming, Feeding, Toileting (specify) Related factor: Psychologic impairment (specify)

Sexuality Patterns, Altered Related factor: Psychologic impairment (specify)

Sleep Pattern Disturbance Related factors: Psychologic impairment (specify), Sleep deprivation

Social Interaction, Impaired Related factor: Psychologic impairment (specify)

Thought Processes, Altered Related factor: Mental disorder (specify)

Violence, Risk for: Self-Directed or Directed at Others Risk factors: Manic excitement, Rage reaction, History of violence, Command hallucinations, Toxic reaction to medications

Paranoid Patient

Associated psychiatric diagnoses include but are not limited to schizophrenia: undifferentiated type, paranoid type; affective disorders: major depression (single episode, recurrent), bipolar disorders (mixed, manic, depressed), schizoaffective disorder; paranoid disorders; substance abuse disorders; organic mental disorders; personality disorders.

Anxiety Related factors: Threat to or change in role functioning, Change in environment, Threat to or change in interaction pattern

Coping, Defensive Related factor: Psychologic impairment (specify)

Coping, Ineffective Individual Related factor: Personal vulnerability in situational crisis

Family Processes, Altered Related factor: Illness/disability of family member

Fear Related factor: Imagined threat to own well-being

Health Maintenance, Altered Related factors: Significant alteration in communication skills, Lack of ability to make deliberate and thoughtful judgments

Home Maintenance Management, Impaired Related factor: Psychologic impairment (specify)

Noncompliance Related factors: Denial of illness, Negative perception of treatment regimen

Nutrition, Altered: Less Than Body Requirements Related factor: Psychologic impairment (specify)

Parenting, Altered Related factor: Psychologic impairment (specify)

Personal Identity Disturbance Related factor: Psychologic impairment (specify)

Post-Trauma Response Related factors: Abuse, Incest

Powerlessness Related factors: Health care environment, Treatment regimen

Role Performance, Altered Related factor: Psychologic impairment (specify)

Self-Care Deficit: Bathing/Hygiene, Dressing/Grooming, Feeding, Toileting (specify) Related factor: Psychologic impairment (specify)

Self-Esteem Disturbance Related factor: Psychologic impairment (specify)

Sexuality Patterns, Altered Related factors: Impaired relationship with significant other, Conflicts with sexual orientation

Sleep Pattern Disturbance Related factor: Psychologic impairment

Social Interaction, Impaired Related factor: Psychologic impairment (specify)

Thought Processes, Altered Related factors: Mental disorder (specify), Organic mental disorder (specify), Personality disorder (specify)

Violence, Risk for: Self-Directed or Directed at Others Risk factors: Panic states, Drug/alcohol intoxication/withdrawal, Paranoid ideation, Organic brain syndrome, Command hallucinations

Phobic Patient

Associated psychiatric diagnoses include but are not limited to agoraphobia, simple phobia, social phobia.

Anxiety Related factors: Threat to or change in role functioning, Threat to or change in environment, Threat to self-concept, Threat to or change in interaction pattern, Unmet needs

Coping, Ineffective Individual Related factors: Personal vulnerability in situational crisis (specify), Personal vulnerability in maturational crisis (specify)

Denial, Ineffective Related factors: Specific to patient

Diversional Activity Deficit Related factor: Impaired perception of reality

Family Processes, Altered Related factor: Illness of family member

Fear Related factor: Real or imagined threat to own well-being

Post-Trauma Response Related factors: Abuse, Assault, Accidents, Disaster, Incest

Powerlessness Related factor: Phobic disorder

Rape-Trauma Syndrome Related factor: Biopsychosocial response to event

Role Performance, Altered Related factor: Psychologic impairment (phobic disorder)

Social Interaction, Impaired Related factor: Psychologic impairment (phobic disorder)

Social Isolation Related factor: Psychologic impairment (phobic disorder)

Thought Processes, Altered Related factor: Mental disorder (phobic disorder)

Psychotic Patient

Associated psychiatric diagnoses include but are not limited to schizophrenia: disorganized type, catatonic type, paranoid type, undifferentiated type; schizophreniform disorder; affective disorders: manic episode, major depressive episode, bipolar disorders (mixed, manic, depressed); organic mental disorders; substance abuse disorders.

Communication, Impaired: Verbal Related factor: Psychologic impairment (specify)

Coping, Defensive Related factor: Psychologic impairment (specify)

Denial, Ineffective Related factors: Specific to patient

Diversional Activity Deficit Related factors: Disturbance in motivation, Impaired perception of reality

Family Processes, Altered Related factors: Hospitalization/change in environment, Illness/disability of family member

Health Maintenance, Altered Related factors: Lack of ability to make deliberate and thoughtful judgments

Home Maintenance Management, Impaired Related factor: Psychologic impairment (specify)

Injury: Risk for Risk factors: *Psychologic:* Affective factors, Orientation; *Chemical:* Drugs (alcohol, caffeine, nicotine); *Physical:* Cognitive, affective, and psychomotor factors

Noncompliance Related factors: Denial of illness, Negative perception of treatment regimen

Parenting, Altered Related factor: Psychologic impairment (specify)

Personal Identity Disturbance Related factor: Psychologic impairment (specify)

Role Performance, Altered Related factor: Psychologic impairment (specify)

Self-Care Deficit: Bathing/Hygiene, Dressing/Grooming, Feeding, Toileting (specify) Related factor: Psychologic impairment (specify)

Self-Esteem Disturbance Related factor: Psychologic impairment (specify)

Self-Mutilation: Risk for Risk factors: Fluctuating emotions, Command hallucinations, Clients in psychotic state—frequently males in young adulthood

Sleep Pattern Disturbance Related factor: Psychologic impairment (specify)

Social Interaction, Impaired Related factor: Psychologic impairment (specify)

Thought Processes, Altered Related factors: Mental disorder (specify), Organic mental disorder (specify)

Violence, Risk for: Self-Directed or Directed at Others Risk factors: Paranoid ideation, Suicide ideation, History of violence, Substance abuse (specify)

Severely Depressed Patient

Associated psychiatric diagnoses include but are not limited to bipolar disorder, depressed; major depression; dysthymic disorder.

Activity Intolerance Related factors: Weakness/fatigue, Depression

Anxiety Related factors: Change in role functioning, Change in interaction patterns, Threat to self-concept

Constipation Related factors: Decreased activity, Medication (specify)

Coping, Ineffective Individual Related factors: Personal vulnerability in situational crisis, Personal vulnerability in maturational crisis

Denial, Ineffective Related factors: Specific to patient

Diversional Activity Deficit Related factor: Disturbance in motivation

Family Processes, Altered Related factor: Illness/disability of family member

Fatigue Related factor: Overwhelming psychologic demands

Fear Related factors: Real or imagined threat to own well-being, Powerlessness

Fluid Volume Deficit: Risk for Risk factor: Deviations affecting access to or intake of fluids

Grieving, Dysfunctional Related factors: Actual loss (specify), Anticipated loss (specify), Perceived loss (specify)

Health Maintenance, Altered Related factors: Lack of ability to make deliberate and thoughtful judgments, Significant alteration in communication skills

Home Maintenance Management, Impaired Related factor: Psychologic impairment (specify)

Hopelessness Related factor: Long-term stress

Injury: Risk for Risk factors: *Psychologic:* Affective factors, Orientation; *Chemical:* Drugs (alcohol, caffeine, nicotine); *Physical:* Cognitive, affective, and psychomotor factors

Nutrition, Altered: Less Than Body Requirements Related factor: Psychologic impairment (specify)

Nutrition, Altered: More Than Body Requirements Related factor: Psychologic impairment (specify)

Oral Mucous Membrane, Altered Related factor: Medication (antidepressants)

Parenting, Altered Related factor: Psychologic impairment (specify)

Personal Identity Disturbance Related factor: Psychologic impairment (specify)

Post-Trauma Response Related factors: Abuse, Accidents, Assault, Disaster, Epidemic, Incest, Kidnapping, Rape, Torture, Catastrophic illness or accident, Participation in combat

Powerlessness Related factor: Psychologic impairment (specify)

Rape-Trauma Syndrome Related factor: Biopsychosocial response by patient to event

Role Performance, Altered Related factor: Psychologic impairment (specify)

Self-Care Deficit: Bathing/Hygiene, Dressing/Grooming, Feeding, Toileting (specify) Related factor: Depression

Self-Esteem, Low: Chronic Related factors: Psychologic impairment (specify), Repeatedly unmet expectations

Self-Mutilation: Risk for Risk factors: Inability to cope with increased psychologic/physiologic tension in a healthy manner; Feelings of depression, rejection, self-hatred, separation anxiety, guilt, and depersonalization

Sexuality Patterns, Altered Related factor: Disturbance in self-esteem, lack of energy

Sleep Pattern Disturbance Related factors: Anxiety, Psychologic impairment (depression)

Social Interaction, Impaired Related factor: Psychologic impairment (depression)

Thought Processes, Altered Related factor: Mental disorder (specify)

Violence, Risk for: Self-Directed or Directed at Others Risk factor: Suicidal ideation/intent

Substance Abuse Patient

Alcohol/drug intoxication/withdrawal/dependence.

Anxiety Related factors: Change in health status, Change in role functioning, Situational crisis, Unmet needs

Body Temperature, Altered: Risk for Risk factor: Dehydration

Coping, Defensive Related factor: Psychologic impairment (substance abuse)

Coping, Ineffective Family: Compromised Related factors: Temporary family disorganization and role changes, Unrealistic expectations/demands, Lack of mutual decision-making skills, Inadequate information/understanding by family member

Coping, Ineffective Family: Disabling Related factors: Arbitrary disregard for patient's needs, Chronically unresolved feelings (specify guilt, anxiety, hostility, despair, and so on), Conflicting coping styles, Highly ambivalent family relationships, Violence used to manage conflict

Coping, Ineffective Individual Related factors: Personal vulnerability in situational crisis (specify), Personal vulnerability in maturational crisis (specify)

Decisional Conflict Related factor: Chemical dependence

Denial, Ineffective Related factors: Specific to patient

Diarrhea Related factors: Excessive alcohol intake, Excessive substance abuse

Fluid Volume Deficit: Risk for Risk factor: Excessive, continuous consumption of alcohol

Fluid Volume Excess Related factor: Increased fluid intake secondary to thirst

Grieving, Dysfunctional Related factors: Actual loss (specify), Anticipated loss (specify), Perceived loss (specify)

Health Maintenance, Altered Related factor: Lack of ability to make deliberate and thoughtful judgments

Home Maintenance Management, Impaired Related factors: Insufficient family organization or planning, Psychologic impairment (substance abuse)

Injury: Risk for Risk factors: *Psychologic:* Affective factors, Orientation; *Chemical:* Drugs (alcohol, caffeine, nicotine)

Noncompliance Related factors: Denial of illness, Negative perception of treatment regimen

Nutrition, Altered: Less Than Body Requirements Related factor: Chemical dependence (specify)

Pain, Chronic Related factors: Specific to patient

Parenting, Altered Related factors: Dysfunctional relationship between parents, Change in marital status, Psychologic impairment (substance abuse)

Post-Trauma Response Related factors: Abuse, Accidents, Assault, Disaster, Epidemic, Incest, Kidnapping, Torture, Terrorism, Participation in combat

Powerlessness Related factor: Pattern of helplessness

Rape-Trauma Syndrome Related factor: Biopsychosocial response of patient to event

Role Performance, Altered Related factor: Psychologic impairment (substance abuse)

Self-Esteem, Low: Chronic Related factor: Repeatedly unmet expectations

Self-Mutilation: Risk for Risk factors: Inability to cope with increased psychologic/physiologic tension in a healthy manner, Drug/alcohol abuse

Sensory/Perceptual Alterations: Visual, Auditory, Kinesthetic, Tactile Related factors: Alcohol intoxication, Substance intoxication (specify)

Sexuality Patterns, Altered Related factors: Disturbance in self-esteem, Substance abuse

Sleep Pattern Disturbance Related factor: Chemical dependence (specify)

Social Interaction, Impaired Related factor: Chemical dependence (specify)

Therapeutic Regimen Management, Ineffective Individual Related factors: Decisional Conflict, Family patterns of health care, Inadequate number and types of cues to action, Knowledge deficit, Perceived seriousness, Perceived benefits, Powerlessness, Social support deficits

Violence, Risk for: Self-Directed or Directed at Others Risk factors: Substance intoxication (specify), Substance withdrawal (specify)

Suicidal Patient

Associated psychiatric diagnoses include but are not limited to schizophrenia: disorganized type, catatonic type, paranoid type, undifferentiated type; schizophreniform disorder; affective disorders: manic episode, major depressive episode, bipolar disorders (mixed, manic, depressed), major depression (single episode, recurrent); panic disorders; post-traumatic stress disorder; organic mental disorders: primary degenerative dementia with depression, multi-infarct dementia with depression, alcohol/substance intoxication/withdrawal/dependence; personality disorders: borderline personality disorder, schizoid personality disorder.

Anxiety Related factors: Threat to self-concept, Threat to/change in role functioning, Situational/maturational crises, Unmet needs

Coping, Ineffective Family: Compromised Related factors: Temporary family disorganization and role changes, Unrealistic expectations/demands, Lack of mutual decision-making skills, Inadequate understanding by family member

Coping, Ineffective Family: Disabling Related factor: Highly ambivalent family relationships

Coping, Ineffective Individual Related factors: Personal vulnerability in situational crisis (specify), Personal vulnerability in maturational crisis (specify)

Decisional Conflict Related factors: Perceived threat to value system, Lack of support system

Denial, Ineffective Related factors: Specific to patient

Fear Related factors: Powerlessness, Real or imagined threat to own well-being

Hopelessness Related factors: Abandonment, Lack of social supports, Lost spiritual belief

Personal Identity Disturbance Related factor: Situational crisis (specify)

Post-Trauma Response Related factors: Abuse, Accidents, Assault, Disaster, Epidemic, Incest, Kidnapping, Terrorism, Torture, Catastrophic illness or accident, Participation in combat

Rape-Trauma Syndrome Related factor: Patient's biopsychosocial response to event

Role Performance, Altered Related factors: Situational crisis (specify), Psychologic impairment (specify)

Self-Esteem, Low: Chronic Related factors: Psychologic impairment (specify), Repeatedly unmet expectations

Self-Esteem, Low: Situational Related factor: Situational crisis (specify)

Self-Mutilation: Risk for Risk factors: Inability to cope with increased psychologic/physiologic tension in a healthy manner; Feelings of depression, rejection, self-hatred, separation anxiety, guilt, and depersonalization; Fluctuating emotions; Drug/alcohol abuse

Sensory/Perceptual Alterations: Visual, Auditory, Kinesthetic, Gustatory, Tactile, Olfactory (specify) Related factor: Alcohol/substance abuse (specify)

Thought Processes, Altered Related factors: Mental disorder (specify), Organic mental disorder (specify), Personality disorder (specify), Substance abuse

Violence, Risk for: Self-Directed or Directed at Others Risk factors: History of suicide attempt, Command hallucinations, Battered women, Panic states, History of abuse by others, Suicidal ideation, Substance abuse

Withdrawn Patient

Associated psychiatric diagnoses include but are not limited to major depression; schizophrenia: disorganized type, catatonic type, paranoid type, undifferentiated type; schizophreniform disorder; phobic disorders; schizoid personality disorder; avoidant personality disorder; substance abuse disorders; organic mental disorders.

Anxiety Related factors: Threat to role functioning, Change in role functioning

Communication, Impaired: Verbal Related factor: Psychologic impairment (specify)

Coping, Ineffective Individual Related factors: Personal vulnerability in situational crisis (specify), Personal vulnerability in maturational crisis (specify)

Denial, Ineffective Related factors: Specific to patient

Diversional Activity Deficit Related factors: Disturbance in motivation, Deficit in social skills, Impaired perception of reality

Family Processes, Altered Related factor: Illness/disability of family member

Fear Related factors: Powerlessness, Real or imagined threat to own well-being

Grieving, Dysfunctional Related factors: Actual loss (specify), Anticipated loss (specify), Perceived loss (specify)

Health Maintenance, Altered Related factors: Lack of ability to make thoughtful and deliberate judgments, Significant alteration in communication skills

Hopelessness Related factors: Lack of social supports, Long-term stress

Parenting, Altered Related factors: Psychologic impairment (specify), Situational crisis (specify)

Post-Trauma Response Related factors: Abuse, Accidents, Assault, Disaster, Epidemic, Incest, Kidnapping, Terrorism, Torture, Catastrophic illness or event, Participation in combat

Rape-Trauma Syndrome: Silent Reaction Related factor: Patient's biopsychosocial response to event

Role Performance, Altered Related factor: Psychologic impairment (specify)

Self-Esteem, Low: Chronic Related factors: Psychologic impairment (specify), Repeatedly unmet expectations

Self-Esteem, Low: Situational Related factor: Situational crisis

Self-Mutilation: Risk for Risk factors: Inability to cope with increased psychologic/physiologic tension in a healthy manner; Feelings of depression, rejection, self-hatred, separation anxiety, guilt, and depersonalization; Need for sensory stimuli

Sleep Pattern Disturbance Related factor: Psychologic impairment (specify)

Social Interaction, Impaired Related factor: Psychologic impairment (specify)

Social Isolation Related factor: Psychologic impairment (specify)

Thought Processes, Altered Related factors: Mental disorder (specify), Organic mental disorder (specify), Personality disorder (specify)

Antepartum and Postpartum Conditions

Abortion, induced or elective
Change in birthing plans
Gestational diabetes
Hyperemesis gravidarum
Maternal infection
Painful breast
Perinatal loss
Postpartum care, uncomplicated
Pregnancy-induced hypertension
Suppression of preterm labor
Uterine bleeding

Abortion, Induced or Elective

Coping, Ineffective Individual Related factor: Unresolved feelings about elective abortion

Fluid Volume Deficit Related factor: Abnormal blood loss secondary to incomplete abortion

Infection: Risk for Risk factors: Invasive procedures, Broken skin, Traumatized tissue

Knowledge Deficit (specify) Related factor: Limited exposure to information (contraception)

Pain [Acute] Related factor: Strong uterine contractions

Powerlessness Related factor: Treatment regimen

Self-Esteem Disturbance Related factors: Unmet expectations for pregnancy, Unmet expectations for child

Sexual Dysfunction Related factor: Disturbance in self-esteem

Spiritual Distress Related factor: Test of spiritual beliefs

Change in Birthing Plans

May include any deviation from a couple's original birthing plans. Includes but is not limited to use of analgesia, anesthesia, or forceps, limitation of visitors, episiotomy, cesarean birth.

Body Image Disturbance Related factor: Surgery

Family Processes, Altered Related factor: Unmet expectations for childbirth

Fear Related factors: Real or imagined threat to child, Real or imagined threat to own well-being

Knowledge Deficit (specify) Related factor: Limited exposure to information

Pain [Acute] Related factors: Surgery, Episiotomy

Powerlessness Related factor: Complication threatening pregnancy

Role Performance, Altered Related factor: Unmet expectations for childbirth

Self-Esteem Disturbance Related factor: Unmet expectations for childbirth

Gestational Diabetes

Family Processes, Altered Related factors: Hospitalization/change in environment, Illness/disability of family member

Fear Related factors: Environmental stressors/hospitalization, Powerlessness, Real or imagined threat to own well-being, Real or imagined threat to child, Implications for future pregnancies

Injury: Risk for (Maternal or Fetal) Risk factors: Hypoglycemia, Hyperglycemia

Knowledge Deficit (specify) Related factors: Limited exposure to information (specify), Signs and symptoms of premature labor, Premature rupture of membranes, Blood glucose testing, Insulin dosage and administration

Nutrition, Altered: Less Than Body Requirements Related factor: Limited exposure to new basic nutritional knowledge

Nutrition, Altered: More Than Body Requirements Related factor: Limited exposure to new basic nutritional knowledge

Self-Esteem Disturbance Related factor: Unmet expectations for pregnancy

Therapeutic Regimen Management, Ineffective Individual Related factors: Complexity of therapeutic regimen, Knowledge deficits, Perceived seriousness, Social supports deficits

Hyperemesis Gravidarum

Coping, Ineffective Individual Related factor: Personal vulnerability during health crisis

Family Processes, Altered Related factors: Hospitalization/change in environment, Illness/disability of family member

Fatigue Related factor: Disease process

Fear Related factor: Real or imagined threat to child

Fluid Volume Deficit Related factors: Inadequate fluid intake, Abnormal fluid loss secondary to vomiting

Knowledge Deficit (specify) Related factor: Limited exposure to information (specify)

Nutrition, Altered: Less Than Body Requirements Related factor: Nausea and/or vomiting

Powerlessness Related factor: Complications threatening pregnancy

Role Performance, Altered Related factors: Unmet expectations for pregnancy, Nausea

Self-Esteem Disturbance Related factor: Unmet expectations for pregnancy

Maternal Infection

Includes but is not limited to active genital herpes, amnionitis, acquired immune deficiency syndrome, hepatitis B.

Body Image Disturbance Related factors: Pregnancy, Infection

Breast-Feeding, Interrupted Related factors: Maternal illness, Maternal medications that are contraindicated for the infant

Family Processes, Altered Related factors: Change in family roles, Hospitalization/change in environment

Fatigue Related factor: Disease process

Fear Related factor: Real or imagined threat to child

Knowledge Deficit (specify) Related factor: Limited exposure to information (specify)

Pain [Acute] Related factors: Cesarean birth, Infection

Parenting, Altered: Risk for Risk factor: Delayed parent/infant attachment

Self-Esteem Disturbance Related factors: Cesarean birth, Assumption of new role

Social Interaction, Impaired Related factor: Therapeutic isolation

Painful Breast

Includes but is not limited to sore, cracked nipples, engorgement, mastitis.

Breast-Feeding, Ineffective Related factor: Breast pain

Breast-Feeding, Interrupted Related factors: Engorgement; Sore, cracked nipples; Mastitis; Maternal medications that are contraindicated for the infant

Knowledge Deficit (specify) Related factors: Limited exposure to information about breast hygiene, Limited exposure to information about care of nipples, Limited exposure to information about signs and symptoms of infection

Pain [Acute] Related factors: Sore nipples, Breast engorgement, Infection

Role Performance, Altered Related factors: Assumption of new role, Unmet expectations for childbirth

Skin Integrity, Impaired: Risk for Risk factors: Inadequate breast care, Breast-feeding

Perinatal Loss

Includes but is not limited to less than perfect baby, miscarriage, stillbirth, adoption, elective abortion.

Coping, Ineffective Family: Disabling Related factor: Chronically unresolved feelings about loss

Coping, Ineffective Individual Related factor: Personal vulnerability in a situational crisis

Family Processes, Altered Related factors: Illness/disability of baby, Lack of adequate support system

Fear Related factors: Real or imagined threat to child, Environmental stressors/hospitalization, Powerlessness, Implications for future pregnancies

Grieving, Anticipatory Related factors: Imminent loss of child, Anticipated loss of perfect child

Grieving, Dysfunctional Related factors: Actual or anticipated loss of child, Actual or anticipated loss of perfect child

Knowledge Deficit (specify) Related factors: Limited exposure to information (specify), Limited practice of skill (specify), Information misinterpretation

Parenting, Altered Related factors: Interruption in bonding process, Unrealistic expectations of self or partner

Powerlessness Related factor: Complication threatening pregnancy

Role Performance, Altered Related factors: Loss of child, Birth of less than perfect baby

Self-Esteem Disturbance Related factor: Unmet expectations for child

Sexual Dysfunction Related factors: Medically imposed restrictions, Fear of harming fetus, Disturbance in self-esteem

Spiritual Distress Related factor: Test of spiritual beliefs

Postpartum Care, Uncomplicated

Activity Intolerance Related factor: Weakness/fatigue

Anxiety Related factor: Change in role functioning

Body Image Disturbance Related factor: Lack of or inaccurate information about body's adjustment after delivery

Breast-Feeding, Effective (Potential for Enhanced) Related factors: Basic breast-feeding knowledge, Normal breast structure, Normal infant oral structure, Gestational age of more than 34 weeks, Supportive resources, Maternal confidence

Constipation Related factors: Painful defecation, Decreased activity, Decreased fluid intake

Coping, Ineffective Individual Related factor: Personal vulnerability in a maturational crisis

Family Processes, Altered Related factors: Change in family roles, Change in family structure, Lack of adequate support systems

Fluid Volume Deficit Related factors: Abnormal fluid loss secondary to diuresis, Decreased fluid intake

Home Maintenance Management, Impaired Related factor: Inadequate support system

Infection: Risk for Risk factors: Broken skin, Traumatized tissue, Invasive procedures

Knowledge Deficit (specify) Related factor: Lack of exposure to information about self-care, baby care, bonding, family-planning methods, infant growth and development

Nutrition, Altered: Less Than Body Requirements Related factor: Lack of basic nutritional knowledge concerning lactation

Pain [Acute] Related factors: Pain secondary to episiotomy, Sore nipples, Breast engorgement, Hemorrhoids, Spinal headache

Parenting, Altered: Risk for Risk factors: Lack of knowledge/skill regarding effective parenting; Unrealistic expectations of self, infant, partner

Role Performance, Altered Related factor: Assumption of new role

Sexual Dysfunction Related factors: Pain, Recent childbirth, Disturbance in self-esteem

Sleep Pattern Disturbance Related factors: Excessive social demands, Role demands, Pain

Pregnancy-Induced Hypertension

Also known as toxemia of pregnancy, preeclampsia, eclampsia.

Activity Intolerance Related factors: Imbalance between oxygen supply and demand, Weakness/fatigue

Body Image Disturbance Related factors: Pregnancy and edema

Cardiac Output, Decreased Related factor: Increased ventricular workload

Diversional Activity Deficit Related factor: Prolonged bed rest

Family Processes, Altered Related factors: Hospitalization/change in environment, Illness/disability of family member

Fatigue Related factor: Disease process

Fear Related factors: Changes in birthing plans, Real or imagined threat to child, Environmental stressors/hospitalization, Real or imagined threat to own well-being, Implications for future pregnancies

Fluid Volume Excess Related factors: Sodium and water retention

Home Maintenance Management, Impaired Related factor: Inadequate support system

Injury: Risk for (Maternal and Fetal) Risk factors: Seizure activity, Inadequate placental perfusion

Knowledge Deficit (specify) Related factor: Limited exposure to information (specify)

Nutrition, Altered: Less Than Body Requirements Related factors: Lack of basic nutritional knowledge, Loss of appetite, Nausea/vomiting

Powerlessness Related factor: Complications threatening pregnancy

Therapeutic Regimen Management, Ineffective Individual Related factors: Knowledge deficits, Perceived seriousness, Perceived benefits

Tissue Perfusion, Altered: Cerebral, Renal, Placental Related factors: Vasospasm, Edema, Decreased intravascular volume

Suppression of Preterm Labor

Anxiety Related factor: Outcome of pregnancy

Coping, Ineffective Individual Related factor: Personal vulnerability in situational crisis

Diversional Activity Deficit Related factor: Prolonged bed rest

Family Processes, Altered Related factors: Illness/disability of family member, Change in family roles, Lack of adequate support systems

Fear Related factor: Possibility of early labor and delivery

Home Maintenance Management, Impaired Related factor: Inadequate support system

Knowledge Deficit (specify) Related factor: Limited exposure to information about causes, identification, and treatment of preterm labor

Powerlessness Related factor: Complications threatening pregnancy

Self-Care Deficit: Bathing/Hygiene, Dressing/Grooming, Feeding, Toileting (specify) Related factor: Medically imposed restrictions

Self-Esteem Disturbance Related factor: Unmet expectations for childbirth

Sexual Dysfunction Related factors: Medically imposed restrictions, Fear of harming fetus

Sleep Pattern Disturbance Related factors: Frequency of medication and monitoring

Therapeutic Regimen Management, Ineffective Individual Related factors: Knowledge deficits, Excessive demands made on individual/family, Social support deficits

Uterine Bleeding

Includes but is not limited to the following: antepartal: first trimester spotting, placenta previa, abruptio placentae, uterine rupture, hydatidiform mole; postpartal: postpartum hemorrhage/shock, uterine atony.

Breast-Feeding, Interrupted Related factors: Maternal illness, Fatigue

Cardiac Output, Decreased Related factor: Hypovolemia

Diversional Activity Deficit Related factors: Prolonged bed rest

Family Processes, Altered Related factors: Change in family roles, Hospitalization/change in environment, Illness/disability of family member

Fear Related factors: Real or imagined threat to child, Real or imagined threat to own well-being, Powerlessness, Environmental stressors/hospitalization, Implications for future pregnancies

Fluid Volume Deficit Related factor: Abnormal blood loss

Home Maintenance Management, Impaired Related factor: Inadequate support system

Infection: Risk for Risk factors: Traumatized tissue, Invasive procedures

Knowledge Deficit (specify) Related factor: Limited exposure to information regarding recovery

Pain [Acute] Related factors: Nausea and/or vomiting, Surgical procedure, Uterine contractions

Powerlessness Related factor: Complications threatening pregnancy

Self-Care Deficit: Bathing/Hygiene, Dressing/Grooming, Feeding, Toileting (specify) Related factor: Medically imposed restrictions

Self-Esteem Disturbance Related factor: Unmet expectations for childbirth

Sexual Dysfunction Related factors: Medically imposed restrictions, Fear of harming fetus

Tissue Perfusion, Altered: Placental Related factor: Imbalance between oxygen supply/demand to the fetus secondary to hypovolemia, hypotension, placental separation

Newborn Conditions

Bleeding/obstruction of urinary tract postcircumcision
Drug withdrawal
Feeding problems
High-risk infant
Hyperbilirubinemia
Hypoglycemia
Hypothermia
Inability to adapt to extrauterine life
Low birth weight
Respiratory distress

Bleeding/Obstruction of Urinary Tract Postcircumcision

Fluid Volume Deficit Related factor: Abnormal blood loss

Pain [Acute] Related factor: Surgery

Urinary Retention Related factor: Urethral obstruction

Drug Withdrawal

Breast-Feeding, Ineffective Related factor: Infant fatigue

Breathing Pattern, Ineffective Related factor: Depression of respiratory center secondary to ____ (specify drug)

Coping, Ineffective Family: Disabling Related factor: Arbitrary disregard for patient's needs

Fluid Volume Deficit Related factor: Inadequate fluid intake secondary to inadequate sucking reflex

Growth and Development, Altered Related factor: Unhealthy maternal life-style during pregnancy

Home Maintenance Management, Impaired Related factors: Physical/psychologic impairment of family member other than patient, Inadequate support system, Insufficient family organization or planning

Infant Feeding Pattern, Ineffective Related factor: Neurological impairment/delay

Injury: Risk for Risk factors: Psychomotor hyperactivity, Seizure activity

Nutrition, Altered: Less Than Body Requirements Related factors: Chemical dependence, Inadequate sucking reflex in infant, Vomiting, Food intolerance

Parenting, Altered Related factors: Psychologic impairment, Substance abuse

Sleep Pattern Disturbance Related factors: Sleep deprivation secondary to ____ (specify), Effect of depressants or stimulants

Feeding Problems

Include but are not limited to the infant with food allergies or intolerances, malabsorption, or abnormal motor problems that affect the infant's ability to consume food.

Breast-Feeding, Ineffective Related factors: Inadequate sucking reflex in infant, Infant fatigue, Inability of infant to "latch on"

Constipation Related factor: Decreased fluid intake

Diarrhea Related factor: Food intolerance

Family Processes, Altered Related factors: Illness/disability of family member, Separation of family members

Fluid Volume Deficit Related factor: Inadequate fluid intake

Infant Feeding Pattern, Ineffective Related factors: Prematurity, Neurological impairment/delay, Oral hypersensitivity, Prolonged NPO, Anatomical abnormalities

Nutrition, Altered: Less Than Body Requirements Related factors: Difficulty in swallowing, Inadequate sucking reflex in the infant, Vomiting, Food intolerance

Swallowing, Impaired Related factor: Abnormal motor problem (specify)

High-Risk Infant

Includes but is not limited to birth asphyxia, meconium aspiration, prematurity, premature rupture of membranes, maternal infection, infant of diabetic mother, intrauterine growth retardation, infant of adolescent mother, infant of chemically dependent mother, lack of prenatal care.

Airway Clearance, Ineffective Related factors: Meconium aspiration, Tracheobronchial secretions

Aspiration: Risk for Risk factor: Presence of enteral or tracheal tubes

Body Temperature, Altered: Risk for Risk factor: Immaturity of newborn's temperature-regulating system

Breast-Feeding, Ineffective Related factors: Infant fatigue, Inadequate sucking reflex, Interrupted or infrequent feeding

Breast-Feeding, Interrupted Related factors: Infant illness, Prematurity, Maternal obligations outside the home, Abrupt weaning of infant

Breathing Pattern, Ineffective Related factor: Decreased energy/fatigue

Cardiac Output, Decreased Related factors: Increased ventricular workload, Hypovolemia, Cardiac anomaly (specify)

Caregiver Role Strain (Actual/Risk for) Related factors/risk factors: Illness severity of the care receiver; Premature birth/congenital defect; Unpredictable illness course; Situational stressors within the family; Chronicity of caregiving; Caregiver's health, developmental readiness, knowledge, skills, experience, competing role commitments, coping styles, isolation, opportunity for respite and recreation

Diarrhea Related factor: Increased intestinal motility secondary to inflammation

Dysfunctional Ventilatory Weaning Response (DVWR) Related factors: Pulmonary immaturity, Impaired gas exchange, Ineffective airway clearance, Ventilator dependence > 1 week

Family Processes, Altered Related factors: Illness/disability of family member, Separation of family members

Fatigue Related factor: Disease process

Fear (Parental) Related factor: Threat to child

Fluid Volume Deficit Related factors: Abnormal blood loss, Abnormal fluid loss (specify), Inadequate fluid intake secondary to ____ (specify)

Fluid Volume Excess Related factor: Decreased urinary output secondary to heart failure

Gas Exchange, Impaired Related factor: Decreased functional lung tissue secondary to pneumonia, chronic lung disease, atelectasis

Grieving, Anticipatory (Parental) Related factor: Imminent loss of child

Growth and Development, Altered Related factors: Congenital anomaly, Fetal distress, Prematurity, Unhealthy maternal life-style during pregnancy, Serious illness

Home Maintenance Management, Impaired Related factors: Inadequate support system, Insufficient family organization or planning

Infant Feeding Pattern, Ineffective Related factors: Prematurity, Neurological impairment/delay, Prolonged NPO, Anatomical abnormalities

Infection: Risk for Risk factors: Inadequate immune system, Insufficient family organization or planning

Nutrition, Altered: Less Than Body Requirements Related factors: Inadequate sucking reflex in the infant, Vomiting, Food intolerance, High metabolic rate

Spontaneous Ventilation, Inability to Sustain Related factors: Metabolic factors, Respiratory muscle fatigue, Pulmonary immaturity

Hyperbilirubinemia

Breast-Feeding, Interrupted Related factor: Infant illness

Diarrhea Related factor: Dietary changes

Family Processes, Altered Related factor: Separation of family members

Fluid Volume Deficit Related factors: Abnormal fluid loss (specify), Inadequate fluid intake secondary to ___ (specify)

Nutrition, Altered: Less Than Body Requirements Related factors: Lethargy, Inadequate sucking reflex in infant

Parenting, Altered Related factor: Interruption in bonding process

Sensory/Perceptual Alterations: Visual Related factor: Sensory deficit secondary to use of eye patches for protection of eyes during phototherapy

Skin Integrity, Impaired: Risk for Risk factors: Incontinence of stool, Drying of skin secondary to phototherapy, Pruritus

Sleep Pattern Disturbance Related factor: Sleep deprivation

Hypoglycemia

Cardiac Output, Decreased Related factor: Poor cardiac contractility

Family Processes, Altered Related factors: Illness/disability of family member, Separation of family members

Injury: Risk for Risk factor: Seizure activity

Nutrition, Altered: Less Than Body Requirements Related factors: Inadequate sucking reflex in infant, High metabolic rate/physiologic stress

Hypothermia

Breathing Pattern, Ineffective Related factor: Decreased energy/fatigue

Cardiac Output, Decreased Related factor: Bradycardia

Family Processes, Altered Related factor: Separation of family members

Nutrition, Altered: Less Than Body Requirements Related factor: Loss of/decreased appetite

Tissue Perfusion, Altered: Peripheral Related factor: Imbalance between oxygen supply/demand

Inability to Adapt to Extrauterine Life

Includes but is not limited to premature infants and infants with serious congenital anomalies.

Activity Intolerance Related factor: Imbalance between oxygen supply and demand

Body Temperature, Altered: Risk for Risk factor: Immaturity of newborn's temperature-regulating system

Breast-Feeding, Ineffective Related factors: Infant fatigue, Inadequate sucking reflex, Interrupted or infrequent feeding

Breathing Pattern, Ineffective Related factor: Decreased energy/fatigue

Cardiac Output, Decreased Related factors: Increased ventricular workload, Hypovolemia, Cardiac anomaly (specify)

Caregiver Role Strain (Actual/Risk for) Related factors/risk factors: Illness severity of the care receiver; Premature birth/congenital defect; Unpredictable illness course; Situational stressors within the family; Chronicity of caregiving; Caregiver's health, developmental readiness, knowledge, skills, experience, competing role commitments, coping styles, isolation, opportunity for respite and recreation

Dysfunctional Ventilatory Weaning Response (DVWR) Related factors: Pulmonary immaturity, Impaired gas exchange, Ineffective airway clearance, Ventilator dependence > 1 week

Family Processes, Altered Related factors: Unmet expectations for child, Separation of family members, Illness/disability of family member

Fatigue Related factor: Disease process

Fear Related factor: Real threat to child

Fluid Volume Deficit Related factors: Abnormal blood loss, Abnormal fluid loss (specify), Inadequate fluid intake secondary to ____ (specify)

Gas Exchange, Impaired Related factors: Decreased pulmonary blood supply secondary to pulmonary hypertension, congestive heart failure, respiratory distress syndrome; Decreased functional lung tissue secondary to respiratory distress syndrome, atelectasis

Grieving, Anticipatory Related factor: Anticipatory loss of child

Growth and Development, Altered Related factors: Congenital anomaly, Fetal distress, Prematurity, Unhealthy maternal life-style during pregnancy, Serious illness

Infant Feeding Pattern, Ineffective Related factors: Prematurity, Neurological impairment/delay, Prolonged NPO, Anatomical abnormalities

Nutrition, Altered: Less Than Body Requirements Related factors: Difficulty in swallowing, Inadequate sucking reflex in infant, Vomiting, Food intolerance

Skin Integrity, Impaired: Risk for Risk factors: Impaired circulation, Immobility, Altered nutritional status

Sleep Pattern Disturbance Related factor: Sleep deprivation secondary to frequent therapeutic interventions

Spontaneous Ventilation, Inability to Sustain Related factors: Metabolic factors, Respiratory muscle fatigue, Pulmonary immaturity

Tissue Perfusion, Altered: Peripheral Related factor: Imbalance between oxygen supply/demand secondary to high metabolic rate

Urinary Retention Related factor: Congenital anomaly (specify)

Low Birth Weight

Activity Intolerance Related factor: Weakness/fatigue

Airway Clearance, Ineffective Related factors: Decreased energy/fatigue

Body Temperature, Altered: Risk for Risk factor: Immaturity of newborn's temperature-regulating system

Breast-Feeding, Ineffective Related factors: Infant fatigue, Inadequate sucking reflex, Interrupted or infrequent feeding

Breast-Feeding, Interrupted Related factor: Prematurity

Breathing Pattern, Ineffective Related factor: Decreased energy/ fatigue

Constipation Related factor: Decreased fluid intake

Family Processes, Altered Related factors: Illness/disability of family member, Separation of family members

Fatigue Related factor: Decreased energy

Fluid Volume Deficit Related factor: Inadequate fluid intake

Gas Exchange, Impaired Related factors: Decreased pulmonary blood supply secondary to respiratory distress syndrome; Decreased functional lung tissue secondary to atelectasis, respiratory distress syndrome

Grieving, Dysfunctional Related factor: Anticipated or perceived loss of the perfect child

Home Maintenance Management, Impaired Related factors: Inadequate support system, Insufficient family organization or planning

Infant Feeding Pattern, Ineffective Related factor: Prematurity

Nutrition, Altered: Less Than Body Requirements Related factors: Inadequate sucking reflex in infant, Food intolerance, High metabolic rate

Skin Integrity, Impaired: Risk for Risk factors: Fragile skin, Lack of subcutaneous fat

Sleep Pattern Disturbance Related factor: Sleep deprivation secondary to frequent therapeutic interventions

Spontaneous Ventilation, Inability to Sustain Related factors: Metabolic factors, Respiratory muscle fatigue, Pulmonary immaturity

Tissue Perfusion, Altered: Peripheral Related factor: Imbalance between oxygen supply/demand

Respiratory Distress

Includes but is not limited to broncho-pulmonary dysplasia, respiratory distress syndrome/hyaline membrane disease, meconium aspiration, pneumonia, pneumothorax, transient tachypnea.

Activity Intolerance Related factor: Weakness/fatigue

Airway Clearance, Ineffective Related factors: Decreased energy/ fatigue, Tracheobronchial secretions

Aspiration: Risk for Risk factor: Presence of enteral or tracheal tubes

Breast-Feeding, Interrupted Related factors: Prematurity, Infant illness

Breathing Pattern, Ineffective Related factors: Decreased energy/ fatigue, Dependence on ventilator

Cardiac Output, Decreased Related factors: Increased ventricular workload, Cardiac anomaly (specify)

Caregiver Role Strain (Actual/Risk for) Related factors/risk factors: Illness severity of the care receiver; Premature birth/congenital defect; Unpredictable illness course; Situational stressors within the family; Chronicity of caregiving; Caregiver's health, developmental readiness, knowledge, skills, experience, competing role commitments, coping styles, isolation, opportunity for respite and recreation

Constipation Related factor: Decreased fluid intake

Dysfunctional Ventilatory Weaning Response (DVWR) Related factors: Pulmonary immaturity, Impaired gas exchange, Ineffective airway clearance, Ventilator dependence > 1 week

Family Processes, Altered Related factors: Illness/disability of family member, Separation of family members

Fatigue Related factor: Disease process

Fear (Parental) Related factor: Real threat to child

Fluid Volume Deficit Related factors: Inadequate fluid intake secondary to fatigue with oral feedings, Abnormal fluid loss (insensible water loss secondary to rapid respiratory rate)

Gas Exchange, Impaired Related factors: Decreased pulmonary blood supply secondary to pulmonary hypertension/persistent fetal circulation, respiratory distress syndrome; Decreased functional lung tissue secondary to pneumonia, atelectasis, respiratory distress syndrome; Diaphragmatic hernia

Grieving, Anticipatory (Parental) Related factor: Anticipated or perceived loss of child

Home Maintenance Management, Impaired Related factors: Inadequate support system, Insufficient family planning or organization

Infant Feeding Pattern, Ineffective Related factors: Prematurity, Anatomical abnormalities

Infection: Risk for Risk factors: Inadequate immune system, Invasive monitoring

Nutrition, Altered: Less Than Body Requirements Related factors: Inadequate sucking reflex in infant, Food intolerance, High metabolic rate, Lethargy

Skin Integrity, Impaired: Risk for Risk factor: Decreased peripheral perfusion

Sleep Pattern Disturbance Related factor: Sleep deprivation secondary to frequent therapeutic interventions

Spontaneous Ventilation, Inability to Sustain Related factors: Metabolic factors, Respiratory muscle fatigue, Pulmonary immaturity

Tissue Perfusion, Altered: Peripheral Related factor: Imbalance between oxygen supply/demand

Pediatric Conditions

Burns

Cancer, see *Medical Conditions:* Cancer, pp. 346–349

Casts and traction

Child abuse

Chronic illness: Developmental problems/needs

Cleft lip/cleft palate: Surgical repair

Coagulation disorders

Congenital malformations of the central nervous system: Surgical repair

Diabetes mellitus, see *Medical Conditions:* Endocrine disorders, pp. 352–353

Failure to thrive

Gastroenteritis

Gastrointestinal obstruction: Surgical repair

Infection of central nervous system

Ingestion/accidental poisoning

Juvenile rheumatoid arthritis, see *Medical Conditions:* Arthritis, pp. 342–343

Obese child

Osteomyelitis

Pregnancy in adolescence

Renal failure, Acute, see *Medical Conditions:* Renal failure, Acute, pp. 361–362

Renal failure, Chronic, see *Medical Conditions:* Renal failure, Chronic, pp. 362–364

Respiratory disorder, Chronic

Respiratory infection, Acute

Rheumatic fever, see *Medical Conditions:* Pericarditis/endocarditis, p. 360

Seizure disorders

Sepsis

Sickle cell crisis

Suicidal adolescent, see *Psychiatric Conditions:* Suicidal patient, pp. 395–396

Tonsillectomy

Burns

Activity Intolerance Related factor: Acute pain

Body Image Disturbance Related factor: Burns, Scarring

Body Temperature, Altered: Risk for Risk factor: Dehydration secondary to impairment in skin integrity

Constipation Related factors: Decreased gastrointestinal motility, Dehydration

Coping, Ineffective Individual Related factor: Severe injury

Diversional Activity Deficit Related factors: Long-term hospitalization, Prolonged bed rest

Family Processes, Altered Related factors: Hospitalization/change in environment, Illness/disability of family member

Fear Related factors: Painful therapeutic procedures, Environmental stressors/hospitalization, Real threat to own well-being

Fluid Volume Deficit Related factor: Abnormal fluid loss secondary to loss of skin integrity

Infection: Risk for Risk factors: Malnutrition, Broken skin

Nutrition, Altered: Less Than Body Requirements Related factor: High metabolic needs

Pain [Acute] Related factor: Injury

Parental Role Conflict Related factor: Intimidation with invasive or restrictive modalities

Self-Care Deficit: Bathing/Hygiene, Dressing/Grooming, Feeding, Toileting (specify) Related factor: Pain with movement

Skin Integrity, Impaired Related factor: Burns

Social Interaction, Impaired Related factors: Self-concept disturbance, Limited physical mobility, Reactions of others

Casts and Traction

Includes but is not limited to orthopedic trauma, congenital hip dysplasia.

Body Image Disturbance Related factors: Surgery, Congenital defects

Diversional Activity Deficit Related factors: Forced inactivity, Prolonged bed rest, Long-term hospitalization

Family Processes, Altered Related factors: Hospitalization/change in environment, Illness/disability of family member

Fear Related factors: Environmental stressors/hospitalization

Infection: Risk for Risk factors: Trauma, Broken skin

Mobility, Impaired Physical Related factors: Pain/discomfort, Medically imposed restrictions, Musculoskeletal impairment

Pain [Acute] Related factors: Pain secondary to injury, Pain secondary to surgery, Pruritus

Peripheral Neurovascular Dysfunction Related factor: Immobilization

Self-Care Deficit: Bathing/Hygiene, Dressing/Grooming, Feeding, Toileting (specify) Related factors: Pain/discomfort, Musculoskeletal impairment, Medically imposed restrictions

Skin Integrity: Risk for Risk factors: Altered circulation, Physical immobilization

Tissue Perfusion, Altered: Peripheral Related factors: Interruption of venous flow to ____ (specify) secondary to constriction pressure, Interruption of arterial flow to ____ (specify) secondary to compartment syndrome

Urinary Incontinence, Functional Related factor: Mobility deficits

Child Abuse

Caregiver Role Strain (Actual/Risk for) Related factor/risk factor: Presence of abuse or violence

Coping, Ineffective Family: Disabling Related factors: Chronically unresolved feelings (specify), Highly ambivalent family relationships, Substance-abusing family member, Emotionally disturbed family member, Use of violence to manage conflict, Child sexual/physical abuse

Coping, Ineffective Individual Related factor: Personal vulnerability in situational crisis

Fear Related factors: Real threat to own well-being, Powerlessness

Growth and Development, Altered Related factor: Abuse

Home Maintenance Management, Impaired Related factors: Physical/psychologic impairment of family member other than patient, Inadequate support system, Developmental disability, Psychologic impairment, Lack of knowledge

Hopelessness Related factor: Long-term stress

Injury: Risk for Risk factors: Physical/psychologic abuse, Parental neglect

Knowledge Deficit (specify) Related factors: Limited exposure to information about normal growth and development of children, Limited practice of parenting skills, Cognitive limitations

Nutrition, Altered: Less Than Body Requirements Related factor: Parental neglect

Pain [Acute] Related factor: Trauma

Parental Role Conflict Related factors: Change in marital status, Relocation, Financial or legal crisis

Parenting, Altered Related factors: Absent or ineffective role model; Interruption in bonding process; Lack of knowledge/skill; Lack of or inappropriate response of child to parent; Lack of support for nurturing figure(s); Psychologic impairment; Physical illness; Unrealistic expectations of self, infant, partner; Dysfunctional relationship between parents/nurturing figures; Situational crisis (specific to family)

Post-Trauma Response Related factors: Abuse, Assault, Torture, Accidents, Incest

Self-Esteem Disturbance Related factor: Abuse

Sleep Pattern Disturbance Related factors: Anxiety, Emotional state

Social Interaction, Impaired Related factor: Concept disturbance

Violence, Risk for: Directed at Others Risk factor: History of physical/mental abuse by others

Chronic Illness: Developmental Problems/Needs

Activity Intolerance Related factors: Decreased strength and endurance, Weakness/fatigue, Imbalance between oxygen supply and demand, Pain (acute or chronic)

Activity Intolerance: Risk for Risk factors: Limited mobility, Frail or debilitated states, Chronic illness, Pain

Adjustment, Impaired Related factors: Incomplete grieving, Necessity for major life-style/behavior change, Pattern of dependence, Inadequate support systems

Anxiety Related factors: Threat to or change in role functioning, Threat to or change in interaction patterns, Unmet needs

Body Image Disturbance Related factors: Chronic illness, Chronic pain, Treatment side-effects

Caregiver Role Strain (Actual/Risk for) Related factors/risk factors: Illness severity of the care receiver, Premature birth/congenital defect, Developmental delay or retardation of the care receiver, Marginal caregiver's coping patterns, Duration of caregiving required, Caregiver's competing role commitments, Complexity/amount of caregiving tasks, Lack of respite and recreation for caregiver

Family Processes, Altered Related factors: Change in family roles, Illness/disability of family member, Unmet expectations for child, Lack of adequate support systems

Fear Related factors: Powerlessness, Real threat to own well-being

Grieving, Dysfunctional Related factors: Loss (actual or anticipated), Chronic illness

Growth and Development, Altered Related factors: Serious illness, Prescribed dependence/limitations

Home Maintenance Management, Impaired Related factors: Home environment obstacles, Inadequate support system, Insufficient family organization or planning, Insufficient finances, Lack of familiarity with community resources, Developmental disability

Hopelessness Related factor: Failing or deteriorating physical condition

Knowledge Deficit (specify) Related factors: Specific to patient, Specific to parent

Noncompliance Related factors: Denial of illness, Negative consequence of treatment regimen, Perceived benefits of continued illness

Nutrition, Altered: Less Than Body Requirements Related factor: Chronic illness

Pain, Chronic Related factors: Specific to patient

Parenting, Altered Related factors: Interruption in bonding process, Treatment-imposed separation, Lack of knowledge/skill necessary to address the child's special needs

Powerlessness Related factor: Chronic illness

Role Performance, Altered Related factors: Chronic illness, Chronic pain

Self-Care Deficit: Bathing/Hygiene, Dressing/Grooming, Feeding, Toileting (specify) Related factors: Depression, Pain/discomfort, Intolerance to activity, Decreased strength and endurance

Self-Esteem Disturbance Related factors: Chronic illness, Chronic pain

Social Interaction, Impaired Related factors: Self-concept disturbance, Limited physical mobility

Spiritual Distress Related factor: Test of spiritual beliefs

Cleft Lip/Cleft Palate: Surgical Repair

Airway Clearance, Ineffective Related factor: Edema secondary to surgery

Body Image Disturbance Related factor: Obvious congenital anomaly

Family Processes, Altered Related factors: Hospitalization/change in environment, Illness/disability of family member, Separation of family members

Fear Related factors: Environmental stressors/hospitalization, Separation from parent

Fluid Volume Deficit: Risk for Risk factor: Deviation affecting access to or intake of fluids secondary to difficult handling of oral fluids

Infant Feeding Pattern, Ineffective Related factors: Anatomical abnormalities, Oral hypersensitivity

Infection: Risk for Risk factor: Trauma secondary to surgery

Injury: Risk for (Disruption of Surgical Site) Risk factors: Limitations of maturational age, Tension on suture line secondary to crying

Nutrition, Altered: Less Than Body Requirements Related factors: Difficulty in chewing, Difficulty in swallowing secondary to acute pain

Oral Mucous Membrane, Altered Related factor: Surgery in oral cavity

Pain [Acute] Related factor: Surgical repair of cleft lip/palate

Parenting, Altered Related factors: Interruption in bonding process, Lack of knowledge/skill in special needs of child, Treatment-imposed separation

Self-Care Deficit: Feeding Related factors: Age of child and need for adapted feeding

Coagulation Disorders

Include but are not limited to hemophilia, von Willebrand's disease, idiopathic thrombocytopenic purpura.

Activity Intolerance: Risk for Risk factors: Limited mobility, Pain, Fatigue, Decreased hemoglobin

Coping, Ineffective Individual Related factors: Chronic illness and limitations

Family Processes, Altered Related factors: Illness/disability of family member, Environmental stressors/hospitalization

Fear Related factors: Risks associated with diagnosis (uncontrollable bleeding, potential joint degeneration, risk of transfusion-acquired diseases)

Growth and Development, Altered Related factors: Serious illness, Prescribed dependence/limitations

Injury: Risk for Risk factor: Uncontrolled bleeding

Knowledge Deficit (specify) Related factors: Lack of exposure to information about prevention of bleeding and injury and early recognition of bleeding, Cognitive limitations, Unreadiness to learn

Pain [Acute] Related factor: Joint hemorrhage

Parenting, Altered Related factors: Lack of knowledge/skill in care of special child, Treatment-imposed separation

Powerlessness Related factor: Chronic illness

Role Performance, Altered Related factor: Chronic illness

Self-Esteem Disturbance Related factor: Chronic illness

Congenital Malformations of the Central Nervous System: Surgical Repair

Include but are not limited to spina bifida, meningocele, myelomeningocele, hydrocephalus.

Caregiver Role Strain (Actual/Risk for) Related factors/risk factors: Illness severity of the care receiver, Congenital defect, Developmental delay of care receiver, Caregiver's competing role commitments, Lack of respite and recreation for caregiver

Diversional Activity Deficit Related factors: Forced inactivity, Prolonged bed rest, Long-term hospitalization

Family Processes, Altered Related factors: Hospitalization/change in environment, Illness/disability of family member, Separation of family members

Fear (Parental) Related factor: Real threat to child

Infection: Risk for Risk factor: Broken skin secondary to surgery

Injury: Risk for Risk factor: Increased intracranial pressure/seizures secondary to shunt malfunction in hydrocephalus

Knowledge Deficit (Parental) Related factor: Limited exposure to information (home care)

Mobility, Impaired Physical Related factor: Neuromuscular impairment secondary to spinal cord involvement

Pain [Acute] Related factor: Surgery

Parenting, Altered Related factors: Interruption in bonding process, Lack of knowledge/skill in needs of special child, Treatment-imposed separation

Self-Care Deficit: Bathing/Hygiene, Dressing/Grooming, Feeding, Toileting (specify) Related factor: Neuromuscular impairment

Sensory/Perceptual Alterations: Kinesthetic, Tactile Related factor: Sensory deficits secondary to spinal cord involvement

Skin Integrity, Impaired: Risk for Risk factors: Immobility, Incontinence of stool/urine

Failure to Thrive

Activity Intolerance Related factor: Weakness/fatigue

Coping, Ineffective Family: Disabling Related factors: Chronically unresolved feelings, Highly ambivalent family relationships

Family Processes, Altered Related factors: Unmet expectations for child, Hospitalization/change in environment

Fluid Volume Deficit Related factors: Inadequate fluid intake secondary to disinterest in eating/drinking, Abnormal fluid loss (loose stools)

Infant Feeding Pattern, Ineffective Related factor: Prolonged NPO

Infection: Risk for Risk factor: Malnutrition

Nutrition, Altered: Less Than Body Requirements Related factors: Food intolerance, Malabsorption, Loss of appetite, Parental neglect

Parenting, Altered Related factors: Lack of or inappropriate response of child to parent, Lack of knowledge/skill, Absent or ineffective role model, Interruption in bonding process

Skin Integrity, Impaired: Risk for Risk factor: Altered nutritional status

Social Interaction, Impaired Related factors: Developmental disability, Limited physical mobility

Gastroenteritis

Diarrhea Related factors: Food intolerance, Stress, Dietary changes, Increased intestinal motility

Family Processes, Altered Related factors: Hospitalization/change in environment, Separation of family members

Fear Related factors: Environmental stressors/hospitalization, Real or imagined threat to own well-being

Fluid Volume Deficit Related factors: Abnormal fluid loss (diarrhea) secondary to infection, Food intolerance, Inflammatory disease, Malabsorption

Nutrition, Altered: Less Than Body Requirements Related factors: Loss of appetite, Nausea/vomiting

Oral Mucous Membrane, Altered Related factor: Dehydration

Pain [Acute] Related factor: Muscle cramps (abdominal)

Sensory/Perceptual Alterations: Visual, Auditory, Kinesthetic, Tactile (specify) Related factor: Electrolyte imbalance

Skin Integrity, Impaired: Risk for Risk factors: Incontinence of stool, Diarrhea

Gastrointestinal Obstruction: Surgical Repair

Includes but is not limited to gastroschisis, omphalocele, intestinal atresia, meconium ileus, imperforate anus, Hirschsprung's disease, pyloric stenosis, intussusception, inguinal hernia, and hydrocele.

Activity Intolerance Related factors: Acute pain, Decreased strength and endurance

Breathing Pattern, Ineffective Related factor: Acute pain

Family Processes, Altered Related factors: Illness/disability of family member, Hospitalization/change in environment, Separation of family members

Fear Related factors: Environmental stressors/hospitalization, Real threat to well-being

Fluid Volume Deficit Related factors: Abnormal blood loss, Abnormal fluid loss

Nutrition, Altered: Less Than Body Requirements Related factors: Loss of appetite, Nausea/vomiting

Pain [Acute] Related factor: Surgery

Parenting, Altered Related factors: Lack of knowledge/skill in special needs of child

Skin Integrity, Impaired: Risk for Risk factors: Altered nutritional status, Surgical wound

Infection of Central Nervous System

Includes but is not limited to meningitis, encephalitis, rabies, Reye's syndrome, Guillain-Barré syndrome.

Caregiver Role Strain (Actual/Risk for) Related factors/risk factors: Illness severity of the care receiver, Duration of caregiving required, Caregiver's competing role commitments

Communication, Impaired: Verbal Related factor: Inability to speak secondary to coma

Family Processes, Altered Related factors: Illness of child, Separation of family members

Fear (Parental) Related factor: Real threat to child

Fluid Volume Deficit Related factors: Inadequate fluid intake secondary to nausea, Abnormal fluid loss secondary to vomiting

Grieving, Anticipatory (Parental) Related factor: Anticipated loss of child

Injury: Risk for Risk factor: Seizure activity

Mobility, Impaired Physical Related factors: Neuromuscular impairment, Coma

Pain [Acute] Related factors: Nausea/vomiting, Headache, Paresthesia

Self-Care Deficit: Bathing/Hygiene, Dressing/Grooming, Feeding, Toileting (specify) Related factors: Neuromuscular impairment, Coma

Sensory/Perceptual Alterations: Visual, Auditory, Kinesthetic, Gustatory, Tactile, Olfactory (specify) Related factor: Sensory deficits secondary to coma

Ingestion/Accidental Poisoning

Breathing Pattern, Ineffective Related factor: Depression of respiratory center secondary to ____ (specify drug)

Family Processes, Altered Related factors: Hospitalization/change in environment, Illness/disability of family member, Separation of family members, Parental guilt

Fluid Volume Excess Related factor: Decreased urine output secondary to renal dysfunction

Gas Exchange, Impaired Related factor: Anemia secondary to lead poisoning

Home Maintenance Management, Impaired Related factors: Lack of knowledge about prevention of accidental poisoning, Insufficient family organization or planning

Injury: Risk for Risk factor: Seizures secondary to lead poisoning, aspirin toxicity

Sensory/Perceptual Alterations: Visual, Auditory, Kinesthetic, Gustatory, Tactile, Olfactory (specify) Related factors: Decreased consciousness, Encephalopathy

Obese Child

Body Image Disturbance Related factor: Eating disorder (obesity)

Coping, Ineffective Family: Disabling Related factors: Arbitrary disregard for child's needs, Conflicting coping styles, Highly ambivalent relationships

Health Maintenance, Altered Related factors: Cultural beliefs, Lack of social supports, Lack of ability to make deliberate and thoughtful judgments secondary to maturational age

Nutrition, Altered: More Than Body Requirements Related factors: Psychologic impairment, Sedentary life-style, Lack of basic nutritional knowledge, Ethnic/cultural norms

Self-Esteem Disturbance Related factor: Obesity

Social Interaction, Impaired Related factor: Self-concept disturbance

Social Isolation Related factor: Obesity

Osteomyelitis

Activity Intolerance Related factor: Acute pain

Diversional Activity Deficit Related factors: Long-term hospitalization, Forced inactivity

Family Processes, Altered Related factors: Illness/disability of family member, Hospitalization/change in environment, Separation of family members

Mobility, Impaired Physical Related factors: Pain/discomfort, Musculoskeletal impairment

Nutrition, Altered: Less Than Body Requirements Related factor: High metabolic state

Pain [Acute] Related factor: Inflammation

Self-Care Deficit: Bathing/Hygiene, Dressing/Grooming, Feeding, Toileting (specify) Related factors: Pain/discomfort, Decreased strength and endurance, Neuromuscular impairment

Social Interaction, Impaired Related factor: Limited physical mobility

Pregnancy in Adolescence

Includes pregnancy, antepartum and postpartum periods, and parenting.

Body Image Disturbance Related factor: Pregnancy

Coping, Ineffective Individual Related factors: Adolescent pregnancy, Adolescent parenthood

Family Processes, Altered Related factors: Lack of adequate support systems, Change in family roles

Fear Related factors: Threat to own well-being, Powerlessness

Health Maintenance, Altered Related factors: Lack of social supports, Lack of material resources, Cultural beliefs, Lack of ability to make deliberate and thoughtful judgments secondary to maturational age

Home Maintenance Management, Impaired Related factors: Inadequate support system, Insufficient family organization or planning, Insufficient finances, Lack of familiarity with community resources

Knowledge Deficit (specify) Related factors: Limited exposure to information (birth control, parenting), Limited practice of skills, Information misinterpretation

Nutrition, Altered: Less Than Body Requirements Related factors: High metabolic needs, Lack of basic nutritional knowledge, Limited access to food, Nausea/vomiting

Nutrition, Altered: More Than Body Requirements Related factors: Ethnic/cultural norms, Lack of basic nutritional knowledge

Parenting, Altered Related factors: Lack of knowledge/skill, Lack of support for nurturing figure, Unrealistic expectations of self/infant/partner, Situational crisis

Role Performance, Altered Related factors: Assumption of new role, Unmet expectations for pregnancy, Unmet expectations for childbirth

Social Interaction, Impaired Related factors: Sociocultural conflict, Self-concept disturbance

Social Isolation Related factors: Alteration in physical appearance, Life-style changes

Violence, Risk for: Directed at Child Risk factors: Rage reaction, History of physical/mental abuse by others, Substance abuse

See also *Antepartum and Postpartum Conditions,* pp. 398–405.

Respiratory Disorder, Chronic

Includes but is not limited to asthma, bronchopulmonary dysplasia, cystic fibrosis.

Activity Intolerance Related factors: Imbalance between oxygen supply and demand, Anxiety, Weakness/fatigue, Decreased strength and endurance

Adjustment, Impaired Related factors: Necessity for major lifestyle/behavior changes, Pattern of dependence

Airway Clearance, Ineffective Related factors: Tracheobronchial secretions, Spasms of the bronchi and bronchioles

Body Image Disturbance Related factor: Chronic illness

Breathing Pattern, Ineffective Related factors: Anxiety, Pulmonary infection, Decreased energy/fatigue

Caregiver Role Strain (Actual/Risk for) Related factors/risk factors: Illness severity of the care receiver, Caregiver's competing role commitments, Complexity/amount of caregiving tasks, Duration of the caregiving required, Lack of respite and recreation for caregiver

Coping, Ineffective Individual Related factor: Stressors of chronic illness

Fluid Volume Deficit: Risk for Risk factors: Inadequate fluid intake secondary to difficulty in breathing, Abnormal fluid loss secondary to increased insensible water loss from rapid respirations

Gas Exchange, Impaired Related factor: Decreased functional lung tissue secondary to fibrotic, nonventilated areas of lung parenchyma in bronchopulmonary dysplasia

Infection: Risk for Risk factors: Malnutrition, Stasis of respiratory secretions

Knowledge Deficit (specify) Related factors: Limited exposure to information, Limited practice of skill

Nutrition, Altered: Less Than Body Requirements Related factors: Loss of appetite with chronic illness, High metabolic needs secondary to pulmonary infection, Malabsorption of nutrients secondary to cystic fibrosis

Parenting, Altered Related factors: Lack of knowledge/skill in care of special child, Treatment-imposed separation

Powerlessness Related factor: Chronic illness

Role Performance, Altered Related factor: Chronic illness

Self-Care Deficit: Bathing/Hygiene, Dressing/Grooming, Feeding, Toileting (specify) Related factors: Intolerance to activity, Developmental disability

Self-Esteem Disturbance Related factor: Chronic illness

Social Interaction, Impaired Related factors: Developmental disability, Self-concept disturbance

Social Isolation Related factors: Medical condition, Alteration in physical appearance, Life-style changes

Respiratory Infection, Acute

Includes but is not limited to tonsillitis, pharyngitis, croup, laryngotracheobronchitis, epiglottitis, bronchitis, pneumonia.

Activity Intolerance Related factors: Imbalance between oxygen supply/demand, Weakness/fatigue

Airway Clearance, Ineffective Related factors: Edema, Tracheobronchial secretions

Diversional Activity Deficit Related factor: Time spent in croupette

Family Processes, Altered Related factors: Illness/disability of family member, Hospitalization/change in environment, Separation of family members

Fear Related factors: Real threat to well-being, Environmental stressors/hospitalization, Separation from parent

Fluid Volume Deficit: Risk for Risk factors: Inadequate fluid intake secondary to difficulty in breathing, Abnormal fluid loss secondary to increased insensible water loss from rapid respirations

Gas Exchange, Impaired Related factor: Decreased functional lung tissue secondary to pneumonia

Nutrition, Altered: Less Than Body Requirements Related factors: Loss of appetite, High metabolic needs

Pain [Acute] Related factors: Sore throat, Pain with inspiration

Sensory/Perceptual Alterations: Visual, Auditory, Kinesthetic, Tactile (specify) Related factor: Sensory deficit secondary to time spent in croupette

Skin Integrity, Impaired: Risk for Risk factors: Altered nutritional status, Hyperthermia, Damp therapeutic environment

Seizure Disorders

Adjustment, Impaired Related factors: Assault to self-esteem, Incomplete grieving

Anxiety Related factors: Threat to role functioning, Change in role functioning

Family Processes, Altered Related factors: Hospitalization/change in environment, Illness/disability of family member, Separation of family members

Fear Related factor: Real threat to own well-being

Injury: Risk for Risk factor: Seizure activity

Knowledge Deficit (specify) Related factors: Specific to patient, Specific to parent

Noncompliance Related factors: Denial of illness, Negative perception of treatment regimen, Perceived benefits of continued illness

Powerlessness Related factor: Chronic illness

Self-Esteem Disturbance Related factor: Chronic illness

Social Interaction, Impaired Related factor: Self-concept disturbance

Sepsis

Breathing Pattern, Ineffective Related factors: Decreased energy/fatigue

Constipation Related factor: Decreased fluid intake

Diarrhea Related factor: Increased intestinal motility

Family Processes, Altered Related factors: Illness/disability of family member, Separation of family members

Fluid Volume Deficit: Risk for Risk factors: Decreased fluid intake, Fever

Injury: Risk for Risk factor: Seizure activity secondary to high fever

Nutrition, Altered: Less Than Body Requirements Related factors: Inadequate sucking reflex in infant, Vomiting, Food intolerance, High metabolic state, Lethargy

Skin Integrity, Impaired: Risk for Risk factors: Decreased peripheral perfusion, Hyperthermia

Sleep Pattern Disturbance Related factor: Sleep deprivation secondary to frequent therapeutic interventions

Sickle Cell Crisis

Activity Intolerance Related factor: Imbalance between oxygen supply/demand

Family Processes, Altered Related factors: Illness of family member, Hospitalization/change in environment

Fear Related factors: Environmental stressors/hospitalization, Real threat to well-being of child

Fluid Volume Deficit Related factor: Increased need for fluid volume in blood to prevent sickling and thrombosis

Gas Exchange, Impaired Related factor: Decreased pulmonary blood supply secondary to anemia

Infection: Risk for Risk factor: Chronic illness

Knowledge Deficit (specify) Related factors: Limited exposure to information about prevention of sickle cell crisis by minimizing oxygen needs of body, Cognitive limitations, Unreadiness to learn

Pain [Acute] Related factor: Sickle cell crisis

Tissue Perfusion, Altered: Peripheral Related factors: Imbalance between oxygen supply/demand secondary to anemia, Thrombosis secondary to clumping of red blood cells in sickle cell crisis

Tonsillectomy

Airway Clearance, Ineffective Related factors: Trauma, Edema, Pain, Tracheobronchial secretions

Family Processes, Altered Related factors: Hospitalization/change in environment, Separation of family members

Fear Related factors: Environmental stressors/hospitalization, Surgical procedure

Nutrition, Altered: Less Than Body Requirements Related factor: Loss of appetite

Oral Mucous Membrane, Altered Related factor: Surgery in oral cavity

Pain [Acute] Related factor: Surgery

Bibliography

Acute Pain Management Guideline Panel. (Feb. 1992). *Acute Pain Management: Operative or Medical Procedures and Trauma. Clinical Practice Guideline.* AHCPR Publication No. 92-0032. Rockville, MD: Agency for Health Care Policy and Research, Public Health Service, U.S. Department of Health and Human Services.

Anderson, L., and Price, C. (1986). Nursing care of patients with pulmonary insufficiency. *Critical Care Nursing Currents.* Vol. 4, No. 4, 19–34.

Auerbach, K. G. (1990). Assisting the employed breastfeeding mother. *Journal of Nurse-Midwifery,* Vol. 35, No. 1, 26–34.

Ballard, P. (1983). Breast-feeding for the working mother. *Issues in Comprehensive Pediatric Nursing,* Vol. 6, 249–259.

Bowers, K. (1991). Introduction to case management: A three-hour workshop. El Camino Hospital, Mountain View, CA.

Bowers, B. (1987). Intergenerational caregiving: Adult caregivers and their aging parents. *Advances in Nursing Science,* Vol. 9, No. 2, 20–31.

Carnevali, Doris. (1984). Nursing diagnosis: An evolutionary view. *Topics in Clinical Nursing.* Vol. 5, No. 4, 10–20.

Carpenito, Lynda J. (1993). *Nursing Diagnosis: Application to Clinical Practice,* 5th ed. Philadelphia, PA: J. B. Lippincott.

Carroll, J., Schaffer, C. B., Spensley, J., and Abramowitz, S. (1981). Family antecedents of adult self-mutilators. *International Journal of Family Psychiatry,* Vol. 2, Nos. 1 and 2, 147–161.

Chilman, C., Nunnally, E., and Cox, F. (1988). *Chronic Illness and Disability.* Beverly Hills, CA: Sage Publications. 30–31.

Conn, L. M., and Lion, J. R. (1983). Self-mutilation: A review. *Psychiatric Medicine,* Vol. 1, No. 1, 21–33.

Cook, J. S., and Fontaine, K. L. (1987). Violence against others—Rape. *Essentials of Mental Health Nursing.* Menlo Park, CA: Addison-Wesley. 522–530.

Cox, C. (1985). The health self-determinism index. *Nursing Research,* Vol. 34, No. 3, 177–183.

Doughty, D. (Ed.). (1991). *Urinary and Fecal Incontinence: Nursing Management.* St. Louis, MO: Mosby-Yearbook.

El Camino Hospital Care Delivery Task Force. (1991). Objectives for new care delivery system. El Camino Hospital, Mountain View, CA.

El Camino Hospital Clinical Practice Council. (1992). *Management of the Adult Patient Being Weaned.* El Camino Hospital, Mountain View, CA.

Favazza, A. R. (1989). Why patients mutilate themselves. *Hospital and Community Psychiatry,* Vol. 40, No. 2, 137–145.

Figueroa, M. (1988). A dynamic taxonomy of self-destructive behavior. *Psychotherapy,* Vol. 25, No. 2, 280–287.

Fitzpatrick, Joyce J., et al. (1989). Translating nursing diagnosis into ICD code. *American Journal of Nursing,* Vol. 89, No. 4, 483–495.

Forte, A., Mayberry, L. J., and Ferketich, S. (1987). Breast milk collection and storage practices among mothers of hospitalized neonates. *Journal of Perinatology,* Vol. 7, No. 1, 35–39.

Geissler, E. (1991). Transcultural nursing and nursing diagnoses. *Nursing and Health Care,* 12 (4): 190-92, 203.

Gordon, M. (1985). Practice based data set for a nursing information system. *Journal of Medical Systems,* 9:43–55.

Gordon, M. (1987) *Nursing Process and Application,* 2d ed. New York: McGraw-Hill.

Gray, M. (1992). *Genitourinary Disorders.* St. Louis, MO: Mosby-Yearbook.

Gyulay, Jo-Eileen. (1989). Grief responses. *Issues in Comprehensive Pediatric Nursing,* Vol. 12, No. 1, 1–31.

Halpern, J. S., (1989). Clinical notebook: Lower extremity peripheral nerve assessment. *Journal of Emergency Nursing,* Vol. 15, No. 4, 333–337.

Hawkins-Walsh, E. (1988). Breastfeeding the premature infant. *Pediatric Nursing Forum,* Vol. 3, No. 4, 3–13.

Henneman, E. A. (1991). The art and science of weaning from mechanical ventilation. *AACN Focus on Critical Care,* Vol. 18, No. 6, 490–501.

Hilt, N. E., and Cogburn, S. B. (1980). *Manual of Orthopaedics.* St. Louis, MO: C. V. Mosby. 487–537.

Hurley, Mary (Ed.). (1986). *Classification of Nursing Diagnoses: Proceedings of the Sixth Conference, North American Nursing Diagnosis Association.* St. Louis, MO: C. V. Mosby.

International Association of Enterostomal Therapy. (1987). *Standards of Care, Dermal Wounds: Pressure Sores.* Irvine, CA.

Jenny, J., and Logan, J. (1991). Analyzing expert nursing practice to develop a new nursing diagnosis: Dysfunctional ventilatory weaning response. In R. M. Carroll-Johnson (Ed.). *Classification of Nursing Diagnoses: Proceedings of the Ninth Conference.* Philadelphia, PA: J. B. Lippincott, 133–140.

Johnson, Sharon E. (1988). Alteration in temperature regulation: Hypothermia. *Classifications of Nursing Diagnoses: Proceedings of the Eighth Conference, North American Nursing Diagnosis Association.* St. Louis, MO: C. V. Mosby. 378–380.

Jones, E., et al. (Nov. 1974). *Patient Classification for Long-Term Care: User's Manual.* HEW Publication No. HRA-74-3107.

Knebel, A. F. (1991). Weaning from mechanical ventilation: Current controversies. *Heart & Lung,* Vol. 20, No. 4, 321–333.

Kritek, Phyllis. (1986). Diagnostics: The struggle to classify our diagnoses. *American Journal of Nursing,* Vol. 86, No. 6, 722–723.

Laffrey, S. C., and Crabtree, M. K. (1988). Health and health behavior of persons with chronic cardiovascular disease. *International Journal of Nursing Studies,* Vol. 25, No. 1, 41–52.

Lambert, M. and Jones, P. (1989). Nursing diagnoses recorded in nursing situations encountered in a Department of Public Health. In Carroll-Johnson, R., ed., *Classification of Nursing Diagnoses: Proceedings of the Eighth Conference.* North American Nursing Diagnosis Association. Philadelphia, PA: J. B. Lippincott.

Logan, J., and Jenny, J. (1991). Interventions for the nursing diagnosis, Dysfunctional Ventilatory Weaning Response: A qualitative study. In R. M. Carroll-Johnson (Ed.). *Classification of Nursing Diagnoses: Proceedings of the Ninth Conference,* Philadelphia, PA: J. B. Lippincott. 141–147.

Loomis, M., et al. (1986). *Classification of Individual Human Responses of Concern for Psychiatric/Mental Health Nursing*

Practice. Unpublished draft. American Nurses' Association Subcommittee.

Lubkin, I. M. (1986). Compliance. In *Chronic Illness: Impact and Interventions.* Boston, MA: Jones and Bartlett, 126–149.

McCaffrey, M. (1979). *Nursing Management of the Patient with Pain,* 2d ed. Philadelphia, PA: J. B. Lippincott.

McCloskey, J. C., and Bulechek, G. M. (1992). *Nursing Interventions Classification (NIC).* St. Louis, MO: C. V. Mosby.

McLane, A. (Ed.). (1987). *Classification of Nursing Diagnoses: Proceedings of the Seventh Conference, North American Nursing Diagnosis Association.* St. Louis, MO: C. V. Mosby.

Marculescu, Gail. (1986). *The Nursing Diagnosis Disturbance in Self-Concept, Related to a Change in Body Image in Post-Surgical Patients: A Descriptive Study.* Unpublished Master's Thesis. San Jose State University.

Marini, J. J. (1986). The physiologic determinants of ventilator dependency. *Respiratory Care,* Vol. 31, 271–282.

Matz, R. (1986). Hypothermia: Measures and countermeasures. *Hospital Practice,* Vol. 21, No. 1A, 45–71.

Mirotznik, J., and Ruskin, A. P. (1985). Inter-institutional relocation and its effects on psychosocial status. *The Gerontologist,* Vol. 25, No. 3, 265–270.

Mott, S., James, S., and Sperhac, A. (1990). *Nursing Care of Children and Families.* Menlo Park, CA: Addison-Wesley.

Neifert, M., and Seacat, J. (1986). Medical management of successful breastfeeding. *Pediatric Clinics of North America,* Vol. 33, No. 4, 743–762.

NIC Interventions Linked to NANDA Diagnoses. (1993). Iowa City: Iowa Intervention Project.

North American Nursing Diagnosis Association. (1986). Seventh Conference on Classification of Nursing Diagnoses. *Syllabus of Conference Proceedings.* NANDA, St. Louis, MO.

North American Nursing Diagnosis Association. (1988). Eighth Conference on Classification of Nursing Diagnoses. *Syllabus of Conference Proceedings.* NANDA, St. Louis, MO.

North American Nursing Diagnosis Association. (1988). *Nursing Diagnosis Newsletter,* Vol. 31, No. 1.

North American Nursing Diagnosis Association. (1992). NANDA Nursing Diagnoses: Definitions and Classification 1992. NANDA, St. Louis, MO.

North American Nursing Diagnosis Association. (1992). *Taxonomy I, Revised.* NANDA, St. Louis, MO.

North American Nursing Diagnosis Association. (1994). NANDA approved nursing diagnoses. NANDA, Philadelphia, PA.

Norton, L. C., and Neureuter, A. (1989). Weaning the long-term ventilator dependent patient: Common problems and management. *Critical Care Nurse,* Vol. 9, No. 1, 42–51.

Orzeck, S., and Ouslander, J. (1987). Urinary incontinence: An overview of causes and treatment. *Journal of Enterostomal Therapy,* Vol. 14, No. 1, 20–27.

Panel for the Prediction and Prevention of Pressure Ulcers in Adults. (May 1992). *Pressure Ulcers in Adults: Prediction and Prevention. Clinical Practice Guideline Number 3.* AHCPR Publication No. 92-0047. Rockville, MD: Agency for Health Care Policy and Research, Public Health Service, U.S. Department of Health and Human Services.

Pattison, E. M., and Kahan, J. (1983). The deliberate self-harm syndrome. *American Journal of Psychiatry,* Vol. 140, No. 7, 867–872.

Rakel, B. and Bulechek, G. (1990). Development of alterations in learning: Situational learning disabilities. *Nursing Diagnosis,* 1(4):134–145.

Rantz, K. E. (1987). Reducing death from translocation syndrome. *American Journal of Nursing,* Vol. 87, 1351–1352.

Reuler, J. (1978). Hypothermia: Pathophysiology, clinical settings, and management. *Annals of Internal Medicine,* Vol. 89, 519–527.

Rhynsburger, J. (1989). How to fight MG fatigue. *American Journal of Nursing,* Vol. 89, 337–340.

Schactman, M. (1987). Transfer stress in patients after myocardial infarction. *Focus on Critical Care,* Vol. 14, No. 2, 34–37.

Schainen, J. S. (1991). Environments for nursing care of the older client. In W. C. Chenitz, J. T. Stone, and S. A. Salisbury,

Clinical Gerontological Nursing. Philadelphia, PA: W. B. Saunders.

Seifert, P., and Grandsky, R. (1990). Nursing diagnoses: Their use in developing care plans. *AORN Journal,* Vol. 51, No. 4, 1008–1021.

Shaker, C. (1990). Nipple feeding premature infants: A different perspective. *Neonatal Network,* Vol. 8, No. 5, 9–17.

Sheppard, K. (1987). Alterations in protective mechanisms. *Classification of Nursing Diagnoses: Proceedings of the Seventh Conference, North American Nursing Diagnosis Association.* St. Louis, MO: C. V. Mosby. 239–246.

Sheppard, K. (1988). Validation of the nursing diagnosis "Alterations in Protective Mechanisms." *Classification of Nursing Diagnoses: Proceedings of the Eighth Conference, North American Nursing Diagnosis Association.* St. Louis, MO: C. V. Mosby. 281–283.

Smith, L. (1987). Sexual assault: The nurse's role. *AD Nurse,* Vol. 2, No. 2, 24–28.

Stevens, S. A., and Becker, K. L. (Sept. 1988). A simple, step-by-step approach to neurologic assessment, part 1. *Nursing,* 53–61.

Stine, M. J. (1990). Breastfeeding the premature newborn: A protocol without bottles. *Journal of Human Lactation,* Vol. 6, No. 4, 167–170.

Stuart, G., and Sundeen, S. (1991). *Principles and Practices of Psychiatric Nursing,* 4th ed. St. Louis, MO: Mosby.

Taylor, C., and Cress, S. (1992). *The Indispensable Care Plan Guide—Nursing Diagnosis Cards.* Springhouse, PA: Springhouse Corporation.

Thompson, J., et al. (1989). *Mosby's Manual of Clinical Nursing,* 2d ed. St. Louis, MO: C. V. Mosby.

Urinary Incontinence Guideline Panel. (March 1992). *Urinary Incontinence in Adults: Clinical Practice Guideline.* AHCPR Publication No. 92-0038. Rockville, MD: Agency for Health Care Policy and Research, Public Health Service, U.S. Department of Health and Human Services.

Voith, A. (1986). A conceptual framework for nursing diagnoses: Alterations in urinary elimination. *Rehabilitation Nurs-*

ing, Vol. 11, No. 1, 18–20.

Walsh, B. W., and Rosen, P. M. (1988). *Self-Mutilation: Theory, Research, and Treatment.* New York, NY: The Guilford Press.

Wilkinson, J. (1992). *Nursing Process in Action: A Critical Thinking Approach.* Redwood City, CA: Addison-Wesley.

Yang, K. L., and Tobin, M. J. (1991). A prospective study of indexes predicting the outcome of trials of weaning from mechanical ventilation. *New England Journal of Medicine,* Vol. 324, No. 21, 1445–1451.

Youll, J. W. (1989). The bridge beyond: Strengthening nursing practice in attitudes towards death, dying, and the terminally ill, and helping the spouses of critically ill patients. *Intensive Care Nursing,* Vol. 5, No. 2, 88–94.

Appendix A
Diagnoses in Progress–1994

The following diagnostic labels are still in early stages of development and should be used with caution for other than testing purposes.

Decreased Adaptive Capacity: Intracranial (1.7.1)

Definition: A clinical state in which intracranial fluid dynamic mechanisms that normally compensate for increases in intracranial volumes are compromised, resulting in repeated disproportionate increases in intracranial pressure (ICP) over baseline in response to a variety of noxious and non-noxious stimuli.

Defining Characteristics

Major

Repeated increases in ICP of greater than 10 mm Hg for more than 5 minutes following any of a variety of external stimuli

Minor

Disproportionate increase in ICP following single environmental or nursing maneuver stimulus; elevated P_2ICP waveform; volume pressure response test variation (Volume-pressure ratio > 2, Pressure-volume index < 10); baseline ICP equal to or greater than 10 mm Hg; wide amplitude ICP waveform

Related Factors

Brain injuries; sustained increase in ICP greater than or equal to 10 to 15 mm Hg; decreased cerebral perfusion pressure less than or equal to 50 to 60 mm Hg; systemic hypotension with intracranial hypertension

Energy Field Disturbance (1.8)

Definition: A disruption of the flow of energy surrounding a person's being which results in a disharmony of the body, mind and/or spirit.

Defining Characteristics

Temperature change (warmth/coolness); visual changes (image/color); disruption of the field (vacant/hold/spike/bulge); movement (wave/spike/tingling/dense/flowing); sounds (tone/words)

Risk for Loneliness (3.1.3)

Definition: A subjective state in which an individual is at risk of experiencing vague dysphoria.

Risk Factors

Affectional deprivation; physical isolation; cathectic deprivation; social isolation

Risk for Altered Parent/ Infant/Child Attachment (3.2.1.1.2.1)

Definition: Disruption of the interactive process between parent/significant other and infant that fosters the development of a protective and nurturing reciprocal relationship.

Risk Factors

Inability of parents to meet their personal needs; anxiety associated with the parent role; substance abuse; premature infant; ill infant/child who is unable to effectively initiate parental contact due to altered behavioral organization; separation; physical barriers; lack of privacy

Altered Family Process: Alcoholism (3.2.2.3.1)

Definition: The state in which the psychosocial, spiritual and physiological functions of a family unit are chronically disorganized, leading to conflict, denial of problems, resistance to change, ineffective problem-solving, and a series of self-perpetuating crises.

Defining Characteristics

Major

Feelings

Decreased self-esteem/worthlessness; frustration; powerlessness; anger/suppressed rage; anxiety/tension/distress; insecurity; repressed emotions; responsibility for alcoholic's behavior; lingering resentment; shame/embarrassment; hurt; unhappiness; guilt; emotional isolation/loneliness; vulnerability; mistrust; hopelessness; rejection

Roles and Relationships

Deterioration in family relationships/disturbed family dynamics; ineffective communication with spouse/marital problems; altered role function/disruption of family roles; inconsistent parenting/low perception of parental support; family denial; intimacy dysfunction; chronic family problems; closed communication systems

Behaviors

Inappropriate expression of anger; difficulty with intimate relationships; loss of control of drinking; impaired communication; ineffective problem-solving skills; partner's support of continued drinking; inability to meet emotional needs of family members; manipulation; dependency; criticizing; alcohol abuse; broken promises; rationalization/denial of problems; refusal to get help/inability to accept and receive help appropriately; blaming; inadequate understanding or knowledge of alcoholism

Minor

Feelings

Differentness from other people; depression; hostility; fear; emotional control by others; confusion; dissatisfaction; loss; misunderstanding by others; abandonment; confusion between love and pity; moodiness; failure; being unloved; lack of identity

Roles and Relationships

Triangulating family relationships; reduced ability of family members to relate to each other for mutual growth and maturation; lack of skills necessary for relationships; lack of cohesiveness; disrupted family rituals; inability to meet security needs of family members; lack of demonstrated respect for individuality and autonomy of family members; pattern of rejection; economic problems; neglected obligations

Behaviors

Inability to meet spiritual needs of family members; inability to express or accept wide range of feelings; orientation toward tension relief rather than achievement of goals; alcohol centered special occasions; escalating conflict; lying; contradictory, paradoxical communication; lack of dealing with conflict; harsh self-judgment; isolation; nicotine addiction; difficulty having fun; self-blaming; unresolved grief; controlling communication/power struggles; inability to adapt to change; immaturity; stress-related physical illnesses; inability to deal with traumatic experiences constructively; seeking approval and affirmation; lack of reliability; disturbances in academic performance in children; disturbances in concentration; chaos; substance abuse other than alcohol; failure to accomplish current or past developmental tasks/difficulty with life cycle transitions; verbal abuse of spouse or parent; agitation; diminished physical contact

Related Factors

Abuse of alcohol; family history of alcoholism; resistance to treatment; inadequate coping skills; genetic predisposition; addictive personality; lack of problem-solving skills; biochemical influences

Potential for Enhanced Spiritual Well-Being (4.2)

Definition: Spiritual well-being is the process of an individual's developing/unfolding of mystery through harmonious interconnectedness that springs from inner strengths.

Defining Characteristics

Inner strengths: A sense of awareness, self-consciousness, sacred source, unifying force, inner core, and transcendence

Unfolding mystery: One's experience about life's purpose and meaning, mystery, uncertainty, and struggles

Harmonious interconnectedness: Relatedness, connectedness, harmony with self, others, higher power/God, and the environment

Potential for Enhanced Community Coping (5.1.3.1)

Definition: A pattern of community activities for adaption and problem solving that is satisfactory for meeting the demands or needs of the community but can be improved for management of current and future problems/stressors.

Defining Characteristics

Major

Deficits in one or more characteristics that indicate effective coping

Minor

Active planning by community for predicted stressors; active problem solving by community when faced with issues; agreement that community is responsible for stress management; positive communication among community members; positive communication between community/aggregates and larger community; programs available for recreation and relaxation; resources sufficient for managing stressors

Related Factors

Available social supports; available resources for problem solving; sense of power to manage stressors

Ineffective Community Coping (5.1.3.2)

Definition: A pattern of community activities for adaption and problem solving that is unsatisfactory for meeting the demands or needs of the community.

Defining Characteristics

Major

None

Minor

Community does not meet its own expectations; deficits in community participation; deficits in communication methods; excessive community conflicts; expressed difficulty in meeting demands for change; expressed vulnerability; high illness rates; stressors perceived as excessive

Related Factors

Deficits in social support; inadequate resources for problem solving; powerlessness

Ineffective Management of Therapeutic Regimen: Families (5.2.2)

Definition: A pattern of regulating and integrating into family processes a program for treatment of illness and the sequelae of illness that is unsatisfactory for meeting health goals.

Defining Characteristics

Major

Inappropriate family activities for meeting the goals of a treatment or prevention program

Minor

Acceleration (expected or unexpected) of illness symptoms of a family member; lack of attention to illness and its sequelae; verbalized desire to manage the treatment of illness and prevention of the sequelae; verbalized difficulty with regulation/integration of one or more effects or prevention of complication; verbalizes that family did not take action to reduce risk factors for progression of illness and sequelae

Related Factors

Complexity of health care system; complexity of therapeutic regimen; decisional conflicts; economic difficulties; excessive demands made on individual or family; family conflict

Ineffective Management of Therapeutic Regimen: Community (5.2.3)

Definition: A pattern of regulating and integrating into community processes programs for treatment of illness and the sequelae of illness that are unsatisfactory for meeting health-related goals.

Defining Characteristics

Deficits in persons and programs accountable for illness care of aggregates; deficits in advocates for aggregates; deficits in community activities for secondary and tertiary prevention; illness symptoms above the norm expected for the number and type of population; insufficient number of health care resources for the incidence or prevalence of illness(es); unavailable health care resources for illness care; unexpected acceleration of illness(es).

Effective Management of Therapeutic Regimen: Individual (5.2.4)

Definition: A pattern of regulating and integrating into daily living a program for treatment of illness and its sequelae that is satisfactory for meeting specific health goals.

Defining Characteristics

Appropriate choices of daily activities for meeting the goals of a treatment or prevention program; illness symptoms within a normal range or expectation; verbalized desire to manage the treatment of illness and prevention of sequelae; verbalized intent to reduce risk factors for progression of illness and sequelae

Risk for Perioperative Positioning Injury (6.1.1.2)

Definition: A state in which the client is at risk for injury as a result of the environmental conditions found in the perioperative setting.

Risk Factors

Disorientation; immobilization, muscle weakness; sensory/perceptual disturbances due to anesthesia; obesity; emaciation; edema

Risk for Disorganized Infant Behavior (6.8.1)

Definition: Risk for alteration in integration and modulation of the physiological and behavioral systems of functioning (ie, autonomic, motor, state, organizational, self-regulatory, and attentional-interactional systems).

Risk Factors

Pain; oral/motor problems; environmental overstimulation; lack of containment/boundaries; prematurity; invasive/painful procedures

Disorganized Infant Behavior (6.8.2)

Definition: Alteration in integration and modulation of the physiological and behavioral systems of functioning (ie, autonomic, motor, state, organizational, self-regulatory, and attentional-interactional systems).

Defining Characteristics

Major

Change from baseline physiologic measures; tremors, startles, twitches; hyperextension of arms and legs; diffuse/unclear sleep; deficient self-regulatory behaviors; deficient response to visual/auditory stimuli

Minor

Yawning; apnea

Potential for Enhanced Organized Infant Behavior (6.8.3)

Definition: A pattern of modulation of the physiological and behavioral systems of functioning (ie, autonomic, motor, state, organizational, self-regulatory, and attentional-interactional systems) that is satisfactory but that can be improved, resulting in higher levels of integration in response to environmental stimuli.

Defining Characteristics

Stable physiologic measures; definite sleep-wake states; use of some self-regulatory behaviors; response to visual/auditory stimuli

Related Factors

Prematurity; pain

Impaired Environmental Interpretation Syndrome (8.2.1)

Definition: Consistent lack of orientation to person, place, time, or circumstances over more than three to six months necessitating a protective environment.

Defining Characteristics

Major

Consistent disorientation in known and unknown environments; chronic confusional states

Minor

Loss of occupation or social functioning from memory decline; inability to follow simple directions, instructions; inability to reason; inability to concentrate; slow in responding to questions

Related Factors

Dementia (Alzheimer's disease, multi-infarct dementia, Pick's disease, AIDS dementia); Parkinson's disease; Huntington's disease; depression; alcoholism

Acute Confusion (8.2.2)

Definition: The abrupt onset of a cluster of global, transient changes and disturbances in attention, cognition, psychomotor activity, level of consciousness, and/or sleep-wake cycle.

Defining Characteristics

Major

Fluctuation in cognition; fluctuation in sleep-wake cycle; fluctuation in level of consciousness; fluctuation in psychomotor activity; increased agitation or restlessness; misperceptions; lack of motivation to initiate and/or follow through with goal-directed or purposeful behavior

Minor

Hallucinations

Related Factors

Over 60 years of age; dementia; alcohol abuse; drug abuse; delirium

Chronic Confusion (8.2.3)

Definition: An irreversible, long-standing, and/or progressive deterioration of intellect and personality characterized by decreased ability to interpret environmental stimuli, decreased capacity for intellectual thought processes, and manifested by disturbances of memory, orientation, and behavior.

Defining Characteristics

Major

Clinical evidence of organic impairment; altered interpretation/response to stimuli; progressive/long-standing cognitive impairment

Minor

No change in level of consciousness; impaired socialization; impaired memory (short term, long term); altered personality

Related Factors

Alzheimer's disease; Korsakoff's psychosis; multi-infarct dementia; cerebral vascular accident; head injury

Impaired Memory (8.3.1)

Definition: The state in which an individual experiences an inability to remember or recall bits of information or behavioral skills. Impaired memory may be attributed to pathophysiological or situational causes that are either temporary or permanent.

Defining Characteristics

Major

Observed or reported experiences of forgetting; inability to determine if a behavior was performed; inability to learn or retain new skills or information; inability to perform a previously learned skill; inability to recall factual information; inability to recall recent or past events

Minor

Forgetting to perform a behavior at a scheduled time

Related Factors

Acute or chronic hypoxia; anemia; decreased cardiac output; fluid and electrolyte imbalance; neurological disturbances; excessive environmental disturbances

Appendix B NANDA's Taxonomy I, Revised: Proposed ICD-10 Version

Conditions That Necessitate Nursing Care

Human Response Pattern: Choosing

(A human response pattern involving the selection of alternatives)

*Y00 Family Coping, Impaired

Y00.0 Compromised

Y00.1 Disabled

Y01 [Health-Seeking Behaviors]

Y01.0–9 Health Seeking Behaviors (Specify)

*Y02 Individual Coping, Impaired

Y02.0 Adjustment, Impaired

Y02.1 Conflict: Decisional

Y02.2 Coping: Defensive

*Y02.3 Denial, Impaired

Y02.4 Noncompliance

Human Response Pattern: Communicating

(A human response pattern involving the sending of messages)

Y10 [Communication, Impaired]

Y10.0 Verbal

Human Response Pattern: Exchanging

(A human response pattern involving mutual giving and receiving)

Y20 [Bowel Elimination, Altered]

Y20.0 Bowel Incontinence

Y20.1 Constipation: Colonic

Y20.2 Constipation: Perceived
Y20.3 Diarrhea
*Y21 Cardiac Output, Altered
Y22 [Fluid Volume, Altered]
Y22.0 Deficit
Y22.1 Deficit: Risk
Y22.2 Excess
*Y23 Injury: Risk
*Y23.0 Aspiration
*Y23.1 Disuse Syndrome
*Y23.2 Poisoning
*Y23.3 Suffocation
*Y23.4 Trauma
Y24 [Nutrition, Altered]
Y24.0 Less Than Body Requirement
Y24.1 More Than Body Requirement
Y24.2 More Than Body Requirement: Risk
Y25 [Physical Regulation, Altered]
Y25.0 Dysreflexia
Y25.1 Hyperthermia
Y25.2 Hypothermia
*Y25.3 Infection: Risk
*Y25.4 Thermoregulation, Impaired
Y26 [Respiration, Altered]
*Y26.0 Airway Clearance, Impaired
*Y26.1 Breathing Pattern, Impaired
Y26.2 Gas Exchange, Impaired
Y27 Tissue Integrity, Altered
*Y27.0 Oral Mucous Membrane, Impaired
Y27.1 Skin Integrity, Impaired
Y27.2 Skin Integrity, Impaired: Risk
Y28 [Tissue Perfusion, Altered]
Y28.0 Cardiopulmonary
Y28.1 Cerebral
Y28.2 Gastrointestinal
Y28.3 Peripheral
Y28.4 Renal

Y29 Urinary Elimination, Altered

Y29.0 Incontinence: Functional

Y29.1 Incontinence: Reflex

Y29.2 Incontinence: Stress

Y29.3 Incontinence: Urge

Y29.4 Incontinence: Total

*Y29.5 Retention

Human Response Pattern: Feeling

(A human response pattern involving the subjective awareness of information)

Y30 Anxiety

Y31 [Comfort, Altered]

Y31.0 Pain [Acute]

Y31.1 Pain, Chronic

Y32 Fear

Y33 [Grieving]

Y33.0 Anticipatory

Y33.1 Dysfunctional

Y34 Post-Trauma Response

Y34.0 Rape-Trauma Syndrome

Y34.1 Rape-Trauma Syndrome: Compound Reaction

Y34.2 Rape-Trauma Syndrome: Silent Reaction

*Y35 Violence: Risk

Human Response Pattern: Knowing

(A human response pattern involving the meaning associated with information)

Y40 [Knowledge Deficit]

Y40.0–9 Knowledge Deficit (Specify)

Y41 Thought Processes, Altered

Human Response Pattern: Moving

(A human response pattern involving activity)

Y50 [Activity, Altered]

Y50.0 Activity Intolerance

Y50.1 Activity Intolerance: Risk

Y50.2 Diversional Activity Deficit

Y50.3 Fatigue
Y50.4 Physical Mobility, Impaired
Y50.5 Sleep Pattern Disturbance
*Y51 Bathing/Hygiene Deficit
*Y52 Dressing/Grooming Deficit
*Y53 Feeding Deficit
*Y53.0 Breast-feeding, Impaired
Y53.1 Swallowing, Impaired
Y54 Growth and Development, Altered
Y55 Health Maintenance, Altered
Y56 Home Maintenance Management, Impaired
*Y57 Toileting Deficit

Human Response Pattern: Perceiving

(A human response pattern involving the reception of information)

Y60 [Meaningfulness, Altered]
Y60.0 Hopelessness
Y60.1 Powerlessness
Y61 [Self-Concept, Altered]
Y61.0 Body Image Disturbance
Y61.1 Personal Identity Disturbance
Y61.2 Self-Esteem Disturbance: Chronic Low
Y61.3 Self-Esteem Disturbance: Situational
*Y62 [Sensory Perception, Altered]
Y62.0 Auditory
Y62.1 Gustatory
Y62.2 Kinesthetic
Y62.3 Olfactory
Y62.4 Tactile
Y62.5 Visual
Y62.6 Unilateral Neglect

Human Response Pattern: Relating

(A human response pattern involving establishment of bonds)

Y70 Family Processes, Altered
Y71 Role Performance, Altered

Y71.0 Parental Role Conflict
Y71.1 Parenting, Altered
Y71.2 Parenting, Altered: Risk
Y71.3 Sexual Dysfunction
Y72 Sexuality Patterns, Altered
Y73 [Socialization, Altered]
Y73.0 Social Interaction, Impaired
Y73.1 Social Isolation

Human Response Pattern: Valuing

(A human response pattern involving the assigning of relative worth)

Y80 [Spiritual State, Altered]
Y80.0 Spiritual Distress

Note: Items in brackets are not diagnoses accepted by NANDA. Items with an asterisk (*) are changes in terminology from NANDA diagnostic labels.

Reference: NANDA Nursing Diagnoses: Definitions and Classification 1992

Appendix C Diagnosis Qualifiers

(Suggested/not limited to the following)

Qualifier	*Definition*
Acute	Severe but of short duration
Altered	A change from baseline
Chronic	Lasting a long time; recurring; habitual; constant
Decreased	Lessened, lesser in size, amount, or degree
Deficient	Inadequate in amount, quality, or degree; defective; not sufficient; incomplete
Depleted	Emptied wholly or in part; exhausted of
Disturbed	Agitated; interrupted, interfered with
Dysfunctional	Abnormal, incomplete functioning
Excessive	Characterized by an amount or quantity that is greater than necessary, desirable, or useful
Impaired	Made worse, weakened; damaged, reduced; deteriorated
Increased	Greater in size, amount, or degree
Ineffective	Not producing the desired effect
Intermittent	Stopping or starting again at intervals; periodic; cyclic
Potential for Enhanced	Made greater, to increase in quality, or more desired (for use with wellness diagnoses)

Reference: NANDA Nursing Diagnoses: Definitions & Classification 1995–1996

Appendix D NIC Intervention Labels and Definitions

Analgesic administration Use of pharmacologic agents to reduce or eliminate pain

Anesthesia administration Preparation for and administration of anesthetic agents, and monitoring of patient responsiveness during administration

Anger control assistance Facilitation of the expression of anger in an adaptive nonviolent manner

Animal assisted therapy Purposeful use of animals to provide affection, attention, diversion, and relaxation

Anticipatory guidance Preparation of patient for an anticipated developmental and/or situational crisis

Anxiety reduction Minimizing apprehension, dread, foreboding, or uneasiness related to an unidentified source of anticipated danger

Area restriction Limitation of patient mobility to a specified area for purposes of safety or behavior management

Art therapy Facilitation of communication through drawings or other art forms

Artificial airway management Maintenance of endotracheal and tracheostomy tubes and preventing complications associated with their use

Aspiration precautions Prevention or minimization of risk factors in the patient at risk for aspiration

Assertiveness training Assistance with the effective expression of feelings, needs, and ideas while respecting the rights of others

Attachment promotion Facilitation of the development of the parent-infant relationship

Autogenic Training Assisting with self-suggestions about feelings of heaviness and warmth for the purpose of inducing relaxation

Bathing Cleaning of the body for the purposes of relaxation, cleanliness, and healing

Bed rest care Promotion of comfort and safety and prevention of complications for a patient unable to get out of bed

Behavior management Helping a patient to manage negative behavior

Behavior modification Promotion of a behavior change

Bibliotherapy Use of literature to enhance the expression of feelings and the gaining of insight

Biofeedback Assisting the patient to modify a body function using feedback from instrumentation

Birthing Delivery of a baby

Bleeding precautions Reduction of the risk of blood loss for a patient with reduced coagulability

Bleeding reduction Limitation of the loss of blood volume during an episode of bleeding

Bleeding reduction: Gastrointestinal Limitation of the amount of blood loss from the upper and lower gastrointestinal tract and related complications

Bleeding reduction: Nasal Limitation of the amount of blood loss from the nasal cavity

Bleeding reduction: Wound Limitation of the blood loss from wound that may be a result of trauma, incisions, or placement of a tube or catheter

Blood products administration Administration of blood or blood products and monitoring of patient's response

Body image enhancement Improving a patient's conscious and unconscious perceptions and attitudes toward his/her body

Body mechanics promotion Facilitating the use of posture and movement in daily activities to prevent fatigue and musculoskeletal strain or injury

Bottle feeding Preparation and administration of fluids to an infant via a bottle

Bowel incontinence care Promotion of bowel continence and maintenance of perianal skin integrity

Bowel irrigation Instillation of a substance into the lower gastrointestinal tract

Bowel management Establishment and maintenance of a regular pattern of bowel elimination

Bowel training Assisting the patient to train the bowel to evacuate at specific intervals

Calming technique Reducing anxiety in patient experiencing acute distress

Cardiac care Limitation of complications resulting from an imbalance between myocardial oxygen supply and demand for a patient with symptoms of impaired cardiac function

Cardiac care: Acute Limitation of complications for a patient recently experiencing an episode of an imbalance between myocardial oxygen supply and demand resulting in impaired cardiac function

Cardiac care: Rehabilitative Promotion of maximum functional activity level for a patient who has suffered an episode of impaired cardiac function which resulted from an imbalance between myocardial oxygen supply and demand

Cardiac precautions Prevention of an acute episode of impaired cardiac function by minimizing myocardial oxygen consumption or increasing myocardial oxygen supply

Caregiver support Provision of the necessary information, advocacy, and support to facilitate primary patient care by someone other than a health care professional

Cast care: Maintenance Care of a cast after the drying period

Cast care: Wet Care of a new cast during the drying period

Cerebral edema management Limitation of secondary cerebral injury resulting from swelling of brain tissue

Cesarean section care Preparation and support of patient delivering a baby by cesarean section

Chemotherapy management Assisting the patient and family to understand the action and minimize side effects of antineoplastic agents

Chest physiotherapy Assisting the patient to move airway secretions from peripheral airways to more central airways for expectoration and/or suctioning

Childbirth preparation Providing information and support to facilitate childbirth and to enhance the ability of an individual to develop and perform the role of parent

Circulatory care Promotion of arterial and venous circulation

Circulatory precautions Protection of a localized area with limited perfusion

Code management Coordination of emergency measures to sustain life

Cognitive restructuring Challenging a patient to alter distorted thought patterns and view self and the world more realistically

Cognitive stimulation Promotion of awareness and comprehension of surroundings by utilization of planned stimuli

Communication enhancement Facilitating interaction with a patient who has difficulty delivering or receiving verbal or nonverbal messages

Communication enhancement: Hearing deficit Assistance in accepting and learning alternate methods for living with diminished hearing

Communication enhancement: Visual deficit Assistance in accepting and learning alternate methods for living with diminished vision

Confusion management Provision of a modified environment for the patient who is experiencing a chronic confusional state

Constipation/Impaction management Prevention and alleviation of constipation/impaction

Contact lens care Prevention of eye injury and lens damage by proper use of contact lenses

Coping enhancement Assisting a patient to adapt to perceived stressors, changes, or threats which interfere with meeting life demands and roles

Cough enhancement Promotion of deep inhalation by the patient with subsequent generation of high intrathoracic pressures and compression of underlying lung parenchyma for the forceful expulsion of air

Counseling Use of an interactive helping process focusing on the needs, problems, or feelings of the patient and significant others to enhance or support coping, problem-solving, and interpersonal relationships

Crisis intervention Use of short-term counseling to help the patient cope with a crisis and resume a state of functioning comparable to or better than the precrisis state

Culture brokerage Bridging, negotiating, or linking the orthodox health care system with a patient and family of a different culture

Cutaneous stimulation Stimulation of the skin and underlying tissues for the purpose of decreasing undesirable signs and symptoms such as pain, muscle spasm, or inflammation

Decision-making support Providing information and support for a patient who is making a decision regarding health care

Delirium management Provision of a safe and therapeutic environment for the patient who is experiencing an acute confusional state

Diarrhea management Prevention and alleviation of diarrhea

Diet staging Instituting required diet restrictions with subsequent progression of diet as tolerated

Discharge planning Preparation for moving a patient from one level of care to another within or outside the current health care agency

Distraction Purposeful focusing of attention away from undesirable sensations

Dressing Choosing, putting on, and removing clothes for a person who cannot do this for self

Dying care Promotion of physical comfort and psychological peace in the final phase of life

Dysreflexia management Prevention and elimination of stimuli which cause hyperactive reflexes and inappropriate autonomic responses in a patient with a cervical or high thoracic cord lesion

Dysrhythmia management Preventing, recognizing, and facilitating treatment of abnormal cardiac rhythms

Ear care Prevention or minimization of threats to ear or hearing

Eating disorders management Prevention and treatment of severe diet restriction and overexercising or binging and purging of food and fluids

Electrolyte management Promotion of electrolyte balance and prevention of complications resulting from abnormal or undesired serum electrolyte levels

Electrolyte management: Hypercalcemia Promotion of calcium balance and prevention of complications resulting from serum calcium levels higher than desired

Electrolyte management: Hyperkalemia Promotion of potassium balance and prevention of complications resulting from serum potassium levels higher than desired

Electrolyte management: Hypermagnesemia Promotion of magnesium balance and prevention of complications resulting from serum magnesium levels higher than desired

Electrolyte management: Hypernatremia Promotion of sodium balance and prevention of complications resulting from serum sodium levels higher than desired

Electrolyte management: Hyperphosphatemia Promotion of phosphate balance and prevention of complications resulting from serum phosphate levels higher than desired

Electrolyte management: Hypocalcemia Promotion of calcium balance and prevention of complications resulting from serum calcium levels lower than desired

Electrolyte management: Hypokalemia Promotion of potassium balance and prevention of complications resulting from serum potassium levels lower than desired

Electrolyte management: Hypomagnesemia Promotion of magnesium balance and prevention of complications resulting from serum magnesium levels lower than desired

Electrolyte management: Hyponatremia Promotion of sodium balance and prevention of complications resulting from serum sodium levels lower than desired

Electrolyte management: Hypophosphatemia Promotion of phosphate balance and prevention of complications resulting from serum phosphate levels lower than desired

Electrolyte monitoring Collection and analysis of patient data to regulate electrolyte balance

Embolus care: Peripheral Limitation of complications for a patient experiencing, or at risk for, occlusion of peripheral circulation

Embolus care: Pulmonary Limitation of complications for a patient experiencing, or at risk for, occlusion of pulmonary circulation

Embolus precautions Reduction of the risk of an embolus in a patient with thrombi or at risk for developing thrombus formation

Emergency care Providing life-saving measures in life-threatening situations

Emotional support Provision of reassurance, acceptance, and encouragement during times of stress

Energy management Regulating energy use to treat or prevent fatigue and optimize function

Enteral tube feeding Delivering nutrients and water through an intestinal tube

Environmental management Manipulation of the patient's surroundings for therapeutic benefit

Environmental management: Attachment process Manipulation of the patient's surroundings to facilitate the development of the parent-infant relationship

Environmental management: Comfort Manipulation of the patient's surroundings for promotion of optimal comfort

Environmental management: Safety Monitoring and manipulation of the physical environment to promote safety

Environmental management: Violence prevention Monitoring and manipulation of the physical environment to decrease the potential for violent behavior directed toward self, others, or environment

Epidural analgesia administration Preparation and delivery of narcotic analgesics into the epidural space

Exercise promotion Facilitation of regular physical exercise to maintain or advance to a higher level of fitness and health

Exercise therapy: Ambulation Promotion and assistance with walking to maintain or restore autonomic and voluntary body functions during treatment and recovery from illness or injury

Exercise therapy: Balance Use of specific activities, postures, and movements to maintain, enhance, or restore balance

Exercise therapy: Joint mobility Use of active or passive body movement to maintain or restore joint flexibility

Exercise therapy: Muscle control Use of specific activity or exercise protocols to enhance or restore controlled body movement

Eye care Prevention or minimization of threats to eye or visual integrity

Fall prevention Instituting special precautions with patient at risk for injury from falling

Family integrity promotion Promotion of family cohesion and unity

Family integrity promotion: Childbearing family Facilitation of the growth of individuals or families who are adding an infant to the family unit

Family involvement Facilitating family participation in the emotional and physical care of the patient

Family mobilization Utilization of family strengths to influence patient's health in a positive direction

Family planning: Contraception Facilitation of pregnancy prevention by providing information about the physiology of reproduction and methods to control conception

Family planning: Infertility Management, education, and support of the patient and significant other undergoing evaluation and treatment for infertility

Family planning: Unplanned pregnancy Facilitation of decision-making regarding pregnancy outcome

Family process maintenance Minimization of family process disruption effects

Family support Promotion of family interests and goals

Family therapy Assisting family members to move their family toward a more productive way of living

Feeding Providing nutritional intake for patient who is unable to feed self

Fetal monitoring Measurement and interpretation of the physiologic status of the fetus during labor and delivery

Fever treatment Management of a patient with hyperpyrexia caused by nonenvironmental factors

First aid Providing initial care of a minor injury

Flatulence reduction Prevention of flatus formation and facilitation of passage of excessive gas

Fluid/Electrolyte management Regulation and prevention of complications from altered fluid and/or electrolyte levels

Fluid management Promotion of fluid balance and prevention of complications resulting from abnormal or undesired fluid levels

Fluid monitoring Collection and analysis of patient data to regulate fluid balance

Fluid resuscitation Administering prescribed intravenous fluids rapidly

Foot care Cleansing and inspecting the feet for the purposes of relaxation, cleanliness, and healthy skin

Gastrointestinal intubation Insertion of a tube into the gastrointestinal tract

Genetic counseling Use of an interactive helping process focusing on the prevention of a genetic disorder or on the ability to cope with a family member who has a genetic disorder

Grief work facilitation Assistance with the resolution of a significant loss

Guilt work facilitation Helping another to cope with painful feelings of responsibility, actual or perceived

Hair care Promotion of neat, clean, attractive hair

Hallucination management Interaction with patient experiencing, or at risk for, hallucinations

Health screening Detecting health risks or problems by means of history, examination, and other procedures

Health system guidance Facilitating a patient's location and use of appropriate health services

Heat exposure treatment Management of patient overcome by heat due to excessive environmental heat exposure

Heat/Cold application Stimulation of the skin and underlying tissues with heat or cold for the purpose of decreasing pain, muscle spasms, or inflammation

Hemodialysis therapy Management of extracorporeal passage of the patient's blood through a dialyzer

Hemodynamic regulation Optimization of heart rate, preload, afterload, and contractility

Hemorrhage control Reduction or elimination of rapid and excessive blood loss

Home maintenance assistance Helping the patient/family to maintain the home as a clean, safe, and pleasant place to live

Hope instillation Facilitation of the development of a positive outlook in a given situation

Humor Facilitating the patient to perceive, appreciate, and express what is funny, amusing, or ludicrous in order to establish relationships, relieve tension, release anger, facilitate learning, or cope with painful feelings

Hyperglycemia management Preventing and treating above normal blood glucose levels

Hypervolemia management Reduction in extracellular and/or intracellular fluid volume and prevention of complications in a patient who is fluid overloaded

Hypnosis Assisting a patient to induce an altered state of consciousness to create an acute awareness and a directed focus experience

Hypoglycemia management Preventing and treating below normal blood glucose levels

Hypothermia treatment Rewarming and surveillance of a patient whose core body temperature is below 35 degrees Centigrade

Hypovolemia management Expansion of intravascular fluid volume in a patient who is volume depleted

Immunization/Vaccination administration Provision of immunizations for prevention of communicable disease

Incision site care Cleansing, monitoring, and promotion of healing in a wound that is closed with sutures, clips, or staples

Infant care Provision of developmentally appropriate family-centered care to the child under 1 year of age

Infection control Minimizing the acquisition and transmission of infectious agents

Infection protection Prevention and early detection of infection in a patient at risk

Intracranial pressure (ICP) monitoring Measurement and interpretation of patient data to regulate intracranial pressure

Intrapartal care Monitoring and management of patient during labor and delivery

Intravenous (IV) insertion Insertion of a needle into a peripheral vein for the purpose of administering fluids, blood, or medications

Intravenous (IV) therapy Administration and monitoring of intravenous fluids and medications

Invasive hemodynamic monitoring Measurement and interpretation of invasive hemodynamic parameters to determine cardiovascular function and regulate therapy as appropriate

Lactation management Promotion of successful breast feeding and weaning through information and support

Lactation suppression Facilitating the cessation of milk production and minimizing breast engorgement after giving birth

Learning facilitation Promoting the ability to process and comprehend information

Learning readiness enhancement Improving the ability and willingness to receive information

Limit setting Establishing the parameters of desirable and acceptable patient behavior

Mechanical ventilation Use of an artificial device to assist a patient to breathe

Mechanical ventilatory weaning Assisting the patient to breathe without the aid of a mechanical ventilator

Medication administration Preparing, giving, and evaluating the effectiveness of prescription and nonprescription drugs

Medication administration: Enteral Delivering medications through an intestinal tube

Medication administration: Interpleural Administration of medication through an interpleural catheter for reduction of pain

Medication administration: Oral Preparing and giving medications by mouth and monitoring patient responsiveness

Medication administration: Parenteral Preparing and giving medications via the intravenous, intramuscular, intradermal, and/or subcutaneous route

Medication administration: Topical Preparing and applying medications to the skin and mucous membranes

Medication management Facilitation of safe and effective use of prescription and over-the-counter drugs

Meditation Altering the patient's level of awareness by focusing specifically on an image or thought

Memory training Facilitation of memory

Milieu therapy Use of people, resources, and events in the patient's immediate environment to promote optimal psychosocial functioning

Music therapy Using music to help achieve a specific change in behavior or feeling

Mutual goal setting Collaborating with patient to identify and prioritize care goals, then developing a plan for achieving those goals through the construction and use of goal attainment scaling

Nail care Promotion of clean, neat, attractive nails and prevention of skin lesions related to improper care of nails

Neurologic monitoring Collection and analysis of patient data to prevent or minimize neurologic complications

Newborn care Management of neonate during the transition to extrauterine life and subsequent period of stabilization

Newborn monitoring Measurement and interpretation of physiologic status of the neonate the first 24 hours after delivery

Nonnutritive sucking Provision of sucking opportunities for infant who is gavage fed or who can receive nothing by mouth

Nutrition management Assisting with or providing a balanced dietary intake of foods and fluids

Nutrition therapy Administration of food and fluids to support metabolic processes of a patient who is malnourished or at high risk for becoming malnourished

Nutritional counseling Use of an interactive helping process focusing on the need for diet modification

Nutritional monitoring Collection and analysis of patient data to prevent or minimize malnourishment

Oral health maintenance Maintenance and promotion of oral hygiene and dental health for the patient at risk for developing oral or dental lesions

Oral health promotion Promotion of oral hygiene and dental care for a patient with normal oral and dental health

Oral health restoration Promotion of healing for a patient who has an oral mucosa or dental lesion

Ostomy care Maintenance of elimination through a stoma and care of surrounding tissue

Oxygen therapy Administration of oxygen and monitoring of its effectiveness

Pain management Alleviation of pain or a reduction in pain to a level of comfort that is acceptable to the patient

Parent education: Adolescent Assisting parents to understand and help their adolescent children

Parent education: Childbearing family Preparing another to perform the role of parent

Parent education: Childrearing family Assisting parents to understand and promote the physical, psychological, and social growth and development of their toddler, preschool, or school-aged children

Patient contracting Negotiating an agreement with a patient which reinforces a specific behavior change

Patient controlled analgesia (PCA) assistance Facilitating patient control of analgesic administration and regulation

Patient rights protection Protection of health care rights of a patient, especially a minor, incapacitated, or incompetent patient unable to make decisions

Perineal care Maintenance of perineal skin integrity and relief of perineal discomfort

Peripheral sensation management Prevention or minimization of injury or discomfort in the patient with altered sensation

Peripherally inserted central (PIC) catheter care Insertion and maintenance of a peripherally inserted central catheter

Peritoneal dialysis therapy Administration and monitoring of dialysis solution into and out of the abdominal cavity

Physical restraint Application and monitoring of mechanical restraining devices or manual restraints to limit physical mobility of patient

Play therapy Purposeful use of toys or other equipment to assist a patient in communicating his/her perception of the world and to help in mastering the environment

Positioning Moving the patient or a body part to provide comfort, reduce the risk of skin breakdown, promote skin integrity, and/or promote healing

Positioning: Neurologic Achievement of optimal, appropriate body alignment for the patient with a cervical injury

Positioning: Wheelchair Placement of a patient in a properly selected wheelchair to enhance comfort, promote skin integrity, and foster independence

Postmortem care Providing physical care of the body of an expired patient and support for the family viewing the body

Postpartal care Monitoring and management of the patient who has recently given birth

Pregnancy termination care Management of the physical and psychological needs of the woman undergoing a spontaneous or elective abortion

Prenatal care Monitoring and management of patient during pregnancy to prevent complications of pregnancy and promote a healthy outcome for both mother and infant

Preparatory sensory information Describing both the subjective and objective physical sensations associated with an upcoming stressful health care procedure/treatment

Presence Being with another during times of need

Pressure management Minimizing pressure to body parts

Pressure ulcer care Facilitation of healing in pressure ulcers

Pressure ulcer prevention Prevention of decubitus ulcers for a patient at high risk for developing them

Progressive muscle relaxation Facilitating the tensing and releasing of successive muscle groups while attending to the resulting differences in sensation

Prosthesis care Care of a removable appliance worn by a patient and the prevention of complications associated with its use

Radiation therapy management Assisting the patient to understand and minimize the side effects of radiation treatments

Rape-trauma treatment Provision of emotional and physical support immediately following an alleged rape

Reality orientation Promotion of patient's awareness of personal identity, time, and environment

Recreation therapy Purposeful use of recreation to promote relaxation and enhancement of social skills

Referral Arrangement for services by another care provider or agency

Reminiscence therapy Using the recall of past events, feelings, and thoughts to facilitate adaptation to present circumstances

Respiratory monitoring Collection and analysis of patient data to ensure airway patency and adequate gas exchange

Respite care Provision of short-term care to provide relief for family caregiver

Resuscitation Administering emergency measures to sustain life

Risk identification Analysis of potential risk factors, determination of health risks, and prioritization of risk reduction strategies for an individual or group

Risk identification: Childbearing family Identification of an individual or family likely to experience difficulties in parenting and prioritization of strategies to prevent parenting problems

Role enhancement Assisting a patient, significant other, and/or family to improve relationships by clarifying and supplementing specific role behaviors

Seclusion Solitary containment in a fully protective environment with close surveillance by nursing staff for purposes of safety or behavior management

Security enhancement Intensifying a patient's sense of physical and psychological safety

Seizure management Care of a patient during a seizure and the postictal state

Seizure precautions Prevention or minimization of potential injuries sustained by a patient with a known seizure disorder

Self-awareness enhancement Assisting a patient to explore and understand his/her thoughts, feelings, motivations, and behaviors

Self-care assistance Assisting another to perform activities of daily living

Self-care assistance: Bathing/Hygiene Assisting patient to perform personal hygiene

Self-care assistance: Dressing/Grooming Assisting patient with clothes and makeup

Self-care assistance: Feeding Assisting a person to eat

Self-care assistance: Toileting Assisting another with elimination

Self-esteem enhancement Assisting a patient to increase his/her personal judgment of self worth

Self-modification assistance Reinforcement of self-directed change initiated by the patient to achieve personally important goals

Self-responsibility facilitation Encouraging a patient to assume more responsibility for own behavior

Sexual counseling Use of an interactive helping process focusing on the need to make adjustments in sexual practice or to enhance coping with a sexual event/disorder

Shock management Facilitation of the delivery of oxygen and nutrients to systemic tissue with removal of cellular waste products in a patient with severely altered tissue perfusion

Shock management: Cardiac Promotion of adequate tissue perfusion for a patient with severely compromised pumping function of the heart

Shock management: Vasogenic Promotion of adequate tissue perfusion for a patient with severe loss of vascular tone

Shock management: Volume Promotion of adequate tissue perfusion for a patient with severely compromised intravascular volume

Shock prevention Detecting and treating a patient at risk for impending shock

Sibling support Assisting a sibling to cope with a brother's or sister's illness

Simple guided imagery Purposeful use of imagination to achieve relaxation and/or direct attention away from undesirable sensations

Simple massage Stimulation of the skin and underlying tissues with varying degrees of hand pressure to decrease pain, produce relaxation, and/or improve circulation

Simple relaxation therapy Use of techniques to encourage and elicit relaxation for the purpose of decreasing undesirable signs and symptoms such as pain, muscle tension, or anxiety

Skin care: Topical treatments Application of topical substances or manipulation of devices to promote skin integrity and minimize skin breakdown

Skin surveillance Collection and analysis of patient data to maintain skin and mucous membrane integrity

Sleep enhancement Facilitation of regular sleep/wake cycles

Smoking cessation assistance Helping a patient to stop smoking

Socialization enhancement Facilitation of another person's ability to interact with others

Specimen management Obtaining, preparing, and preserving a specimen for a laboratory test

Spiritual support Assisting the patient to feel balance and connection with a greater power

Splinting Stabilization, immobilization, and/or protection of an injured body part with a supportive appliance

Subarachnoid hemorrhage precautions Reduction of internal and external stimuli or stressors to minimize risk of rebleeding prior to aneurysm surgery

Substance use prevention Prevention of an alcoholic or drug use lifestyle

Substance use treatment Supportive care of patient/family members with physical and psychosocial problems associated with the use of alcohol or drugs

Substance use treatment: Alcohol withdrawal Care of the patient experiencing sudden cessation of alcohol consumption

Substance use treatment: Drug withdrawal Care of a patient experiencing drug detoxification

Substance use treatment: Overdose Monitoring, treatment, and emotional support of a patient who has ingested prescription or over-the-counter drugs beyond the therapeutic range

Suicide prevention Reducing risk of self-inflicted harm for a patient in crisis or severe depression

Support group Use of a group environment to provide emotional support and health-related information for members

Support system enhancement Facilitation of support to patient by family, friends, and community

Surgical assistance: Circulating Coordinating activities in the operating suite to maximize the patient's safety

Surgical assistance: Scrubbing Assisting with operative procedures conducted in the operating room

Surgical preparation Providing care to a patient immediately prior to surgery and verification of required procedures/tests and documentation in the clinical record

Surveillance Purposeful and ongoing acquisition, interpretation, and synthesis of patient data for clinical decision-making

Surveillance: Safety Purposeful and ongoing collection and analysis of information about the patient and the environment for use in promoting and maintaining patient safety

Sustenance support Helping a needy individual/family to locate food, clothing, or shelter

Suturing Approximating edges of a wound using sterile suture material and a needle

Swallowing therapy Facilitating swallowing and preventing complications of impaired swallowing

Teaching: Disease process Assisting the patient to understand information related to a specific disease process

Teaching: Group Development, implementation, and evaluation of a patient teaching program for a group of individuals experiencing the same health condition

Teaching: Individual Planning, implementation, and evaluation of a teaching program designed to address a patient's particular needs

Teaching: Infant care Instruction on nurturing and physical care needed during the first year of life

Teaching: Preoperative Assisting a patient to understand and mentally prepare for surgery and the postoperative recovery period

Teaching: Prescribed Activity/Exercise Preparing a patient to achieve and/or maintain a prescribed level of activity

Teaching: Prescribed diet Preparing a patient to correctly follow a prescribed diet

Teaching: Prescribed medication Preparing a patient to safely take prescribed medications and monitor for their effects

Teaching: Procedure/Treatment Preparing a patient to understand and mentally prepare for a prescribed procedure or treatment

Teaching: Psychomotor skill Preparing a patient to perform a psychomotor skill

Teaching: Safe sex Providing instruction concerning sexual protection during sexual activity

Technology management Use of technical equipment and devices to monitor patient condition or sustain life

Temperature regulation Attaining and/or maintaining body temperature within a normal range

Therapeutic touch Directing one's own interpersonal energy to flow through the hands to help or heal another

Therapy group Use of the emotional reactions of members of a group to help individual group members work out interpersonal conflicts

Total parenteral nutrition (TPN) administration Preparation and delivery of nutrients intravenously and monitoring of patient responsiveness

Touch Providing comfort and communication through purposeful tactile contact

Traction care Management of a patient who has a device to immobilize and stabilize a body part

Transcutaneous electrical nerve stimulation (TENS) Stimulation of skin and underlying tissues with controlled, low-voltage electrical vibration via electrodes

Transport Moving a patient from one location to another

Triage Establishing priorities of care in an emergency or disaster situation

Truth telling Use of whole truth, partial truth, or decision delay to promote the patient's self-determination and well-being

Tube care Management of a patient with an external drainage device exiting the body

Tube care: Chest Management of a patient with an external water-seal drainage device exiting the chest cavity

Tube care: Gastrointestinal Management of a patient with a gastrointestinal tube

Tube care: Urinary Management of a patient with urinary drainage equipment

Tube care: Ventriculostomy/Lumbar drain Management of a patient with an external cerebrospinal fluid drainage system

Urinary catheterization Insertion of a catheter into the bladder for temporary or permanent drainage of urine

Urinary catheterization: Intermittent Regular periodic use of a catheter to empty the bladder

Urinary elimination management Maintenance of an optimum urinary elimination pattern

Urinary incontinence care Institution of a program to promote continence and to maintain perineal skin integrity

Urinary retention care Assistance in relieving bladder distention

Values clarification Assisting another to clarify her/his own values in order to facilitate effective decision-making

Ventilation assistance Promotion of an optimal spontaneous breathing pattern that maximizes oxygen and carbon dioxide exchange in the lungs

Visitation facilitation Promoting beneficial visits by family and friends

Vital signs monitoring Collection and analysis of cardiovascular, respiratory, and body temperature data to determine and prevent complications

Weight gain assistance Facilitating gain of body weight

Weight management Facilitating maintenance of optimal body weight and percent body fat

Weight reduction assistance Facilitating loss of weight and/or body fat

Wound care Prevention of wound complications and promotion of wound healing

Wound care: Closed drainage Maintenance of a pressure drainage system at the wound site

Wound irrigation Flushing of an open wound to cleanse and remove debris and excessive drainage

Appendix E
Care Planning Checklist

Nursing Diagnosis

Nursing diagnosis = Problem + Etiology

1. What is the patient's problem (NANDA label)?
2. What is the etiology of the problem (patient's related/risk factors)?

Assessment Data

1. What signs and symptoms (defining characteristics) does the patient have?
   a. Major (subjective, objective)
   b. Critical (subjective, objective)
   c. Other (subjective, objective)
2. Does patient data match the nursing diagnosis definition?
3. What are the "major" or "critical" defining characteristics necessary in order to use this diagnostic label? Do they match the patient data in question 1?

Patient Outcomes and Evaluation Criteria

1. Have you included target times and evaluation intervals?
2. Are the outcomes measurable?
3. Are the outcomes realistic?
4. Does achievement of at least one outcome indicate resolution of the stated problem?

Nursing Actions

1. Are the nursing actions prioritized to address the NIC treatments of choice?
2. Are the nursing actions individualized to meet the patient's specific needs?

3. Are the nursing actions explicit and detailed so that another nurse could use them to provide care?
4. Have you included ongoing assessments, patient teaching, collaborative activities, and other nursing treatments as needed?
5. Have you considered prevention and health promotion, as well as treatment, for the existing problem?

Documentation

1. Did you document the care given for the nursing diagnosis?
2. Did you document the patient's response to the care using the evaluation criteria?

Evaluation

1. Were the desired outcomes achieved (evaluation criteria met)?
2. If not, do you need to revise, modify, or discontinue:
   a. The nursing diagnosis?
   b. The patient outcomes/evaluation criteria?
   c. The nursing actions?

Appendix F NANDA Approved Nursing Diagnoses

This taxonomically organized list represents the NANDA approved nursing diagnoses for clinical use and testing (1994).

**Diagnoses in progress (in early stages of development). Added in 1994.*

Pattern 1. Exchanging

1.1.2.1 Altered Nutrition: More Than Body Requirements
1.1.2.2 Altered Nutrition: Less Than Body Requirements
1.1.2.3 Altered Nutrition: Potential for More Than Body Requirements
1.2.1.1 Risk for Infection
1.2.2.1 Risk for Altered Body Temperature
1.2.2.2 Hypothermia
1.2.2.3 Hyperthermia
1.2.2.4 Ineffective Thermoregulation
1.2.3.1 Dysreflexia
1.3.1.1 Constipation
1.3.1.1.1 Perceived Constipation
1.3.1.1.1 Colonic Constipation
1.3.1.2 Diarrhea
1.3.1.3 Bowel Incontinence
1.3.2 Altered Urinary Elimination
1.3.2.1.1 Stress Incontinence
1.3.2.1.4 Functional Incontinence
1.3.2.1.5 Total Incontinence
1.3.2.2 Urinary Retention
1.4.1.1 Altered (Specify Type) Tissue Perfusion (Renal, Cerebral, Cardiopulmonary, Gastrointestinal, Peripheral
1.4.1.2.1 Fluid Volume Excess
1.4.1.2.2.1 Fluid Volume Deficit

1.4.1.2.2.2 Risk for Fluid Volume Deficit
1.4.2.1 Decreased Cardiac Output
1.5.1.1 Impaired Gas Exchange
1.5.1.2 Ineffective Airway Clearance
1.5.1.3 Ineffective Breathing Pattern
1.5.1.3.1 Inability to Sustain Spontaneous Ventilation
1.5.1.3.2 Dysfunctional Ventilatory Weaning Response (DVWR)
1.6.1 Risk for Injury
1.6.1.1 Risk for Suffocation
1.6.1.2 Risk for Poisoning
1.6.1.3 Risk for Trauma
1.6.1.4 Risk for Aspiration
1.6.1.5 Risk for Disuse Syndrome
1.6.2 Altered Protection
1.6.2.1 Impaired Tissue Integrity
1.6.2.1.1 Altered Oral Mucous Membrane
1.6.2.1.2.1 Impaired Skin Integrity
1.6.2.1.2.2 Risk for Impaired Skin Integrity
1.7.1 Decreased Adaptive Capacity: Intracranial
1.8 Energy Field Disturbance

Pattern 2. Communicating
2.1.1.1 Impaired Verbal Communication

Pattern 3. Relating
3.1.1 Impaired Social Interaction
3.1.2 Social Isolation
3.1.3 Risk for Loneliness
3.2.1 Altered Role Performance
3.2.1.1.1 Altered Parenting
3.2.1.1.2 Risk for Altered Parenting
3.2.1.1.2.1 Risk for Altered Parent/Infant/Child Attachment
3.2.1.2.1 Sexual Dysfunction
3.2.2 Altered Family Processes
3.2.2.1 Caregiver Role Strain
3.2.2.2 Risk for Caregiver Role Strain

**3.2.2.3.1 Altered Family Process: Alcoholism*
3.2.3.1 Parental Role Conflict
3.3 Altered Sexuality Patterns

Pattern 4. Valuing
4.1.1 Spiritual Distress (Distress of the Human Spirit)
**4.2 Potential for Enhanced Spiritual Well Being*

Pattern 5. Choosing
5.1.1.1 Ineffective Individual Coping
5.1.1.1.1 Impaired Adjustment
5.1.1.1.2 Defensive Coping
5.1.1.1.3 Ineffective Denial
5.1.2.1.1 Ineffective Family Coping: Disabling
5.1.2.1.2 Ineffective Family Coping: Compromised
5.1.2.2 Family Coping: Potential for Growth
**5.1.3.1 Potential for Enhanced Community Coping*
**5.1.3.2 Ineffective Community Coping*
5.2.1 Ineffective Management of Therapeutic Regimen (Individuals)
5.2.1.1 Noncompliance (specify)
**5.2.2 Ineffective Management of Therapeutic Regimen: Families*
**5.2.3 Ineffective Management of Therapeutic Regimen: Community*
**5.2.4 Effective Management of Therapeutic Regimen: Individual*
5.3.1.1 Decisional Conflict (Specify)
5.4 Health Seeking Behaviors (Specify)

Pattern 6. Moving
6.1.1.1 Impaired Physical Mobility
6.1.1.1.1 Risk for Peripheral Neurovascular Dysfunction
**6.1.1.1.2 Risk for Perioperative Positioning Injury*
6.1.1.2 Activity Intolerance
6.1.1.2.1 Fatigue
6.1.1.3 Risk for Activity Intolerance
6.2.1 Sleep Pattern Disturbance

6.3.1.1 Diversional Activity Deficit
6.4.1.1 Impaired Home Maintenance Management
6.4.2 Altered Health Maintenance
6.5.1 Feeding Self Care Deficit
6.5.1.1 Impaired Swallowing
6.5.1.2 Ineffective Breastfeeding
6.5.1.2.1 Interrupted Breastfeeding
6.5.1.3 Effective Breastfeeding
6.5.1.3 Ineffective Infant Feeding Pattern
6.5.2 Bathing/Hygiene Self Care Deficit
6.5.3 Dressing/Grooming Self Care Deficit
6.5.4 Toileting Self Care Deficit
6.6 Altered Growth and Development
6.7 Relocation Stress Syndrome
**6.8.1 Risk for Disorganized Infant Behavior*
**6.8.2 Disorganized Infant Behavior*
**6.8.3 Potential for Enhanced Organized Infant Behavior*

Pattern 7. Perceiving
7.1.1 Body Image Disturbance
7.1.2 Self Esteem Disturbance
7.1.2.1 Chronic Low Self Esteem
7.1.2.2 Situational Low Self Esteem
7.1.3 Personal Identity Disturbance
7.2 Sensory/Perceptual Alterations (Specify) (Visual, Auditory, Kinesthetic, Gustatory, Tactile, Olfactory)
7.2.1.1 Unilateral Neglect
7.3.1 Hopelessness
7.3.2 Powerlessness

Pattern 8. Knowing
8.1.1 Knowledge Deficit (Specify)
**8.2.1 Impaired Environmental Interpretation Syndrome*
**8.2.2 Acute Confusion*
**8.2.3 Chronic Confusion*
8.3 Altered Thought Processes
**8.3.1 Impaired Memory*

Pattern 9. Feeling

9.1.1 Pain

9.1.1.1 Chronic Pain

9.2.1.1 Dysfunctional Grieving

9.2.1.2 Anticipatory Grieving

9.2.2 Risk for Violence: Self-directed or Directed at Others

9.2.2.1 Risk for Self-Mutilation

9.2.3 Post-Trauma Response

9.2.3.1 Rape-Trauma Syndrome

9.2.3.1.1 Rape-Trauma Syndrome: Compound Reaction

9.2.3.1.2 Rape-Trauma Syndrome: Silent Reaction

9.3.1 Anxiety

9.3.2 Fear

Index

D

T